T0286268

Encyclopedia of Cancer Prevention and Management: Researches in Cancer Therapy

Volume VII

Encyclopedia of Cancer Prevention and Management: Researches in Cancer Therapy Volume VII

Edited by **Karen Miles and Richard Gray**

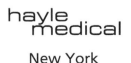

hayle
medical

New York

Published by Hayle Medical,
30 West, 37th Street, Suite 612,
New York, NY 10018, USA
www.haylemedical.com

Encyclopedia of Cancer Prevention and Management:
Researches in Cancer Therapy
Volume VII
Edited by Karen Miles and Richard Gray

International Standard Book Number: 978-1-63241-132-7 (Hardback)

Contents

Permissions

List of Contributors

Preface

The world is advancing at a fast pace like never before. Therefore, the need is to keep up with the latest developments. This book was an idea that came to fruition when the specialists in the area realized the need to coordinate together and document essential themes in the subject. That's when I was requested to be the editor. Editing this book has been an honour as it brings together diverse authors researching on different streams of the field. The book collates essential materials contributed by veterans in the area which can be utilized by students and researchers alike.

This book offers an in-depth understanding of cancer, its prevention and management. The advances as well as researches in cancer therapy are described in this all-inclusive book. This book aims to provide the clinicians and scientists with a descriptive analysis of the state of present knowledge and latest research findings in the field of cancer therapy. It includes sections on anticancer plants, inflammation, immune system and cancer, and diagnostic technologies. The book is believed to enhance the readers' understanding of cancer therapy advancements or/and to keep them updated with the current progresses in this field. This book will serve as a valuable source of information for physicians, researchers as well as patients.

Each chapter is a sole-standing publication that reflects each author's interpretation. Thus, the book displays a multi-facetted picture of our current understanding of application, resources and aspects of the field. I would like to thank the contributors of this book and my family for their endless support.

Editor

Part 1

Promising Anticancer Plants

1

Anticancer Properties of Curcumin

Varisa Pongrakhananon[1,2] and Yon Rojanasakul[2]
[1]Chulalongkorn University, Department of Pharmacology and Physiology
Faculty of Pharmaceutical Sciences, Bangkok,
[2]West Virginia University
Department of Basic Pharmaceutical Sciences, Morgantown, West Virginia
[1]Thailand
[2]USA

1. Introduction

Curcumin is a major biological active compound from turmeric or *Curcuma longa*. This non-toxic natural compound has been reported to possess several biological activities that are therapeutically beneficial to cancer treatment. It has been reported to increase the efficacy of other chemotherapeutic agents and to reduce their toxic side effects which are the major drawback of most chemotherapeutic agents. Curcumin is also well known for its anti-inflammatory activity (Amanda and Robert, 2008). Since cancer often develops under chronic inflammatory conditions, curcumin has the potential to be a preventive treatment agent against cancer. Furthermore, unlike most chemotherapeutic agents which act on a specific process of cancer development, i.e., cell growth or apoptosis, curcumin exerts its effect on various stages of cancer development, i.e., oncogene activation (Singh and Singh, 2009), cancer cell proliferation (Simon et al., 1998), apoptosis evasion (Han et al., 1999), anoikis resistance (Pongrakhananon et al., 2010), and metastasis (Chen et al., 2008) (Figure 1). Therefore, curcumin has the potential to overcome chemoresistance which is a major problem in cancer chemotherapy. This chapter will provide an overview of the anticancer activities of curcumin and present pre-clinical and clinical evidence supporting the use of curcumin as an anticancer agent.

Cancer is known to be associated with genetic instability in which *c-myc* serves as a major modifier of many targeted genes (Mai and Mushinski, 2003). Likewise, the mutation of proto-oncogene *ras* has been identified in many types of tumor (Rajalingam et al., 2007). The dysregulation of these oncogenes is well recognized as an initial step in the development of tumorigenesis. Interestingly, curcumin has been reported to have a suppressive effect on the oncogenes and inhibit their downstream effectors such as cell cycle promoting and proapoptotic proteins (Singh and Singh, 2009). Curcumin also exhibits anticancer properties through its ability to inhibit cell proliferation and induce apoptosis. The anti-proliferative effect of curcumin is dependent on its concentration, duration of treatment, and specific cell type. At low doses, curcumin causes cell cycle arrest, while at higher doses it induces apoptosis. Cell proliferation is controlled by several cell cycle regulating proteins, notably the family of cyclin and cyclin-dependent kinases (Kastan and Bartek, 2004) whose expression is tightly associated with tumorigenesis (Diehl, 2002). Curcumin inhibits cell cycle progression by downregulating cyclin D1 and the transition from G1 to S phase in human head and neck squamous carcinoma cells (Aggarwal et al., 2004). It also inhibits bladder cancer cell proliferation through the downregulation of cyclin A and upregulation of p21 (Park et al., 2006).

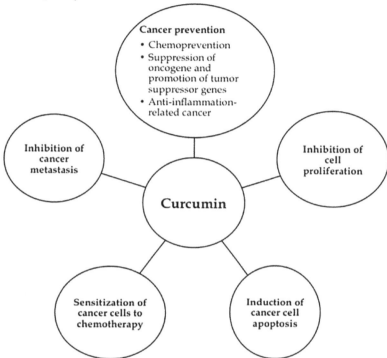

Fig. 1. Anticancer properties of curcumin

Curcumin possesses apoptosis-inducing activity causing cancer cell death primarily through the mitochondrial death pathway. It induces an upregulation of the proapoptotic protein Bax and downregulation of the antiapoptotic protein Bcl-2 in breast cancer cells (Chiu and Su, 2009), resulting in the loss of mitochondrial function, release of cytochrome c, and activation of caspase-9 and -3 (Chen et al., 2010). Curcumin also potentiates the cytotoxic effect of chemotherapeutic agents such as cisplatin (Chanvorachote et al., 2009), doxorubicin (Notarbartolo et al., 2005), tamoxifen (Chuang et al., 2002), and placitaxel (Genta and Amiji, 2009). The use of curcumin as a chemo-sensitizing agent in combination therapy has the potential to overcome chemoresistance which is common in advance staged cancers and is a major cause of cancer-related death.

An increasing number of reports have described the inhibitory effect of curcumin on cancer metastasis. Metastasis is a multi-step process involving tumor vascularization, cancer cell detachment, avoidance of anoikis, and increased cell invasion. The vascularization induced by tumor is an essential step providing nutrients, oxygen, and removing waste products for tumor growth and metastasis. A key mechanism that cancer cells utilize during metastasis is the acquisition of anoikis resistance. Anoikis or detachment-induced apoptosis is recognized as an important mechanism preventing cancer cell dissemination and invasion to form secondary tumors. A recent study by our group has shown that curcumin is able to sensitize lung cancer cells to undergo anoikis through a mechanism that involves post-translational modification of Bcl-2 via the ubiquitin-proteasome pathway (Pongrakhananon et al., 2010). Curcumin also acts as a negative regulator of cancer cell migration and invasion through diverse signaling pathways including MMP-9, MMP-2 and COX-2 (Philip et al., 2004, Lee et al., 2005; Hong et al., 2006; Lin et al., 2009).

Animal and clinical studies of curcumin have been well investigated. In mice, curcumin markedly inhibits DMBA and TPA-induced skin tumor formation (Azuine et al., 1992). In a xenograft model, curcumin administration significantly decreases the incidence of breast cancer metastasis to the lung (Aggarwal et al., 2005). In phase 1 clinical studies, oral administration of curcumin was shown to be well tolerated with no dose-limiting toxicity (Sharma et al., 2004; Lao et al., 2006). In patients with intestinal metaplasia, curcumin treatment showed a significant improvement in the precancerous lesion (Cheng et al., 2001), supporting the clinical use of curcumin as a preventive treatment agent against cancer. Although curcumin has demonstrated promising pharmacological effects and safety both *in vitro* and *in vivo*, poor bioavailability and tissue accumulation have been observed with the compound. Further studies on proper drug delivery, dose optimization, and biodistribution are needed.

2. Chemistry of curcumin

For thousands of years, plants and some parts of animal have been used as dietary agents which have been identified to be biologically active. These natural compounds have gained considerable interest for their potential as treatment and preventive agents for human diseases. Curcumin (diferuloylmethane) is a major biologically active compound extracted from the dried rhizome of turmeric or *Curcuma longa*. It has been widely used for centuries as medicinal plant and food additive due to its yellow color. Its medicinal properties are attributed to curcuminoids, which include curcumin (curcumin I), demethoxycurcumin (curcumin II), and bisdemethoxycurcumin (curcumin III) (Figure 2). Curcumin I (77%) is a

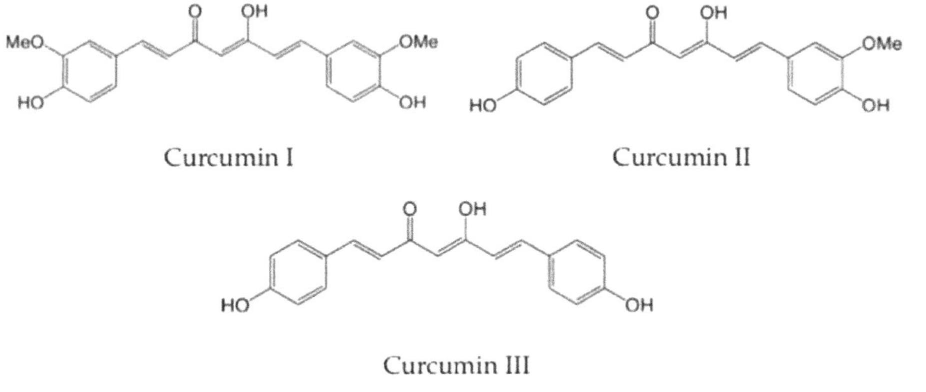

Curcumin I   Curcumin II

Curcumin III

Fig. 2. Chemical structure of curcuminoids

major component found in commercial curcumin, while curcumin II and III constitute approximately 17% and 3% respectively. Cucumin is a water-insoluble compound, but dissolves well in ethanol, dimethylsulfoxide, and other organic solvents. The molecular weight of curcumin is 368.37 and melting point is 183 °C. It shows a spectrophotometric maximum absorption (λmax) at 450 nm in methanol (Prasad and Sarasija, 1997). Fluorescence of curcumin occurs at 524 nm in acetonitrile and 549 nm in ethanol (Chignell et al., 1994). Curcumin undergoes rapid degradation in phosphate buffer and serum-free media, i.e., 90% within 30 minutes (Wang et al., 1997). In serum-containing (10%) media and human blood, curcumin is more stable with less than 20% degradation in 1 hour, and about 50% after 8 hours. Its degradation products are *trans*-6-(4'-hydroxy-3'-methoxyphenyl)-2,4-dioxo-5-hexenal (major) and vanillin, ferulic acid, and feruloyl methane (minor) (Wang et al., 1997).

3. Anticancer properties of curcumin

Curcumin has long been used as a dietary ingredient with known health benefits. Extensive research over the last decade has shown that curcumin possesses anticancer activities and could be used as a preventive or treatment agent against cancers, either as a single or combination therapy with chemotherapeutic agents. Curcumin exhibits biological activities in various stages of carcinogenesis including inhibition of oncogene activation, prevention of cancer-related inflammation, inhibition of cancer cell proliferation, induction of apoptosis and anoikis, prevention of metastasis, and sensitization of cancer cells to chemotherapy.

3.1 Cancer prevention
3.1.1 Chemopreventive properties
Carcinogenesis is a multistep process driven by genetic instability. Continuous exposure to environmental and endogenous genotoxic agents can cause substantial DNA damage. The damaged molecules can be transmitted during cell division producing mutated clones that can give rise to the expansion of premalignant cell population possessing uncontrolled proliferative and invasive properties. Curcumin has been established as a chemopreventive agent that has the ability to suppress or retard the carcinogenic process induced by various chemical carcinogens (Table 1). In animal models of gastric and colon cancer, curcumin inhibits the development of cancerous and precancerous lesions induced by N-methyl-N'-nitro-N-nitrosoguanosine (MNNG), a known mutagenic agent causing DNA methylation (Ikesaka et al., 2001). In the study, MNNG was given in drinking water at the concentration of 100 ppm for 8 weeks, and then 0.2% or 0.5% of curcumin was fed to the rats for 55 weeks. The results showed that the number of atypical hyperplasia in curcumin-treated rats was significantly less than that in the control group. Similarly, the curcumin analog bis-1,7-(2-hydroxyphenyl)-hepta-1,6-diene-3,5-dione was shown to inhibit the tumorigenic effect of 1,2-dimethylhydrazine in rats (Devasena et al., 2003). Furthermore, natural and synthetic curcuminoids exhibit an inhibitory effect on mutagenesis induced by 2-acetamidofluorene (2-AAF) (Anto et al., 1996). In the study, up to 87% of 2-AAF-induced papilloma was inhibited by bis-(p-hydroxycinnamoyl)methane (curcuminoid III), while 70% and 68% of the papilloma were inhibited by feruloyl-p-hydroxycinnamoylmethane (curcuminiod II) and diferuloylmethane (curcuminoid I), respectively. The most potent curcuminoid was salicylcurcuminoid which completely inhibited the papilloma formation.

3.1.2 Suppression of oncogenes and upregulation of tumor suppressor genes
As mentioned earlier, genetic instability is linked to the initiation of carcinogenesis. This irreversible process involves several molecular events that either promote the activity of

oncogenes such as myc and ras or impede the function of tumor suppressor genes such as p53 (Vogelstein and Kinzler, 2004). Curcumin has been shown to suppress oncogenes and activate tumor suppressor genes in various cancer cell types (Table 1). In an *in vivo* study, curcumin suppresses c-fos and c-Ha-ras activation induced by environmental mutagenic agents (Limtrakul et al., 2001). Dietary administration of curcumin (0.1-0.2%) prevents 2-dimethylbenz(α)anthracene (DMBA) and 12-O-tetradecanoylphorbol-13-acetate (TPA)-induced skin tumor in mice. There is an increase in the oncogene (c-fos and ras) expression in this tumor model, which is suppressed by the dietary curcumin. Similarly, c-myc is also a target oncogene attenuated by curcumin in the TPA-induced tumor model (Kakar and Roy, 1994).

Chemopreventive properties			
Cancer	Carcinogen	Animal	References
Stomach cancer	MNNG	Rat	Ikesaki et al., 2001
Colon cancer	DMH	Rat	Devasena et al., 2003
Papilloma	2-AAF	-	Anto et al., 1996
Mammary tumor	DMBA	Rat	Pereira et al., 1996
Skin tumor	TPA	Mouse	Lu et al., 1993
Liver cancer	Diethylnitrosamine	Mouse	Chuang et al., 2000
Oncogene suppression and tumor suppressor gene activation			
Cancer	Mechanism		References
Skin tumor	Suppress c-fos and c-Ha-ras-activation by DMBA		Limtrakul et al., 2001
B cell lymphoma	Suppress c-myc		Han et al., 1999
Mouse skin cancer	Suppress c-myc activated by TPA		Kakar & Roy, 1994
Human colon adenocarcinoma	Enhance p53 activity		Song et al., 2005
Human breast cancer	Enhance p53 activity		Choudhuri et al., 2002
Human glioma	Enhance p53 activity		Liu et al., 2007
Anti-inflammation -related cancer			
Cancer	Mechanism		References
-	Inhibit NO synthase in macrophages		Brouet & Ohshima, 1995
Human mantle cell lymphoma	Inhibit constitutive NF-κB activation		Shishodia et al., 2005
Mouse melanoma	Inhibit constitutive NF-κB activation		Marin et al., 2007
Human oral cancer	Inhibit constitutive NF-κB activation		Sharma et al., 2006
Non-small cell lung carcinoma	Inhibit constitutive NF-κB activation and COX expression		Shishodia et al., 2003

Table 1. Cancer preventive properties of curcumin

3.1.3 Anti-inflammatory activity

Epidemiological studies have supported the concept that cancers frequently originate at the site of chronic inflammation. This event has increasingly been accepted as the seventh hallmark of cancer (Colotta et al., 2009). Inflammation is a vital physiological process in response to injury, which leads to the mediation of inflammatory cells in the presence of enzymes and cytokines for repairing tissue damage. The linkage between cancer and inflammation is generally characterized as being intrinsic or extrinsic (Mantovani et al., 2008). The extrinsic pathway is induced by inflammation that facilitates cancer development, while the intrinsic pathway is driven by genetic instability causing inflammatory environment-related cancer. Both processes mediate the transcription factors involved in cell proliferative function and persistent activation of this event can lead to cancer. A considerable number of reports have described the linkage between cancer preventive properties and anti-inflammatory action of curcumin (Table 1). Mechanistically, curcumin inhibits the induction of nitric oxide synthase (NOS) by activated macrophages (Brouet and Ohshima, 1995). Nitric oxide (NO) and its derivatives such as peroxynitrite play a critical role in the inflammation process causing fibroblast proliferation and fibrosis (Romanska et al., 2002). Treatment of macrophages with lipopolysaccharide (LPS) and IFN-γ induces an inflammatory response that leads to the release of NO, which is inhibited by curcumin. Curcumin also suppresses the transcription of inducible NOS which is activated by LPS and IFN-γ. Since NO is implicated in tumor promotion, the attenuation of NO by curcumin hence suppresses tumor development.

Numerous studies have suggested that NF-κB plays a key role in promoting cancer development during chronic inflammation. NF-κB regulates the expression of several genes involved in the immune and inflammatory responses as well as in cell proliferation and apoptosis (Karin et al., 2002). It is required for the expression of a wide range of inflammatory cytokines and adhesion molecules, and is important in the cellular proliferative function by activating growth factor genes, proto-oncogenes and cell cycle regulators that contribute to carcinogenesis. In a study using human mantle cell lymphoma (MCL), curcumin inhibits constitutive NF-κB activation leading to the suppression of NF-κB regulated genes (Shishodia et al., 2005). MCL expresses a high level of cyclin D1, a cell cycle promoting factor and target transcription of NF-κB, which is a key survival factor of this cancer type. Curcumin treatment causes downregulation of constitutive NF-κB activation, inhibits IκBα kinase (IKK) and phosphorylated IκBα and p65, leading to cell cycle arrest and apoptosis. NF-κB is overexpressed in various tumors and cancer cell lines including melanoma cells. Electrophoretic mobility shift and gene reporter assays have demonstrated that curcumin suppresses constitutive NF-κB activation in melanoma cells and increases the number of cells in the sub G1 phase of cell cycle (Marin et al., 2007). Interestingly, curcumin shows selectivity in inducing apoptosis of melanoma cells but not melanocytes.

Other mechanisms of the anti-inflammatory-related cancer effect of curcumin have been proposed including suppression of cyclooxygenase 2 (COX-2). A wide range of stimuli mediates COX-2 expression and overexpression of this molecule is found in various cancer types in association with accelerated cell growth, antiapoptotic activity, angiogenesis, and metastasis (Prescott and Fitzpatrick, 2000). In a cigarette-smoking (CS) study using non-small cell lung cancer model, CS exposure activates NF-κB and subsequently induces COX-2 expression, which is inhibited by pre-treatment with curcumin (Shishodia et al., 2003). This chemopreventive property of curcumin is also observed in smokeless-tobacco mediated activation of NF-κB and its downstream target COX-2 (Sharma et al., 2006). Since inflammation contributes to tumor initiation, and curcumin possesses anti-inflammatory activity, curcumin could be beneficial in cancer prevention.

3.2 Inhibition of tumor growth and cell proliferation

Excessive proliferation is a hallmark of cancer (Hanahan and Weinberg, 2000). Aberrational cell division is an important basis of cancer development allowing formation and expansion of tumor growth. In normal cells, cell proliferation requires the growth signal that is generated by cell-cell interaction, neighbour cells and extracellular matrix. Cancer cells can further generate their own growth signals, upregulate growth receptors, and be desensitized to antigrowth factors. Upon transmitting the growth signals to their receptors, downstream mediators are activated which drive the quiescent cells to proliferative cycle (Evan and Vousden, 2001). Curcumin has been shown to modulate the expression and activity of growth factors, including epidermal growth factor (EGF) and insulin-like growth factor (IGF) (Table 2). Overexpression of EGF and its receptor, EGFR, was found in human prostate cancer cells undergoing rapid growth expansion (Cai et al., 2008). It has been demonstrated that curcumin blocks the EGF pathway through downregulation of EGFR, suppression of intrinsic EGFR tyrosine kinase activity, and inhibition of ligand-induced EGFR activity in both androgen-dependent and androgen-independent prostate cancer cells (Dorai et al., 2000).

Inhibition of cancer proliferation and tumor growth		
Cancer	Mechanism	References
Prostate cancer cells	Downregulation of EGFR, suppression of intrinsic EGFR tyrosine kinase activity, and inhibition ligand-induced EGFR activity	Dorai et al., 2000
Prostate and breast cancer cells	Downregulation of cyclin D1	Mukhopadhyay et al., 2002
Breast cancer cells	Suppression IGF system	Xia et al., 2007
Breast cancer cells	Induction of cell cycle arrest at S, G2/M phase by upregulation of p21	Chiu & Su, 2009
Human epidermoid carcinoma cells	Inhibit EGFR activity	Korutla & Kumar, 1994
Colon carcinoma cells	Induction of cell cycle arrest at S, G2/M phase	Chen et al., 1999
Human head and neck squamous carcinoma cells	Downregulation of cyclin D1	Aggarwal et al., 2004
Human biliary cancer cells	Downregulation of cyclin D1	Prakobwong et al., 2011
Human hepatocarcinoma cells	Induction of cell cycle arrest at S, G2/M phase	Cheng et al., 2010

Table 2. Inhibition of cancer proliferation and tumor growth

Likewise, insulin-like growth factor has been implicated in the regulation of normal cell growth, in which its atypical expression is found in human cancer cells (Samani et al., 2007). Curcumin abrogates IGF-1 system in MCF-7 human breast carcinoma cells (Xia et al., 2007). It decreases IGF-1 secretion in concomitant with the increasing IGF binding protein IGFBP-3 in a dose-dependent fashion. Furthermore, it abolishes IGF-1-stimulated MCF-7 growth through the suppression of IGF-1 mediated receptor activity and downregulation of IGF receptor mRNA expression.

Deregulation of cell cycle causes limitless replicative potential of cancer. Curcumin exhibits antiproliferative activity via the regulation of cell cycle (Table 2). It disrupts the progression of cell cycle by increasing the number of cancer cells at S, G2/M phase, hence preventing cell entering next cycle (Chen et al., 1999). Additional mechanistic studies indicate that curcumin downregulates cyclin D1 expression through inhibition of its promoter activity and enhanced degradation (Mukhopadhyay et al., 2002). Cyclin D1 is a subunit of cyclin-dependent kinase (Cdk)-4 and Cdk-6 which plays a key role in determining the cell cycle progression from G1 to S phase (Baldin et al., 1993) and overexpression of this gene is a common event in several forms of cancer (Knudsen et al., 2006). Similarly, in the presence of curcumin, cyclin D1 is suppressed as a result of NF-κB inhibition as observed in human head carcinoma, neck squamous carcinoma, and biliary cancer cells (Aggarwal et al., 2004; Prakobwong et al., 2011).

3.3 Induction of cancer cell apoptosis

Apoptosis plays an essential role in various physiological and pathological processes (Hengartner, 2000). Tissue homeostasis maintains the balance of cell proliferation and cell death as part of normal tissue development. Dysregulation of this process can lead to several diseases including cancer. Avoidance of apoptotic cell death is a major characteristic of malignant cells in response to stress conditions, which is achieved by activating the antiapoptotic signals or inhibiting proapoptotic signals (Hanahan and Weinberg, 2000). Several strategies have been developed to overcome this defective mechanism in cancers and curcumin has shown promising activities that modulate this mechanism in favor of cancer cell apoptosis.

Apoptosis generally occurs through two main pathways, intrinsic and extrinsic (Lavrik et al., 2005). The intrinsic pathway is initiated by several cellular stresses such as DNA damage which activates proapoptotic proteins, notably the Bcl-2 family proteins, causing mitochondrial membrane permeabilization and subsequent activation of the caspase cascade. In the extrinsic pathway, the interaction between death ligands and death receptors results in the assembly of death-inducing signaling complex (DISC) and the activation of initiator caspases. Curcumin is known to overcome the apoptosis resistance of cancer cells through both pathways (Table 3). In human acute myelogenous leukemia HL-60 cells, curcumin induces apoptosis by suppressing the expression of antiapoptotic Bcl-2 and Bcl-xL, causing cytochrome c release, caspase-3 activation, and PARP cleavage (Anto et al., 2002). Curcumin also stimulates the death receptor pathway through caspase-8 activation but overexpression of the DISC protein FADD cannot protect the cells from apoptosis in response to curcumin. In A549 lung adenocarcinoma cells, curcumin treatment up-regulates the mitochondrial Bax protein expression, suggesting the intrinsic pathway as a major pathway of curcumin-induced apoptosis in this cell type (Chen et al., 2010).

Molecular mechanisms of curcumin-induced apoptosis

Cancer	Mechanism	References
Human acute myelogenous leukemia cells	Downregulation of Bcl-2 and Bcl-xL	Anto et al., 2002
Lung adenocarcinoma cells	Upregulation of Bax and Downregulation of Bcl-2	Chen et al., 2010
Rat histocytoma cells	Induction of ROS production	Bhaumik et al., 1999
Human gingival fibroblasts and human submandibular gland carcinoma cells	Induction of ROS production	Atsumi et al., 2006
Human breast cancer cells	Downregulation of anti-apoptotic and upregulation of proapoptotic proteins in a p53-dependent manner	Choudhuri et al., 2002
Human breast cancer cells	Inhibition of PI3K/Akt pathway	Squires et al., 2003
Human breast and hepatic cancers cells	Glutathione depletion and ROS production	Syng-Ai et al., 2004
Human ovarian cancer cells	Upregulation of caspase-3 and downregulation of NF-κB expression	Zheng et al., 2002
Human colon cancer cells	Induction of ROS production and deactivation of JNK pathway	Moussavi et al., 2006
Human colon adenocarcinoma cells	Downregulation of anti-apoptotic and upregulation of proapoptotic proteins in a p53-dependent manner	Song et al., 2005
Human melanoma cells	Activation of caspase-3, and -8, Fas receptor aggregation, suppression of NF-κB activation, and downregulation of XIAP expression	Bush et al., 2001
T cell leukemia cells	Inhibition of PI3K/Akt pathway	Hussain et al., 2006
Prostate cancer cells	Inhibition of PI3K/Akt pathway	Shankar & Srivastava, 2007
Human glioblastoma cells	Increasing Bax:Bcl-2 ratio, activation of caspase-8, -9, and -3, downregulation of NF-κB	Karmakar et al., 2006
Breast cancer cells	Inhibition of MAPK and PI3K/Akt pathway	Squires et al., 2003

Table 3. Molecular mechanisms of curcumin-induced apoptosis

In human melanoma cells, curcumin induces apoptosis through the extrinsic pathway by activating caspase-8 (Bush et al, 2001). Inhibition of caspase-8 by specific caspase-8 inhibitor or pan-caspase inhibitor prevents cancer cell apoptosis, whereas specific caspase-9 inhibitor lacks this ability. The underlying apoptosis mechanism involves the induction of Fas receptor oligomerization independent of Fas ligand, supporting the role of death receptor modification in curcumin-induced apoptosis. In some cancers such as human glioblastoma T98G cells, curcumin induces apoptosis through both pathways (Karmakar et al., 2006).

The activation of apoptotic pathwas by curcumin is regulated by reactive oxygen species (ROS). In various cancer cell types including H460 non-small cell lung cancer cells (Chanvorachote et al., 2009), AK5 rat histocytoma cells (Bhaumik et al., 1999), human gingival fibroblasts (HGF), and human submandibular gland carcinoma (HSG) cells (Atsumi et al., 2006), the induction of apoptosis by curcumin requires ROS generation. Likewise, in MCF-7, MDAMB, and HepG2 cells, apoptosis is mediated through oxidative stress induced by curcumin as a result of glutathione depletion (Syng-Ai et al., 2004). In colon cancer cells, curcumin-induced cell death is associated with ROS generation that converges on JNK activation (Moussavi et al., 2006).

Other mechanisms of curcumin-induced apoptosis have been reported. In human HT-29 colon adenocarcinoma (Song et al., 2005) and breast cancer cells (Choudhuri et al., 2002), curcumin upregulates proapoptotic proteins and downregulates antiapoptotic proteins in the Bcl-2 family through p53-dependent mechanism. In T cell leukemia (Hussain et al., 2006) and breast cancer cells (Squires et al., 2003), apoptosis induced by curcumin involves PI3K/Akt signaling pathway. Curcumin inhibits Akt phosphorylation and upregulates p53 expression which induces the proapoptotic Bcl-2 family proteins facilitating cell apoptosis (Shankar and Srivastava, 2007).

3.4 Sensitization of cancer cells to chemotherapy

In addition to its direct apoptosis-inducing effect, curcumin has been reported to sensitize cancer cells to chemotherapy-induced cell death. The main problem of cancer chemotherapy is the acquisition of apoptosis resistance of cancer cells and the cytotoxicity to normal cells. Combination therapy is an alternative approach that can overcome this problem by potentiating the effects of combination drugs and reducing their cytotoxicity by using optimal dosage regimens. Curcumin is one such agent that has been investigated for its effect in combination therapy (Table 4). In non-small cell lung cancer cells, we have recently shown that cotreatment of the cells with cisplatin and curcumin results in a substantial increase in cancer cell death as compared to cisplatin treatment alone (Chanvorachote et al., 2009). Since cisplatin-based therapy is the first line drug for treatment of lung cancer and the efficacy of this drug is frequently attenuated by the development of drug resistance especially in advanced stage cancer (Chang, 2011), curcumin has the potential to overcome this resistance problem. Curcumin promotes the apoptotic effect of cisplatin by inducing superoxide anion and downregulating the anti-apoptotic Bcl-2 protein which facilitates the cancer cell killing by cisplatin.

In pancreatic cancer cells, the acquisition of apoptosis resistance to the combination therapy of gemcitabine and capecitabine (a prodrug of 5-fluorouracil, 5-FU) is frequently observed. It is thought that overexpression of the multidrug resistance-associated protein 5 (MRP5), which promotes cellular efflux of the drugs (Szakacs et al., 2006), contributes to the resistance. Curcumin was shown in a recent study to inhibit MRP5 activity and increase the sensitivity of pancreatic cancer cells to 5-FU-induced toxicity in a dose-dependent manner (Li et al., 2010).

Cancer cells	Chemotherapeutic drugs	References
Non-small cell lung cancer cells	Cisplatin	Chanvorachote et al., 2009
Pancreatic cancer cells	5-Fluorouracil	Li et al., 2010
Hela cells	Taxol	Bava et al., 2005
Human hepatic cancer cells	Doxorubicin	Notarbartolo et al., 2005
Hepatocellular carcinoima cells	Doxorubicin	Chuang et al., 2002
Human ovarian adenocarcinoma cells	Paclitaxel	Ganta & Amiji, 2009
Human melanoma cells	Tamoxifen	Chatterjee & Pandey, 2011
Human colorectal cancer cells	Oxaliplatin	Howells et al., 2010
Bladder cancer cells	Gemcitabine	Tharakan et al., 2010

Table 4. Curcumin potentiates chemotherapeutic agent-induced cancer cell death

Curcumin also augments the therapeutic effect of taxol in Hela cells (Bava et al., 2005). The synergistic mechanism involves the inhibition of NF-κB activation and Akt phosphorylation which results in increased apoptosis and decreased DNA synthesis of cancer cells independent of tubulin polymerization. The increased susceptibility of cancer cells to chemotherapeutic agents by curcumin might overcome the drug resistance problem, thus improving the clinical outcomes.

3.5 Inhibition of cancer metastasis

Cancer metastasis is the spread of cancer cells from the initiation site to other parts of the body, and particularly presented in several advanced stage cancers which are difficult to treat (Gubta and Massagué, 2006). Cancer metastasis is a multistep process involving complex interactions between the disseminating cancer cells and their microenvironment. When transformed cells are initiated and continue to grow at the primary site, angiogenic factors are synthesized for vascularization which increases the likelihood of tumor cells to enter in the blood stream or lymphatic system and colonize at distant sites. Once at the new sites, the extravasation of cancer cells allows the formation and growth of secondary tumors which complete the metastatic process (Fidler, 2003). Agents that inhibit metastasis provide a major advantage in treating cancers. Several studies have shown that curcumin inhibits cancer angiogenesis, migration and invasion by interacting with key regulatory molecules as summarized in Table 5.

It is well established that vascular endothelial growth factor (VEGF) and matrix metallo-proteinase family proteins (MMP) are essential factors in the angiogenesis and invasion of cancer cells (Carmeliet, 2005; Helmestin et al., 1994). In non-small cell lung cancer cells, VEGF, MMP-9 and MMP-2 are inhibited by curcumin through MEKK and ERK-dependent pathways, resulting in inhibition of cell migration and invasion (Lin et al., 2009). Similarly, in a human glioblastoma xenograft mouse model, curcumin inhibits tumor growth, suppresses angiogenesis, and increases animal survival through the inhibition of MMP-9 and neovascularization (Perry et al., 2010). Curcumin also acts as a potent inhibitor of breast cancer cell motility and invasion through the attenuation of MMP-3 which acts as an invasive factor in this cancer cell type (Boonrao et al., 2010).

Cancer	Effects	Mechanism	References
Human non-small cell lung cancer	Inhibition of cell invasion and migration	Inhibition of VEGF, MMP-9, and MMP-2 through MEKK and ERK pathway	Lin et al., 2009
Human glioblastoma	Suppression of angiogenesis	Inhibition of MMP-9	Perry et al., 2010
Human breast cancer	Inhibition of cancer motlity and invasion	Attenuation of MMP-3 activity	Boonrao et al., 2010
Human non-small cell lung cancer	Sensitization of cancer cell anoikis	Downregulation of Bcl-2 through proteasomal degradation	Pongrakhananon et al., 2010
Human lung cancer	Inhibition invasion and metastasis	Activation of tumor suppressor HLJ1 through JNK/JunD pathway	Chen et al., 2008
Human colon cancer	Inhibition of migration	Inhibition of neurotensin-mediated activator protein-1 and NF-κB activation, and suppression of neurotensin-stimulated IL-8 gene induction	Wang et al., 2006
Prostate cancer	Inhibition of invasion	Downregulation of MMP-2 and MMP-9	Hong et al., 2006
Human fribosarcoma	Inhibition of migration and invasion	Downregulation of MMP-2, MMP-9, uPA, MT1-MMP, and TIMP-2	Yodkeeree et al., 2008

Table 5. Antimetastatic properties of curcumin

Several studies have investigated the molecular mechanisms of cancer cell survival during metastasis. Survival of primary cancer cells in the circulation is a key factor determining its metastatic ability. In general, most adherent cells undergo apoptosis when detached due to improper environmental conditions. This detachment-induced apoptosis or anoikis which is often impaired in metastatic cancers (Mehlen and Puisieux, 2006) has increasingly been recognized as an important mechanism for controlling cancer cell dissemination and invasion to secondary sites. A recent study by our group has shown that curcumin can sensitize non-small cell lung cancer cells to anoikis (Pongrakhananon et al., 2010) through a mechanism that involves Bcl-2 downregulation through ubiquitin-proteasomal degradation. This process is dependent on ROS generation, partcularly superoxide anion which mediates the Bcl-2 degradation process, consistent with the previous findings on the pro-oxidant properties of curcumin (Bhaumik et al., 1999; Khar et al., 2001; Wang et al., 2008).

3.6 Animal studies

Several animal studies have been reported on the anticancer and chemopreventive effects of curcumin in various cancer types. Since the *in vivo* chemopreventive effect of curcumin has earlier been described under 3.1.1 and summarized in Table 1, we will focus on the direct *in vivo* anticancer properties of curcumin.

The anticancer property of curcumin in prostate cancer was investigated by using prostate cancer cells implanted into nude mice (Dorai et al., 2001). Dietary curcumin at the concentration of 2% was given to the mice, and after 6 weeks of treatment the animals were examined for tumor growth, apoptosis, and vascularity. The results showed that curcumin was able to decrease tumor volume, increase cancer cell apoptosis, and inhibit vascular angiogenesis as indicated by the reduction in microvessel density. A similar study using a murine xenograft model of human lung carcinoma cells was reported (Su et al., 2010). In this study, NCI-H460 cells were implanted subcutaneously into nude mice, and curcumin (30 and 45 mg/kg of bodyweight) was intraperitoneally injected into the mice every 4 days after the tumor reached 100 mm^3 in size. Curcumin was shown to significantly decrease the tumor size as compared to non-treated control.

The antitumor property of curcumin-encapsulated nanoparticles was investigated in the xenograft mouse model of human pancreatic cancer (Bisht et al., 2010). The nanoparticle formulation was injected twice daily for 3 weeks into the xenografted mice. Plasma concentration of curcumin was sustained in the treated mice at Tmax of 2.75 ± 1.50 h and Cmax of 17,176 ± 5,176 ng/ml. Tumor volume was substantially decreased in curcumin treated group. A greater antitumor effect was observed when curcumin was combined with gemcitabine. Curcumin also exhibited antimetastatic activity which was greatly enhanced by the combination treatment. The underlying mechanism of curcumin action involves NF-κB activation and downregualtion of cyclin D1 and MMP-9.

Curcumin also improves the therapeutic activity of paclitaxel in breast cancer (Aggarwal et al., 2005). Since most metastatic breast cancers acquire apoptosis resistance to paclitaxel, which is the first line therapy for breast cancer, a combination therapy with apoptosis-sensitizing agents such as curcumin could be beneficial. In a mouse model of breast cancer metastasis, curcumin was shown to decrease the incidence of breast cancer metastasis to the lung as compared to paclitaxel treatment alone. Tissue sections from treated animals showed that NF-κB, MMP-9, and COX-2 expression were increased in the paclitaxel-treated group but suppressed in the curcumin co-treatment group, supporting the ability of curcumin to abrogate paclitaxel resistance in this metastatic breast cancer model.

3.7 Clinical studies

Several clinical studies are ongoing to investigate the efficacy and safety of curcumin as a preventive treatment agent for a variety of cancers. In prospective phase I clinical trials, curcumin was shown to be safe even at high doses (Cheng et al., 2001). In this study, patients with premalignant lesions caused by oral leukoplakia, intestinal metaplasia, uterine cervical intraepithelial neoplasia, skin Bowen's disease, and bladder cancer were given a curcumin tablet which was taken orally for the period of three months at the daily dose of 500, 1000, 2000, 4000, and 8000 mg. No toxicity was observed in these patients even the highest dose (8000 mg/day). However, this dose was unacceptable by the patients due to its bulky volume. Peak serum concentration of curcumin after the 4000 mg administration was 0.51±0.11 µM, and 0.63±0.06 µM and 1.77±1.87 µM respectively after the 6000 mg and 8000 mg dosing. A similar study showed that a single dose of curcumin up to 12,000 mg had no dose-limiting toxic effect in healthy volunteers, not even minor adverse effects such as diarrhea (Lao et al., 2006).

Expanding from the above findings, another phase I clinical study was conducted in patients with colon adenocarcinoma to investigate the phamacodynamic of curcumin (Sharma et al., 2004). Curcuminoid, formulated as 500 mg in soft gelatin capsule containing 450 mg of curcumin, 40 mg of desmethoxycurcumin, and 10 mg of bisdesmethoxycurcumin, was taken orally at the dose of 450, 900, 1800, and 3600 mg/day of curcumin for 4 months. Since curcumin is known to induce glutathione S-transferase (GST), suppress prostaglandin E2 (PGE2) production, and inhibit oxidative DNA adduct (M1G) formation, these biomarkers are frequently used to indicate curcumin efficacy. Curcumin and its metabolites were collected from plasma, urine, and feces, and analyzed to assess the pharmacokinetic parameters. The results showed that curcumin was well tolerated by the patients without a dose-limiting toxicity, except in a few cases where patients reported a minor gastrointestinal upset. The result also showed that curcumin at the dose of 3600 mg/day was suitable for phase II evaluation. Curcumin was shown to inhibit PGE2 without affecting GST and M1G, suggesting that GST and M1G may not be useful as indicators for curcumin efficacy. Furthermore, curcumin and its glucuronide and sulfate metabolites were found in the plasma and urine. The presence of these metabolites at all time points indicates that curcumin has poor systemic availability when given orally.

Consistent with the above finding, numerous other studies have demonstrated low systemic bioavailability of curcumin resulting from poor absorption, rapid metabolism, and rapid systemic elimination (Hsu et al., 2007; Ireson et al., 2001; Maiti et al., 2007; Garcea et al., 2004). Glucuronide and sulfate metabolites of curcumin are rapidly detected in the peripheral and portal circulation after curcumin administration (Garcea et al., 2004). In this study, patients with liver metastasis from colorectal adenocarcinoma were administered orally with curcumin at the daily dose of 450, 1800, and 3600 mg for a week. No curcumin or its metabolites was detected in the bile or hepatic tissue, indicating that curcumin is not suitable for treating patients with tumors distant from the absorption site.

In a phase II clinical study conducted in patients with advanced pancreatic cancer, curcumin was administered orally at the dose of 8 g/day for 8 weeks (Dhillon et al., 2008). The treatment was well tolerated by the patients with no systemic side effects, while effectively reducing the tumor size and the activation of NF-κB and COX-2. Mechanistically, curcumin induces cancer cell apoptosis through an upregulation of p53 in the tumor tissues (He et al., 2011).

4. Conclusion

Curcumin has a great potential in cancer therapy and is gaining wide acceptance as a preventive treatment agent due to its safety. It affects multiple steps in the carcinogenic process, which is important in avoiding chemoresistance. Clinical studies have indicated its efficacy as a single agent or in combination therapy; however, more rigorous testing are needed. Furthermore, problems associated with the low bioavailability of curcumin, including poor absorption, rapid metabolism, and limited tissue distribution, must be addressed. Current strategies that have been investigated to overcome these problems include alternative administration routes, chemical modifications, and various drug delivery and formulation strategies. These strategies will likely benefit the development of curcumin as an anticancer agent.

5. Acknowledgment

This work was supported by NIH grants R01-HL076340, R01-HL076340-04S1, and R01-HL095579.

6. References

Aggarwal, S., Takada, Y., Singh, S., Myers, J.N., & Aggarwal, B.B. (2004) Inhibition of growth and survival of human head and neck squamous cell carcinoma cells by curcumin via modulation of nuclear factor-kappaB signaling. *International Journal of Cancer*, Vol. 111, No. 5, (September 2004), pp. 679-692, ISSN 1097-2015

Aggarwal, B.B., Shishodia, S., Takada, Y., Banerjee, S., Newman, R.A., Bueso-Ramos, C.E., & Price, J.E. (2005) Curcumin suppresses the paclitaxel-induced nuclear factor-kappaB pathway in breast cancer cells and inhibits lung metastasis of human breast cancer in nude mice. *Clinical Cancer Research*, Vol. 11, No. 20, (October 2005), pp. 7490-7498, ISSN 1078-0432

Amanda, M.G., & Robert, A.O. (2008) Curcumin and resveratrol inhibit nuclear factor-kappaB-mediated cytokine expression in adipocytes. *Nutrition and Metabolism*, Vol. 12, No. 5, (June 2008), pp. 1-13, ISSN 1743-7075

Anto, R.J., George, J., Babu, K.V., Rajasekharan, K.N., & Kuttan, R. (1996) Antimutagenic and anticarcinogenic activity of natural and synthetic curcuminoids. *Mutation Research*, Vol. 370, No. 2, (September 1996), pp. 127-131, ISSN 1383-5742

Anto, R.J., Mukhopadhyay, A., Denning, K., & Aggarwal, B.B. (2002). Curcumin (diferuloylmethane) induces apoptosis through activation of caspase-8, BID cleavage and cytochrome c release: Its suppression by ectopic expression of bcl-2 and bcl-xl. *Carcinogenesis*, Vol. 23, No. 1, (January 2002), pp. 143-150, ISSN 0143-3334

Atsumi, T., Tonosaki, K., & Fujisawa, S. (2006). Induction of early apoptosis and ROS-generation activity in human gingival fibroblasts (HGF) and human submandibular gland carcinoma (HSG) cells treated with curcumin. *Archives of Oral Biology*, Vol. 51, No. 10, (October 2006), pp. 913-921, ISSN0003-9969

Azuine, M.A., Kayal, J.J., & Bhide, S.V. (1992) Protective role of aqueous turmeric extract against mutagenicity of direct-acting carcinogens as well as benzopyrene-induced genotoxicity and carcinogenicity. *Journal of Cancer Research and Clinical Oncology*, Vol. 118, No. 6, pp. 447-452, ISSN 1432-1335

Baldin, V., Lukas, J., Marcote, M.J., Pagano, M. & Draetta, G. (1993) Cyclin D1 is a nuclear protein required for cell cycle progression in G1. *Genes & Development*, Vol. 7, No. 5, (May 1993), pp. 812-21, ISSN1549-5477

Bava, S.V., Puliappadamba, V.T., Deepti, A., Nair, A., Karunagaran, D., & Anto, R.J. (2005). Sensitization of taxol-induced apoptosis by curcumin involves down-regulation of nuclear factor-kappaB and the serine/threonine kinase akt and is independent of tubulin polymerization. *The Journal of Biological Chemistry*, Vol. 280, No. 8, (February 2005), pp. 6301-6308, ISSN 1083-351X

Bhaumik, S., Anjum, R., Rangaraj, N., Pardhasaradhi, B.V.V., & Khar, A. (1999) Curcumin mediated apoptosis in AK-5 tumor cells involves the production of reactive oxygen intermediates. *FEBS Letters*, Vol. 456, No. 2, (August 1999), pp.311-314, ISSN 0014-5793

Bisht, S., Mizuma, M., Feldmann, G., Ottenhof, N.A., Hong, S.M., Pramanik, D., Chenna, V., Karikari, C., Sharma, R., Goggins, M.G., Rudek, M.A., &Maitra, A. (2010). Systemic administration of polymeric nanoparticle-encapsulated curcumin (NanoCurc) blocks tumor growth and metastases in preclinical models of pancreatic cancer. *Molecular Cancer Therapeutics*, Vol. 9, No. 8, (August 2010), pp. 2255-2264, ISSN 1535-7163

Boonrao, M., Yodkeeree, S., Ampasavate, C., Anuchapreeda, S., & Limtrakul, P. (2010). The inhibitory effect of turmeric curcuminoids on matrix metalloproteinase-3 secretion in human invasive breast carcinoma cells. *Archives of Pharmacal Research*, Vol. 33, No. 7, (July 2010), pp. 989-998, ISSN 1976-3786

Brouet, I., & Ohshima, H. (1995)Curcumin, an anti-tumor promoter and anti-inflammatory agent, inhibits induction of nitric oxide synthase in activated macrophages.*Biochemical and Biophysical Research Communications*, Vol. 206, No. 2, (January 1995), pp. 533-540, ISSN 1090-2104

Bush, J.A., Cheung, K.J.,Jr, & Li, G. (2001). Curcumin induces apoptosis in human melanoma cells through a fas receptor/caspase-8 pathway independent of p53. *Experimental Cell Research*, Vol. 271, No. 2, (December 2001), pp. 305-314, ISSN 0014-4827

Cai, C.Q., Peng, Y., Buckley, M.T., Wei, J., Chen, F., Liebes, L., Gerald, W.L., Pincus, M.R., Osman, I. & Lee, P. (2008). Epidermal growth factor receptor activation in prostate cancer by three novel missense mutations. *Oncogene*, Vol. 27, No. 22, (January 2008), pp. 3201-3210, ISSN 0950-9232

Carmeliet, P. (2005). VEGF as a key mediator of angiogenesis in cancer. *Oncology*, Vol. 69, No. Suppl 3, (November 2005), pp. 4-10, ISSN 1423-0232

Chang, A. (2011). Chemotherapy, chemoresistance and the changing treatment landscape for NSCLC. *Lung Cancer (Amsterdam, Netherlands)*, Vol. 71, No. 1, (January 2011), pp. 3-10, ISSN 0169-5002

Chanvorachote, P., Pongrakhananon, V., Wannachaiyasit, S., Luanpitpong, S., Rojanasakul, Y., & Nimmanit U (2009) Curcumin sensitizes lung cancer cells to cisplatin-induced apoptosis through superoxide anion-mediated Bcl-2 degradation. *Cancer Investigation*, Vol. 26, No. 6, (July 2009), pp. 624-635, ISSN 1532-4192

Chatterjee, S.J., & Pandey, S. (2011). Chemo-resistant melanoma sensitized by tamoxifen to low dose curcumin treatment through induction of apoptosis and autophagy. *Cancer Biology & Therapy*, vol. 11, No. 2, (January 2011), pp. 216-228, ISSN 1555-8576

Chen, H., Zhang, Z.S., Zhang, Y.L., & Zhou, D.Y. (1999). Curcumin inhibits cell proliferation by interfering with the cell cycle and inducing apoptosis in colon carcinoma cells. *Anticancer Research*, Vol. 19, No.5A, (Septober-October 1999), pp. 3675-3680, ISSN 1791-7530

Chen, H.W., Lee, J.Y., Huang, J.Y., Wang, C.C., Chen, W.J., Su, S.F., Huang, C.W., Ho, C.C., Chen, J.J., Tsai, M.F., Yu, S.L., & Yang, P.C. (2008) Curcumin inhibits lung cancer cell invasion and metastasis through the tumor suppressor HLJ1. *Cancer Research*, Vol. 68, No. 18, (September 2008), pp. 7428-7438, ISSN 1538-7445

Chen, Q.Y., Lu, G.H., Wu, Y.Q., Zheng, Y., Xu, K., Wu, L.J., Jiang, Z.Y., Feng, R., & Zhou, J.Y. (2010) Curcumin induces mitochondria pathway mediated cell apoptosis in A549 lung adenocarcinoma cells. *Oncology Report*, Vol. 23, No. 5, (May 2010), pp. 1285-1292, ISSN 1792- 2431

Cheng, A.L., Hsu, C.H., Lin, J.K., Hsu, M.M., Ho, Y.F., Shen, T.S., Ko, J.Y., Lin, J.T., Lin, B.R., Ming-Shiang, W., Yu, H.S., Jee, S.H., Chen, G.S., Chen, T.M., Chen, C.A., Lai, M.K., Pu, Y.S., Pan, M.H., Wang, Y.J., Tsai, C.C., & Hsieh, C.Y. (2001) Phase I clinical trial of curcumin, a chemopreventive agent, in patients with high-risk or pre-malignant lesions. *Anticancer Research*, Vol. 21, No. 4B, (July-August 2001), pp. 2895-2900, ISSN 1791-7530

Cheng, C.Y., Lin, Y.H., & Su, C.C. (2010). Curcumin inhibits the proliferation of human hepatocellular carcinoma J5 cells by inducing endoplasmic reticulum stress and mitochondrial dysfunction. *International Journal of Molecular Medicine*, Vol. 26, No. 5, (November 2010), pp. 673-678, ISSN 1791-244X

Chignell, C.F., Bilski, P., Reszka, K.J., Motten, A.G., Sik, R.H., & Dahl, T.A. (1994). Spectral and photochemical properties of curcumin. *Photochemistry and Photobiology*, Vol. 59, No. 3, (March 1994), pp. 295-302, ISSN 1751-1097

Chiu, T.L., & Su, C.C. (2009) Curcumin inhibits proliferation and migration by increasing the Bax to Bcl-2 ratio and decreasing NF-kappaBp65 expression in breast cancer MDA-MB-231 cells. *International Journal of Molecular Medicine*, Vol. 23, No. 4, (April 2009), pp. 469-475, ISSN 1791- 244X

Choudhuri, T., Pal, S., Agwarwal, M.L., Das, T., & Sa, G. (2002). Curcumin induces apoptosis in human breast cancer cells through p53-dependent bax induction. *FEBS Letters*, Vol. 512, No.1-3, (February 2002), pp. 334-340, ISSN 0014-5793

Chuang, S.E., Cheng, A.L., Lin, J.K., & Kuo, M.L. (2000). Inhibition by curcumin of diethylnitrosamine-induced hepatic hyperplasia, inflammation, cellular gene products and cell-cycle-related proteins in rats.*Food and Chemical Toxicology : An International Journal Published for the British Industrial Biological Research Association*, Vol. 38, No. 11, (November 2000), pp. 991-995, ISSN 1873-6351

Chuang, S.E., Yeh, P.Y., Lu, Y.S., Lai, G.M., Liao, C.M., Gao, M., & Cheng, A.L. (2002) Basal levels and patterns of anticancer drug-induced activation of nuclear factor-kappaB (NF-kappaB), and its attenuation by tamoxifen, dexamethasone, and curcumin in carcinoma cells. *Biochemical Pharmacology*, Vol. 63, No. 9, (May 2002), pp. 1709-1716, ISSN 1873-2968

Colotta, F., Allavena, P., Sica, A., Garlanda, C., &Mantovani, A. (2009)Cancer-related inflammation, the seventh hallmark of cancer: links to genetic instability. *Carcinogenesis*, Vol. 7, No. 30, (May 2009), pp. 1073-1081, ISSN 1460-2180

Devasena, T., Rajasekaran, K.N., Gunasekaran, G., Viswanathan, P., & Menon, V.P. (2003)Anticarcinogenic effect of bis-1,7-(2-hydroxyphenyl)-hepta-1,6-diene-3,5-dione a curcumin analog on DMH-induced colon cancer model. *Pharmacological Research*, Vol. 47, No. 2, (Febrauary 2003), pp. 133-140, ISSN 1096-1186

Dhillon, N., Aggarwal, B.B., Newman, R.A., Wolff, R.A., Kunnumakkara, A.B., Abbruzzese, J.L., Ng, C.H., Badmaev, E., & Kurzrock, R. (2008). Phase II trial of curcumin in patients with advanced pancreatic cancer. *Clinical Cancer Research : An Official*

Journal of the American Association for Cancer Research, Vol. 14, No. 14, (July 2008), pp. 4491-4499, ISSN 1557-3265

Diehl, J.A. (2002) Cycling to cancer with cyclin D1. *Cancer Biology & Therapy*, Vol. 1, No. 3, (May- June 2002), pp. 226-231, ISSN 1555-8576

Dorai, T., Gehani, N., & Katz, A. (2000). Therapeutic potential of curcumin in human prostate cancer. II. curcumin inhibits tyrosine kinase activity of epidermal growth factor receptor and depletes the protein. *Molecular Urology*, Vol. 4, No. 1, pp. 1-6, ISSN 1091-5362

Dorai, T., Cao, Y.C., Dorai ,B., Buttyan, R., &Katz, A.E. (2001) Therapeutic potential of curcumin in human prostate cancer. III. Curcumin inhibits proliferation, induces apoptosis, and inhibits angiogenesis of LNCaP prostate cancer cells in vivo. *The prostate*, Vol. 47, No. 4, (June 2001), pp. 293-303, ISSN 1097-0045

Evan, G.I., & Vousden, K.H. (2001) Proliferation, cell cycle and apoptosis in cancer. *Nature*, Vol. 6835, No. 411, (May 2001), pp. 342-348, ISSN 1476-4687

Fidler, I.J. (2003) The pathogenesis of cancer metastasis: the seed and soil hypothesis revisited. *Nature Reviews Cancer*, Vol. 3, No.6, (June 2003), pp. 453-458, ISSN 1474-1768

Ganta, S., &Amiji, M. (2009) Coadministration of paclitaxel and curcumin in nanoemulsion formulations to overcome multidrug resistance in tumor cells. *Molecular Pharmacology*, Vol. 6, No. 3, (May-June 2009), pp. 928-939, ISSN 1543-8392

Garcea, G., Jones, D.J., Singh, R., Dennison, A.R., Farmer, P.B., Sharma, R.A., Steward, W.P., Gescher, A.J., & Berry, D.P. (2004). Detection of curcumin and its metabolites in hepatic tissue and portal blood of patients following oral administration. *British Journal of Cancer*, Vol. 90, No. 5, (March 2004), pp. 1011-1015, ISSN 0007-0920

Gupta, G.P., & Massague, J. (2006). Cancer metastasis: Building a framework. *Cell*, Vol. 127, No. 4, (November 2006), pp. 679-695, ISSN 0092-8674

Han, S.S., Chung, S.T., Robertson, D.A., Ranjan, D., & Bondada, S. (1999) Curcumin causes the growth arrest and apoptosis of B cell lymphoma by downregulation of egr-1, c-myc, bcl-XL, NF- kappa B, and p53. *Clinical Immunology*, Vol. 93, No. 2, (November 1999), pp. 152-161, ISSN 1521-7035

Hanahan, D.,& Weinberg, R.A. (2000) The Hallmarks of cancer. *Cell*, Vol. 1, No. 100, (January 2000), pp. 57-70, ISSN0092-8674

He, Z.Y., Shi, C.B., Wen, H., Li, F. L., Wang, B.L., & Wang, J. (2011). Upregulation of p53 expression in patients with colorectal cancer by administration of curcumin. *Cancer Investigation*, Vol. 29, No. 3, (March 2011), pp. 208-213, ISSN 0735-7907

Hengartner, M.O. (2000) The biochemistry of apoptosis. *Nature*, Vol. 407, No. 6805, (October 2000), pp. 770–776, ISSN 0028-0836

Himelstein, B.P., Canete-Soler, R., Bernhard, E.J., Dilks, D.W., & Muschel, R.J. (1994). Metalloproteinases in tumor progression: The contribution of MMP-9. *Invasion & Metastasis*, Vol. 14, No. 1-6, pp. 246-258, ISSN 0251-1789

Hong, J.H., Ahn, K.S., Bae, E., Jeon, S.S., & Choi, H.Y. (2006) The effects of curcumin on the invasiveness of prostate cancer in vitro and in vivo. *Prostate Cancer and Prostatic Diseases*, Vol. 9, No. 2, (January 2006), pp. 147-52, ISSN 1476-5608

Howells, L.M., Sale, S., Sriramareddy, S.N., Irving, G.R., Jones, D.J., Ottley, C.J., Pearson, D.G., Mann, C.D., Manson, M.M., Berry, D.P., Gescher, A., Steward, W.P., &Brown,

K. (2010). Curcumin ameliorates oxaliplatin-induced chemoresistance in HCT116 colorectal cancer cells in vitro and in vivo. *International Journal of Cancer.Journal International Du Cancer*, (Septemper 2010), ISSN 1097-0215

Hsu, C.H., & Cheng, A.L. (2007) Clinical studies with curcumin. *Advances in Experimental Medicine and Biology*, Vol. 595, pp. 471-480, ISSN 0065-2598

Hussain, A.R., Al-Rasheed, M., Manogaran, P.S., Al-Hussein, K.A., Platanias, L.C., Al Kuraya, K., & Uddin, S. (2006). Curcumin induces apoptosis via inhibition of PI3'-kinase/AKT pathway in acute T cell leukemias. *Apoptosis : An International Journal on Programmed Cell Death*, Vol. 11, No. 2, (February 2006), pp. 245-254, ISSN 1573-675X

Ikezaki, S., Nishikawa, A., Furukawa, F., Kudo, K., Nakamura, H., Tamura, K., & Mori, H. (2001)Chemopreventive effects of curcumin on glandular stomach carcinogenesis induced by N-methyl-N'-nitro-N-nitrosoguanidine and sodium chloride in rats. *Anticancer Research*,Vol. 21, No. 5, (September-October 2001), pp. 3407-3411, ISSN 1791-7530

Ireson, C., Orr, S., Jones, D.J., Verschoyle, R., Lim, C.K., Luo, J.L,Howells, L., Plummer, S., Jukes, R., Williams, M., Steward, W.P., &Gescher, A. (2001). Characterization of metabolites of the chemopreventive agent curcumin in human and rat hepatocytes and in the rat in vivo, and evaluation of their ability to inhibit phorbol ester-induced prostaglandin E2 production. *Cancer Research*, Vol. 61, No. 3, (February 2001), pp. 1058-1064, ISSN 1538-7445

Jagetia, G.C., & Rajanikant, G.K. (2005) Curcumin treatment enhances the repair and regeneration of wounds in mice exposed to hemibody gamma irradiation. *Plastic and Reconstructive Surgery*, Vol. 115, No. 2, (February 2005), pp. 515-528, ISSN 1529-4242

Kakar, S. S., & Roy, D. (1994). Curcumin inhibits TPA induced expression of c-fos, c-jun and c-myc proto-oncogenes messenger RNAs in mouse skin. *Cancer Letters*, Vol. 87, No. 1, (November 1994), pp. 85-89, ISSN 0304-3835

Karin, M., Cao, Y., Greten, F.R., & Li, Z.W. (2002)NF-kB in cancer: from innocent bystander to major culprit. *Nature Reviews Cancer*, Vol. 4, No. 2, (April 2002), pp. 301-310, ISSN 1474-1768

Karmakar, S., Banik, N.L., Patel, S.J., & Ray, S.K. (2006). Curcumin activated both receptor-mediated and mitochondria-mediated proteolytic pathways for apoptosis in human glioblastoma T98G cells.*Neuroscience Letters*, Vol. 407, No. 1, (October 2006), pp. 53-58, ISSN 0304-3940

Kastan, M.B., & Bartek, J. (2004) Cell-cycle checkpoints and cancer. *Nature*, Vol. 432, No. 7015, (November 2004), pp. 316-23, ISSN 1476-4687

Khar, A., Ali, A.M., Pardhasaradhi, B.V.V., Varalakshmi, C., Anjum, R., & Kumari, A.L. (2001) Induction of stress response renders human tumor cell lines resistant to curcumin-mediated apoptosis: role of reactive oxygen intermediates. *Cell Stress Chaperones*, Vol. 6, No. 4, (October 2006), pp. 368-376, ISSN1466-1268

Knudsen, K.E., Diehl, J.A., Haiman, C.A., & Knudsen, E.S. (2006). Cyclin D1: Polymorphism, aberrant splicing and cancer risk. *Oncogene*, Vol. 25, No. 11, (March 2006), pp. 1620-1628, ISSN1476-5594

Korutla, L., & Kumar, R. (1994). Inhibitory effect of curcumin on epidermal growth factor receptor kinase activity in A431 cells. *Biochimica Et Biophysica Acta*, Vol. 1224, No. 3, (December 1994), pp. 597-600. ISSN 0006-3002

Lao, C.D., Ruffin, M.T. 4th, Normolle, D., Heath, D.D., Murray, S.I., Bailey, J.M., Boggs, M.E., Crowell, J., Rock, C.L., & Brenner, D.E. (2006)   Dose   escalation   of   a curcuminoid formulation.*BMC Complementary and Alternative Medicine*, Vol. 12, No. 6, (March 2006), pp. 10, ISSN 1472-6882

Lavrik, I.N., Golks, A., & Krammer, P.H. (2005) Caspases: pharmacological manipulation of cell death. *The Journal of Clinical Investigation*, Vol. 115, No. 10, (October 2005), pp. 2665-2672, ISSN 1558-8238

Lee, K.W., Kim, J.H., Lee, H.J., & Surh, Y.J. (2005) Curcumin inhibits phorbol ester-induced upregulation of cyclooxygenase-2 and matrix metalloproteinase-9 by blocking ERK1/2 phosphorylation and NF-kappaB transcriptional activity in MCF10A human breast epithelial cells. *Antioxidant and Redox Signaling*, Vol. 7, No. 11-12, (November-December 2005), pp. 1612-1620, ISSN 1523-0864

Li, Y., Revalde, J.L., Reid, G., & Paxton, J.W. (2010). Modulatory effects of curcumin on multi-drug resistance-associated protein 5 in pancreatic cancer cells. *Cancer Chemotherapy and Pharmacology*,(November 2010), ISSN 1432-0843

Limtrakul, P., Anuchapreeda, S., Lipigorngoson, S., & Dunn, F.W. (2001). Inhibition of carcinogen induced c-ha-ras and c-fos proto-oncogenes expression by dietary curcumin. *BMC Cancer*, Vol. 1, No. 1, (Junuary 2011), ISSN 1471-2407

Lin, S.S., Lai, K.C., Hsu, S.C., Yang, J.S., Kuo, C.L., Lin, J.P., Ma, Y.S., Wu, C.C., & Chung, J.G. (2009) Curcumin inhibits the migration and invasion of human A549 lung cancer cells through the inhibition of matrix metalloproteinase-2 and -9 and vascular endothelial growth factor (VEGF). *Cancer Letters*, Vol. 285, No. 2, (May 2009), pp. 127-133, ISSN 1872-7980

Liu, E., Wu, J., Cao, W., Zhang, J., Liu, W., Jiang, X., & Zhang, X. (2007). Curcumin induces G2/M cell cycle arrest in a p53-dependent manner and upregulates ING4 expression in human glioma. *Journal of Neuro-Oncology*, Vol. 85, No. 3, (December 2007), pp. 263-270, ISSN 1573-7373

Lu, Y.P., Chang, R.L., Huang, M.T., & Conney, A.H. (1993). Inhibitory effect of curcumin on 12-O-tetradecanoylphorbol-13-acetate-induced increase in ornithine decarboxylase mRNA in mouse epidermis.*Carcinogenesis*, Vol. 14, No. 2, (February 1993), pp. 293-297, ISSN 1460-2180

Mai, S.,& Mushinski, J.F. (2003) c-Myc-induced genomic instability. *Journal of Environmental Pathology, Toxicology and Oncology*, Vol. 22, No. 3, pp. 179-199, ISSN 0731-8898

Maiti, K., Mukherjee, K., Gantait, A., Saha, B.P., & Mukherjee, P.K. (2007). Curcumin-phospholipid complex: Preparation, therapeutic evaluation and pharmacokinetic study in rats. *International Journal of Pharmaceutics*,Vol. 330, No. 1-2, (February 2007), pp. 155-163, ISSN 0378-5173

Mantovani, A., Allavena, P., Sica, A., & Balkwill, F. (2008) Cancer-related inflammation. *Nature*, Vol. 7203, No. 454, (July 2008), pp. 436-444, ISSN 1476-4687

Marin, Y.E., Wall, B.A., Wang, S., Namkoong, J., Martino, J.J., Suh, J., Lee, H.J., Rabson, A.B., Yang, C.H., Chen, S., & Ryu, J.H. (2007). Curcumin downregulates the constitutive activity of NF-kappaB and induces apoptosis in novel mouse melanoma cells. *Melanoma Research*, Vol. 17, No. 5, (October 2007), pp. 274-283, ISSN 1473-5636

Mehlen, P., & Puisieux, A. (2006) Metastasis: a question of life or death. *Nature Reviews Cancer*, Vol. 6, No. 6, (June 2006), pp. 449-458, ISSN 1474-1768

Moussavi, M., Assi, K., Gómez-Muñoz, A., & Salh, B. (2006) Curcumin mediates ceramide generation via the de novo pathway in colon cancer cells. *Carcinogenesis*, Vol. 27, No. 8, (August 2006), pp. 1636-1644, ISSN 1460-2180

Mukhopadhyay, A., Banerjee, S., Stafford, L.J., Xia, C., Liu, M., & Aggarwal, B.B. (2002). Curcumin-induced suppression of cell proliferation correlates with down-regulation of cyclin D1 expression and CDK4-mediated retinoblastoma protein phosphorylation. *Oncogene*, Vol. 21, No. 57, (December 2002), pp. 8852-8861, ISSN 1476-5594

Notarbartolo, M., Poma, P., Perri, D., Dusonchet, L., Cervello, M., & D'Alessandro, N. (2005) Antitumor effects of curcumin, alone or in combination with cisplatin or doxorubicin, on human hepatic cancer cells. analysis of their possible relationship to changes in NF-kB activation levels and in IAP gene expression. *Cancer Letters*, Vol. 224, No. 1, (June 2005), pp. 53-65, ISSN 1872- 7980

Park, C., Kim, G.Y., Kim, G.D., Choi, B.T., Park, Y.M., & Choi, Y.H. (2006) Induction of G2/M arrest and inhibition of cyclooxygenase-2 activity by curcumin in human bladder cancer T24 cells. *Oncology Reports*, Vol. 15, No. 5, (May 2006), pp. 1225-1231, ISSN 1791-2431

Pereira, M.A., Grubbs, C.J., Barnes, L.H., Li, H., Olson, G.R., Eto, I., Juliana, M., Whitaker, L.M., Kelloff, G.J., Steele, V.E., & Lubet, R.A. (1996). Effects of the phytochemicals, curcumin and quercetin, upon azoxymethane-induced colon cancer and 7,12-dimethylbenz[a]anthracene-induced mammary cancer in rats. *Carcinogenesis*, Vol. 17, No. 6, (June 1996), pp. 1305-1311, ISSN 1460-2180

Perry, M.C., Demeule, M., Regina, A., Moumdjian, R., & Beliveau, R. (2010). Curcumin inhibits tumor growth and angiogenesis in glioblastoma xenografts. *Molecular Nutrition & Food Research*, Vol. 54, No. 8, (August 2010), pp. 1192-1201, ISSN 1613-4133

Philip, S., Bulbule, A., & Kundu, G.C. (2004) Matrix metalloproteinase-2: mechanism and regulation of NF-kappaB-mediated activation and its role in cell motility and ECM-invasion. *Glycoconjugate Journal*, Vol. 21, No. 8-9, (November 2004), pp. 429-441, ISSN 1573-4986

Pongrakhananon, V., Nimmannit, U., Luanpitpong, S., Rojanasakul, Y., & Chanvorachote, P. (2010) Curcumin sensitizes non-small cell lung cancer cell anoikis through reactive oxygen species- mediated Bcl-2 downregulation. *Apoptosis*, Vol. 15, No. 5, (May 2010), pp. 574-585, ISSN 1360- 8185

Prakobwong, S., Gupta, S.C., Kim, J.H., Sung, B., Pinlaor, P., Hiraku, Y., Wongkham, S., Sripa, B., Pinlaor, S., & Aggarwal, B.B. (2011). Curcumin suppresses proliferation and induces apoptosis in human biliary cancer cells through modulation of multiple cell signaling pathways. *Carcinogenesis*, (February 2011), ISSN1460-2180

Prasad, N.S., & Sarasija, S. (1997) Spectrophotometric estimationof curcumin. *Indian Drugs*, vol. 34, pp. 227-228, ISSN 0019-462X

Prescott, S.M., & Fitzpatrick, F.A. (2000) Cyclooxygenase-2 and carcinogenesis. *Biochimica et biophysica acta*, Vol. 1470, No. 2, (March 2000), pp. M69-78, ISSN 0006-3002

Rajalingam, K., Schreck, R., Rapp, U.R., & Albert, S. (2007) Ras oncogenes and their downstream targets. *Biochimica et Biophysica Acta*, Vol. 1773, No. 8, (January 2007), pp. 1177-1195, ISSN 0006-3002

Romanska, H.M., Polak, J.M., Coleman, R.A., James, R.S., Harmer, D.W., Allen, J.C., & Bishop, A.E. (2002)iNOS gene upregulation is associated with the early proliferative response of human lung fibroblasts to cytokine stimulation. *The Journal of Pathology*, Vol. 3, No. 197, (July 2002),pp. 372–379, ISSN 1096-9896

Samani, A.A., Yakar, S., LeRoith, D., & Brodt, P. (2007) The role of the IGF system in cancer growth and metastasis: overview and recent insights. *Endocrine Reviews*, Vol. 28, No. 1, (Febrauary 2007), pp. 20-47, ISSN 1945-7189

Shankar, S., & Srivastava, R.K. (2007). Involvement of bcl-2 family members, phosphatidylinositol 3'-kinase/AKT and mitochondrial p53 in curcumin (diferulolylmethane)-induced apoptosis in prostate cancer.*International Journal of Oncology*, Vol. 30, No.4, (April 2007), pp. 905-918, ISSN 1019-6439

Sharma, C., Kaur, J., Shishodia, S., Aggarwal, B.B., & Ralhan, R. (2006). Curcumin down regulates smokeless tobacco-induced NF-kappaB activation and COX-2 expression in human oral premalignant and cancer cells. *Toxicology*, Vol. 228, No. 1, (November 2006), pp. 1-15, ISSN 0300-483X

Sharma, R.A., Euden, S.A., Platton, S.L., Cooke, D.N., Shafayat, A., Hewitt, H.R., Marczylo, T.H., Morgan, B., Hemingway, D., Plummer, S.M., Pirmohamed, M., Gescher, A.J., & Steward, W.P. (2004) Phase I clinical trial of oral curcumin: biomarkers of systemic activity and compliance. *Clinical Cancer Research*, Vol. 15, No. 20, (October 2004), pp. 6847-6854, ISSN 1078-0432

Shishodia, S., Potdar, P., Gairola, C.G., & and Aggarwal, B.B. (2003)Curcumin (diferuloylmethane) down-regulates cigarette smoke-induced NF-kBactivation through inhibition of IkBa kinase in human lung epithelial cells:correlation with suppression of COX-2, MMP-9 and cyclin D1. *Carcinogenesis*, Vol.24, No.7, pp.1269-1279, ISSN 1460-2180

Shishodia, S., Amin, H.M., Lai, R., & Aggarwal, B.B. (2005). Curcumin (diferuloylmethane) inhibits constitutive NF-kappaB activation, induces G1/S arrest, suppresses proliferation, and induces apoptosis in mantle cell lymphoma. *Biochemical Pharmacology, Vol. 70, No. 5*, (September 2005), pp. 700-713, ISSN 1873-2968

Simon, A., Allais, D.P., Duroux, J.L., Basly, J.P., Durand-Fontanier, S., & Delage, C. (1998) Inhibitory effect of curcuminoids on MCF-7 cell proliferation and structure-activity relationships. *Cancer Letters*, Vol. 129, No. 1, (July 1998), pp. 111-116, ISSN 1872-7980

Singh, M., & Singh, N. (2009) Molecular mechanism of curcumin induced cytotoxicity in human cervical carcinoma cells *Molecular and Cellular Biochemistry*, Vol. 325, No. 1-2, (February 2009), pp. 107-119, ISSN 1573-4919

Song, G., Mao, Y.B., Cai, Q.F., Yao, L.M., Ouyang, G.L., & Bao, S.D. (2005). Curcumin induces human HT-29 colon adenocarcinoma cell apoptosis by activating p53 and regulating apoptosis-related protein expression. *Brazilian Journal of Medical and Biological Research*, Vol. 38,No. 12, (December 2005), pp. 1791-1798, ISSN 1414-431X

Squires, M.S., Hudson, E.A., Howells, L., Sale, S., Houghton, C.E., Jones, J.L., Fox, L.H., Dickens, M., Prigent, S.A. & Manson, M.M. (2003). Relevance of mitogen activated protein kinase (MAPK) and phosphotidylinositol-3-kinase/protein kinase B (PI3K/PKB) pathways to induction of apoptosis by curcumin in breast cells. *Biochemical Pharmacology*, Vol. 65, No. 3, (February 2003), pp. 361-376, ISSN1873-2968

Su, C.C., Yang, J.S., Lu, C.C., Chiang, J.H., Wu, C.L., Lin, J.J., Lai, K.C., Hsia, T.C., Lu, H.F., Fan, M.J., & Chung, G.J. (2010). Curcumin inhibits human lung large cell carcinoma cancer tumour growth in a murine xenograft model. *Phytotherapy Research : PTR*, Vol. 24, No. 2, (February 2010), pp. 189-192, ISSN 1099-1573

Syng-Ai, C., Kumari, A.L., & Khar, A. (2004). Effect of curcumin on normal and tumor cells: Role of glutathione and bcl-2. *Molecular Cancer Therapeutics*, Vol. 3, No. 9, (September 2004), pp. 1101-1108, ISSN 1538-8514

Szakacs, G., Paterson, J.K., Ludwig, J.A., Booth-Genthe, C. & Gottesman, M.M. (2006) Targeting multidrug resistance in cancer. *Nature Reviews. Drug Discovery*, Vol. 5, No. 3, (March 2006), pp. 219-234, ISSN 1474-1784

Tharakan, S.T., Inamoto, T., Sung, B., Aggarwal, B.B., & Kamat, A.M. (2010). Curcumin potentiates the antitumor effects of gemcitabine in an orthotopic model of human bladder cancer through suppression of proliferative and angiogenic biomarkers. *Biochemical Pharmacology*, Vol. 79, No. 2, (January 2010), pp. 218-228, ISSN 0006-2952

Ventura, A., Kirsch, D.G., McLaughlin, M.E., Tuveson, D.A., Grimm, J., Lintault, L., Newman, J., Reczek, E.E., Weissleder, R., & Jacks, T. (2007) Restoration of p53 function leads to tumour regression in vivo. *Nature*, Vol. 445, No.7128, (February 2007), pp. 661-665, ISSN 0028-0836

Vogelstein, B., & Kinzler, K.W. (2004) Cancer genes and the pathways they control. *Nature Medicine*, Vol. 8, No. 10, (August 2004), pp. 789-799, ISSN 1546-170X

Wang, L., Chanvorachote, P., Toledo, D., Stehlik, C., Mercer, R.R., Castranova, V., & Rojanasakul, Y. (2008) Peroxide is a key mediator of Bcl-2 down-regulation and apoptosis induction by cisplatin in human lung cancer cells. *Molcular Pharmacology*, Vol. 73, No. 1, (October 2007), pp. 119-127, ISSN 1521-0111

Wang, X., Wang, Q., Ives, K.L., & Evers, B.M. (2006). Curcumin inhibits neurotensin-mediated interleukin-8 production and migration of HCT116 human colon cancer cells. *Clinical Cancer Research : An Official Journal of the American Association for Cancer Research*, Vol. 12, No. 18, (September 2006), pp. 5346-5355, ISSN 1557-3265

Wang, Y.J., Pan, M.H., Cheng, A.L., Lin, L.I., Ho, Y.S., Hsieh, C.Y., & Lin, J.K. (1997). Stability of curcumin in buffer solutions and characterization of its degradation products. *Journal of Pharmaceutical and Biomedical Analysis*, Vol. 15, No. 12, (August 1997), pp. 1867-1876, ISSN 1873-264X

Xia, Y., Jin, L., Zhang, B., Xue, H., Li, Q., & Xu, Y. (2007). The potentiation of curcumin on insulin-like growth factor-1 action in MCF-7 human breast carcinoma cells. *Life Sciences*, Vol. 80, No. 23, (May 2007), pp. 2161-2169, ISSN 0024-3205

Yang, F., Lim, G.P., Begum, A.N., Ubeda, O.J., Simmons, M.R., Ambegaokar, S.S., Chen, P.P., Kayed, R., Glabe, C.G., Frautschy, S.A., & Cole, G.M. (2005) Curcumin inhibits formation of amyloid beta oligomers and fibrils, binds plaques, and reduces amyloid in vivo. *Journal of Biological Chemistry*, Vol. 280, No. 7, (December 2004), pp. 5892-5901, ISSN 1083-351X

Yodkeeree, S., Garbisa, S., & Limtrakul, P. (2008). Tetrahydrocurcumin inhibits HT1080 cell migration and invasion via downregulation of MMPs and uPA. *Acta Pharmacologica Sinica*, Vol. 29, No.7, (July 2008), pp. 853-860, ISSN 1745-7254

Zheng, L.D., Tong, Q.S., & Wu, C.H. (2002). Inhibitory effects of curcumin on apoptosis of human ovary cancer cell line A2780 and its molecular mechanism. *Ai Zheng Chinese Journal of Cancer*, Vol. 21, No. 12, (December 2002), pp. 1296-1300, ISSN 1000-467X

2

Salograviolide A: A Plant-Derived Sesquiterpene Lactone with Promising Anti-Inflammatory and Anticancer Effects

Isabelle Fakhoury and Hala Gali-Muhtasib
American University of Beirut
Lebanon

1. Introduction

Natural products are chemical substances produced by living organisms of the Biota superdomain, namely plants, animals, fungi and bacteria (G. & C. Merriam Co., 1913). Up to 80% of all drugs discovered prior to 1981 and 50% of all approved drugs between the years 1994 and 2007 are of natural product origin (Harvey, 2008). The contribution of natural products derived from plants, particularly to the well-being of mankind, extends very far back in history. Some of the most famous findings supportive of this fact come from the Middle East region and include documented medical papyri of ancient Egyptians dating back to ca. 1,850 B.C., as well as recent studies revealing their use of medicinal herbs dispensed in grape wine ca. 3,150 B.C. (McGovern et al., 2009). Incidentally, the oldest evidence for the use of herbal medicine to be so far discovered dates back to the prehistoric Neanderthal man who lived also in the Middle East region around 60,000 years ago (Solecki, 1971).

Several world heritages of medicinal plants have also inspired and greatly contributed to the development of modern medicine (Azaizeh et al., 2008). Indeed some of the early drugs were derived from plants. Morphine, for instance, was the first pharmacologically active pure compound to be extracted from a plant over 200 years ago (Jesse et al., 2009). Clinical, pharmacological, and chemical studies have since then led to the identification of a lengthy list of drugs derived from plants covering a wide range of diseases from diabetes, malaria, microbial infections, osteoporosis to inflammation and cancer.

The story of the discovery of plants exhibiting anticancer properties in particular, began almost fifty years ago. With the increase in cancer incidences, there has been an increase of interest in screening for anti-tumor agents from diverse sources including plants. For that purpose, in 1960 the National Cancer Institute (NCI) launched a large-scale screening of 35,000 sample plants. The program resulted among others, in the discovery in 1967 of the best-selling anticancer drug today; Taxol (Cragg, 1998). This breakthrough boosted cancer researchers all over the world and especially those in regions with high diversity to explore the indigenous plants' active ingredients efficacy against cancer. Considering that more than 60% of anticancer drugs available for clinical use today are derived from natural products including plants (Balunas et al., 2005; Newman and Cragg, 2007), one cannot deny that there has been a successful contribution of plants to the fight against cancer (reviewed in Gali-Muhtasib and Bakkar, 2002; Darwiche et al., 2007).

Lebanon falls within the Levantine Uplands center of diversity. Compared to other Mediterranean countries, it stands second after Turkey in its floristic diversity with 2600 plant species distributed around its humble 10452 km^2 (Nehmeh, 1977). About 311 plants corresponding to 12% of the total plant species are endemic to Lebanon and have been used in part by Lebanese folk medicine practitioners and Lebanese people for preventive and therapeutic purposes (Nehmeh, 1977). As members of the Nature Conservation Center for Sustainable Futures (IBSAR), we have been leading research over the past 10 years for the understanding and evaluation of Lebanese indigenous plant properties against various conditions, especially cancer. The following chapter aims at retracing our adventure with "Salograviolide A" (Sal A), and bringing to light this peculiar molecule that exhibits both anti-inflammatory and anticancer effects.

2. Sesquiterpene lactones in traditional and conventional medicine

Sesquiterpene lactones (SLs) are generally colourless bitter phytochemicals of lipophylic nature. Thousands of molecules are classified in the SLs subfamily of the terpenoids group of plant secondary metabolites. They are predominantly isolated from leaves or flowering heads of plants of the sunflower family Asteraceae and to a limited extent from Umbelliferae and Magnoliaciae (Heywood et al., 1977). The percentage of SLs per plant dry weight often exceeds 1% (Heywood et al., 1977).

The benefits of many plants enriched with SLs have been described in depth in Mediterranean folk literature with emphasis on their laxative values as well as their potential for the treatment of sores, wounds, sprains, fever, pain, headaches, malaria, anaemia, microbial infections, arthritis, cough, bronchitis, diabetes, hypertension and inflammation (Awadallah, 1984; Moukarzel, 1997).

Similarly, scientific literature supports most of the SLs activities attributed to their plants of origin in traditional medicine such as the hypoglycemic (Genta et al., 2010), antibacterial (Bach et al., 2011), antifungal (Vajs et al., 1999), antiplasmodial (Medjroubi et al., 2005), antinociceptive, antipyretic (Akkol et al., 2009) and anti-inflammatory (Al-Saghir et al., 2009) effects.

There are to date around 1500 publications that have reported the anticancer and anti-inflammatory properties of SLs. Three major SLs and/or many of their synthetic derivatives have reached phase I-II cancer clinical trials, namely thapsigargin from *Thapsia garganica* (Apiaceae), artemisinin and artesunate from *Artemisia annua,* and parthenolide from *Tanacetum parthenium* (Fig. 1) (reviewed in Ghantous et al., 2010). These SLs have properties that enable them to target tumor cells and cancer stem cells while sparing normal cells. They also affect different cancers or inflammation conditions. For example, thapsigargin demonstrated promising results against advanced solid tumors (breast, kidney and intestine) while parthenolide had an effect on blood and lymph nodes tumors (reviewed in Ghantous et al., 2010). Artemisinin showed efficacy against lupus nephritis, metastatic breast and colorectal cancer while clinical evidence indicated that artesunate is effective against nonsmall cell lung cancer, metastatic uveal melanoma and laryngeal squamous cell carcinoma (Berger et al., 2005; Christensen et al., 2009; Efferth, 2006; Guzman et al., 2007, as cited in Ghantous et al., 2010). The chemical basis for the observed biological activities of SLs has been reviewed by our group recently (Ghantous et al., 2010).

Centaurea is one of the largest genera of the Asteracae family with almost 250 species (Font et al., 2008). Plants belonging to the *Centaurea* genus are native to Eurasia. They were introduced to North America around the late 1800's and can now be found all around the world. *Centaurea* extracts have also been used in traditional medicine for their effects as stimulants, diuretics, analgesics, anti-rheumatics, anti-microbial, anti-diabetics and anti-inflammatory (refer to www.ibsar.org). Anecdotally; the genus' name is a dedication to the centaur Chiron who, according to Greek mythology, had discovered the curative properties of these medicinal plants (Nehmeh, 1977). Scientists eventually investigated the medicinal properties traditionally attributed to the *Centaurea* genus and isolated a multitude of SLs in addition to other various types of compounds such as alkaloids, lignans, acetylenes and flavonoids. When entering on PubMed the search terms "Centaurea and sesquiterpene lactones", and adding to them the hits from the search "Centaurea and cancer", 46 results get displayed. We investigated the number, nature and biological activity of SLs in the different species and summarized some of them in Table 1.

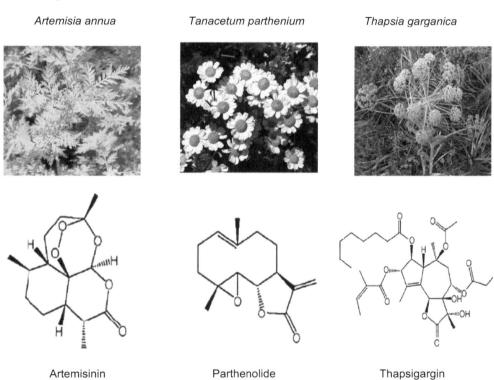

Fig. 1. Illustration of the sesquiterpene lactones that have reached clinical trials, namely thapsigargin extracted from *Thapsia garganica*, artemisinin from *Artemisia annua* L., and parthenolide from *Tanacetum parthenium*. The plants pictures are courtesy of Mr. Luigi Rignanese, Mr. Peter Griffee and Mr. Paul Drobot, respectively.

Table 1 indicates that there are at least 89 SLs in 10 *Centaurea* species. As expected, the amount of the SLs as well as their nature is species-specific. Also, the activities of the represented SLs cover most of those attributed to the plants in traditional medicine. Aside from Sal A, several articles have reported anticancer properties of SLs extracted from *Centaurea* species (Bruno et al., 2005; Chicca et al., 2011; Csupor-Löffler et al., 2009; El-Najjar et al., 2007; Ghantous et al., 2007; González et al., 1980; Koukoulista et al., 2002; Saroglou et al., 2005).

Plant	Number of SLs	Example of SLs	Activity	Reference
C. bella	26	Repin	Anti-tumor	1, 2
C. musimomum	11	Cynaropicrin	Antiplasmodial Cytotoxic	3, 4
C. napifolia	4	Cnicin	Antibacterial Cytotoxic	1, 5
C. nicolai	5	Kandavanolide	Antifungal	6
C. pullata	10	Melitensin	Antibacterial Antifungal	7
C. scoparia	9	Chlorohyssopifolin	Anti-tumor Antiviral Antimicrobial	8, 9, 10
C. solstitialis	7	Solstitialin A	Hypoglycemic Antiviral Antimicrobial	11, 12, 13, 14
C. spinosa	10	Malacitanolide	Antibacterial Cytotoxic	15
C. sulphurea	3	Sulphurein	-	16
C. tweediei	4	Onopordopicrin	Antibacterial Antifungal Cytotoxic	5, 17, 18

1: Bruno et al., 2005 – 2: Nowak et al., 1993– 3: Cho et al., 2004 – 4: Medjroubi et al., 2005– 5: Bach et al., 2011 – 6: Vajs et al., 1999 – 7: Djeddi et al., 2007, 2008 – 8: González et al., 1980 – 9: Ozçelik et al., 2009 – 10: Youssef et al., 1994, 1998 – 11: Akkol et al., 2011 – 12: Cheng et al., 1992 - 13: Gürbüz et al., 2007 – 14: Ozçelik et al., 2009 – 15: Saroglou et al., 2005 – 16: Lakhal et al., 2010 – 17: Fortuna et al., 2001 – 18: Lonergan et al., 1992.

Table 1. Sesquiterpene lactones of different *Centaurea* species and their biological activities.

3. Salograviolide A: Isolation and chemical characterization

In 1992, Daniewski et al. isolated an unusually hydroxylated SL from the aerial parts of the plant *Centaurea salonitana* Vis. of Bulgarian origin collected in the Greek region Gravia (Fig. 2a). The compound was baptised "Salograviolide A" with the prefix "salo" referring to the species *salonitana* from which it was isolated, "gravi" in allusion for the region Gravia and finally the suffix "olide" indicating the presence of a lactone group.

The first procedure used for the isolation and characterization of Sal A (Fig. 2b) included drying the plant and grinding it to a powder. This was followed by dividing the dry material (600 g) into three parts that were each soaked in 1 l of methanol (MeOH) for 24 h. The extracts were afterwards combined, evaporated (7.5 g) and dissolved in a mixture of equal amounts of water and chloroform (H_2O-$CHCl_3$ (1:1)). The aqueous layer was extracted three times with chloroform alone and the final step consisted of evaporating the extract and subjecting it to two separate chromatography techniques for optimal purification, thin layer chromatography (TLC) and column chromatography (CC). Infra Red (IR), high resolution Mass Spectrum (MS) and ^1H and ^{13}C Nuclear Magnetic Resonance (NMR) spectroscopy techniques enabled the identification of the structure of Sal A that was later confirmed by Rychlewska et al. (1992) using crystal X-ray diffraction techniques.

Sal A is a 3β-acetoxy-8α, 9β-dihydroxy-1αH, 5αH, 6βH, 7αH-guaian-4(15), 10(14), 11(13)-trien-6, 12-olide with the molecular formula $C_{17}H_{20}O_6$. It is classified according to its carbocyclic skeleton in the guaianolides group, one of the major groups of SLs. Comprised of 15 carbons (15-C) as indicated by the prefix "sesqui", Sal A has 3 isoprene (5-C) units and a lactone group (cyclic ester) (Fig. 2c). The presence of this α-methylene-γ-lactone is thought to be responsible for the biological activity of Sal A because of its ability to react with nucleophiles by a Michael-type addition (Ghantous et al., 2010).

Sal A was subsequently isolated from other *Centaurea* species, namely from *C. nicolai* Bald (Vajs et al., 1999) and from *C. ainetensis* Bois by bioguided fractionation following an extraction scheme adopted from Harborne (1998) (Saliba et al., 2009).

4. IBSAR efforts for bringing Sal A to the forefront

Ibsar, AUB's nature conservation center for sustainable futures, is an interdisciplinary and interfaculty center founded in the year 2002 by AUB faculty. Ibsar's mission is "to promote the conservation and sustainable utilization of biodiversity in arid and Mediterranean regions by providing an open academic platform for innovative research and development", and its vision is "for societies to become guardians and primary beneficiaries of biodiversity in the region" (www.ibsar.org).

Very early in its establishment, Ibsar recognized that the Lebanese floristic richness also represents an untapped resource for the potential discovery of new therapeutic agents and/or useful dietary supplements. As a result, one of the key program areas in Ibsar has been to integrate traditional knowledge and biotechnology. The objective of this program is to discover useful therapeutic agents that may be hidden in wild Lebanese plants and to develop products attractive to biotechnology industries. Towards this end, plants from the region are collected, extracted and tested for their potential effects on major diseases such as cancer, inflammation, microbial infections, skin diseases and diabetes as well as their value in nutrition and use for general health purposes.

C. ainetensis (Arabic name; Qanturyun Aynata or Shawk al-dardar) whose specimen is deposited at the herbarium of the American University of Beirut (Lebanon), is an endemic plant to Lebanon. It flowers from May to June, has purplish tube of anthers and can only be found growing wild in stony, sterile or bushy places in particular areas in Lebanon, mainly Dayr-ul-Ahmar to Aynata region at elevations of 1200–1800 m above sea level respectively, and in Anti-Lebanon Mountain range above Ayn-Burday at 1250–1300 m (Dinsmore, 1932 as cited in Talhouk et al., 2008).

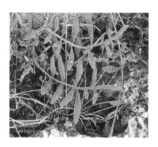 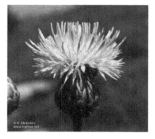

(a) Left: Photo of the plant *Centaurea salonitana* of Portuguese origin. Right:
The aerial part of the plant

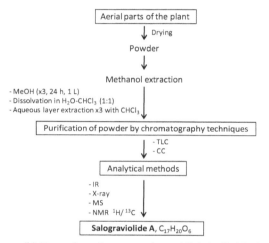

(b) Procedure for extraction of Sal A, $C_{17}H_{20}O_6$

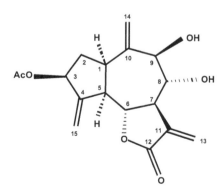

(c) Chemical structure of Sal A.

Fig. 2. Illustration of *Centaurea salonitana*, the procedure of Sal A extraction and its chemical structure.

The plant was collected during its flowering season and water extract was obtained from it by decoction. Briefly, the plant was air dried and soaked either entirely or only its ground flower head in hot boiling water for 20-30 min with a ratio of plant material weight to water volume of 1/8 (1 g of plant for every 8 ml of water). The solution was filtered either through 3 mm Whatman filter or through Sterile Gauze sponges 30x30 cm which yielded a residue and a filtrate named the "crude water extract". The resulting aqueous layer was sterilized using 0.2 μm non-pyrogenic sterile-R filter before storing it at -20°C until use.

C. ainetensis water extract is claimed in Lebanese folk literature to have anti-inflammatory effects. However, no research paper prior to 2004 investigating this plant's biological activity had ever been published. A screening of 29 plants reported by traditional medicine practitioners to have anti-inflammatory effects led to the validation of this activity for C. ainetensis water extract (Talhouk et al., 2008). Moreover, a screening of 109 wild Lebanese plant extracts, including 41 crude water, 34 methanol and 34 chloroform extracts, has resulted in the identification of selective and anti-proliferative bioactivity against several cancer cell lines in four wild Lebanese plant species namely, Achillea damascene also known as Achillea falcata, Centaurea ainetensis, Onopordum cynarocephalum and Ranunculus myosuroudes (Table 2). Although, in vitro, the three other plant extracts showed higher activities than C. ainetensis, the latter extract demonstrated the highest tumor growth inhibition ranging from 73 to 79% when tested in vivo in a mouse model of colorectal cancer (El-Najjar et al, 2007).

It was also shown later, that C. ainestensis water extract was mildly toxic but largely inhibited metastasis of leukemic cells (El-Sabban, unpublished findings).

Finally the extract was tested against the Infectious Bursal Disease (Gumboro) Virus (IBDV) in broilers and showed a mild reduction of IBDV viral antigens in the Bursa of Fabricius as well as a mild reduction in bursal lesions (Barbour, unpublished findings).

In an attempt to unravel the underlying causes for C. ainetensis water extract activity, we isolated the bioactive compound Sal A. The plant was subjected to bio-assay guided fractionation which consisted of testing the anti-tumor, anti-inflammatory and cytotoxicity effects of each fraction of the plant extract. Fractions of the crude water extract were inactive; however, Sal A was obtained from a fractionation of the methanol crude extract. Sal A manifested the same biological activities as the crude water extract with greater efficacy at lower concentrations. A parallel study was conducted to assess the effect of both the water crude extract and methanol crude extract of C. ainetensis along with 26 other indigenous Lebanese plants against nine microbial species. The results showed that the crude water extract was inactive against all microbial species whereas the methanol extract was effective against 88.8% of the tested microorganisms (Barbour et al., 2004).

Fig. 3 summarizes the acid-base extraction procedure used to fractionate the methanol crude extract and isolate Sal A. First the methanol crude extract was obtained by soaking the dried plant flowers in methanol with w/v of 1/10 for 16 h.

The mixture was then incubated on a shaker for 2 h at 20°C. The extract was filtered and yielded a residue and a filtrate named the "methanol crude extract". For further fractionation, the residue issued from the methanol extraction was soaked in EtOAc mixture in a ratio of 10/1 w/v. It was then separated by filtration into a residue and a filtrate consisting of fat and waxes and numbered I.1. To the crude methanol extract, concentrated H_2SO_4 solution was then added drop-wise till the pH reached 2. Following, a mixture of $CHCl_3$-H_2O (2:1 ratio) was added. The $CHCl_3$ phase enriched with terpenoids and phenols was collected and labeled as I.2. The aqueous layer, on the other hand, was basified to pH 10

Plant	Name in Arabic	Concentration (%)*	Growth Inhibition (%)	Cell line
Achillea damascene	Akhilia zat al-alf waraqah	0.5	65	Breast: Scp2
				Colon/intestine:
		3	85	HCT-116
		3	80	HT-29
		3	70	Mode K
Centaurea ainetensis	Quanturyun Aynata/ Shawk	3	60	Breast: Scp2
				Colon/intestine:
	al-dardar	3	60	HCT-116
		3	80	HT-29
		5	50	Mode K
				Skin:
		3	40	PMK
		3	87	SP1
		3	65	308
		3	67	PAM212
		3	40	17
Onopordum cynarocephalum	Aqsun harshafi al ra's	0.1	50	Breast: Scp2
		0.5		Colon/intestine:
		0.5	70	HCT-116
		1.5	50	HT-29
			50	Mode K
Ranunculus myosuroudes	Hawdhan			Skin:
		2	36	PMK
		2	98	SP1
		2	64	308
		2	61	PAM212
		2	20	17

Table 2. Representation of the four Lebanese plant extracts with anticancer potentials. The following results were obtained for the water extracts of *A. damascene*, *C. ainetensis* and *O. cynarocephalum* and the methanol extract of *R. myosuroudes*. Cell proliferation and cytotoxicity were determined using the CellTiter 96 Non-Radioactive Cell Proliferation Assay and the CytoTox 96 Non-Radioactive Cytotoxicity Assay (both kits from Promega, Madison, WI) according to the manufacturer's suggestions.
* % = Volume extract/ Volume media

by adding concentrated NH₄OH drop-wise and then resuspended in a CHCl₃-MeOH mixture (3:1 ratio) to be later separated into two organic and aqueous layers labeled I.3 containing alkaloids and I.4, respectively. I.1, I.2, I.3 and I.4 were evaporated to dryness under reduced pressure and weighed. A known amount of each subfraction was dissolved in a known volume of suitable solvent for further chromatographic and or/bioassays analysis.

Fraction "I.2" was the only of three other fractions to exhibit activity against cancer cells and in models of inflammation. Therefore TLC, thick layer chromatography and CC were used to further subdivide the I.2 bioactive fraction and yielded six subfractions I.2.1-I.2.6. Additional testing showed that only subfraction I.2.2 exhibited the anti proliferative, anti-inflammatory activity observed with the fraction I.2. This subfraction also maintained its bioactivity after it was purified using Solid Phase Extraction.

Finally, UV, IR, NMR and MS enabled the identification of the bioactive compound Sal A.

In conclusion, three research papers on *C. ainetensis* water extracts and three on Sal A anti-inflammatory and anti-tumor activities have been so far published by Ibsar while a fourth one is in progress (Al-Saghir et al., 2009; Barbour et al., 2004; El-Najjar et al., 2007; Ghantous et al., 2007; Saliba et al., 2009; Talhouk et al., 2008). Prior to our work, there was only one published article on Sal A's biological activity since its isolation (Vajs et al., 1999). Therefore, Ibsar has had a major contribution in identifying Sal A's biological activity and determining its mechanisms of action.

5. Salograviolide A: Overview of biological activities

To date, *C. ainetensis* water extract was shown to have antifungal, antibacterial, anti-viral, anticancer and anti-inflammatory activities. Sal A on the other hand, was only shown to have antifungal, anticancer and anti-inflammatory properties. The group of Vajs et al. discovered in 1999 the antifungal activity of Sal A while Ibsar faculty revealed the two others. It is unfortunate that no study has so far assessed whether Sal A is responsible for the antimicrobial and antiviral potentials exhibited by *C. ainetensis* water extract.

Following its isolation from *C. nicolai*, Sal A was tested against seven fungal species: *Aspergillus niger, A. ochraceus, Penicillium ochrochloron, Cladosporium cladosporoides, Fusarium tricinctum, Phomopsis helianthi* and *Trichoderma viride* (Vajs et al., 1999). Each strain was inoculated in the center of a plate with or without Sal A addition to the nutritional agar media. After incubation at 20°C for three weeks, the percentage of fungi inhibition was determined by comparing the diameter of each fungal strain colony inoculated in the presence of Sal A to that of the control inoculated without Sal A. The results showed that Sal A inhibited all the fungi strains except *Trichoderma viride*. Subsequently the use of different concentrations of Sal A enabled the determination of the Minimum Inhibitory Concentration (MICs) to inhibit the mycelial growth of the respective fungal species.

To test for the inflammation potential of *C. ainetensis* water extract, the pro-inflammatory cytokine interleukin-6 (IL-6) was chemically induced in mammary epithelial cells (CID-9 and Scp2) by treatment with endotoxin (ET)). The ability of the extract to reverse or prevent IL-6 production was then assessed and the results demonstrated that *C. ainetensis* water extract inhibited IL-6 in a dose-dependent manner (Talhouk et al., 2008). It was also shown that the extract reversed chemically induced paw edema signs in ET-pretreated Sprague-Dawley rats as well as thermal hyperalgesia in rats subjected to the hot plate test. Sal A was isolated from the water extracts and shown to be responsible for its observed bioactivity. In

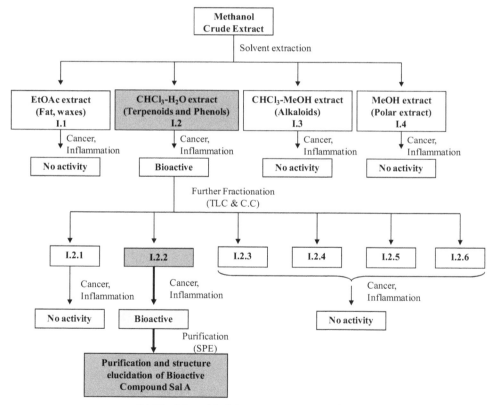

Kigndom	Plantae
Subkingdom	Tracheobionta
Division	Magnioliophyta
Class	Magnoliopside
Subclass	Asteridae
Order	Asterales
Family	Asteraceae
Genus	*Centaurea* L.
Species	*ainetensis*

(a) *Centaurea ainetensis* and its taxonomy

(b) The bioguided fractionation procedure

Fig. 3. Illustration of the indigenous Lebanese plant *Centaurea ainetensis* and the bioguided fractionation procedure that enabled the isolation of Salograviolide A. The plant picture is courtesy of Mr. Khaled Sleem.

parallel, the anti-inflammatory property of Sal A was demonstrated in a murine intestinal epithelial cell model (Mode K cells) treated with IL-1 and in *vivo* in a rat model of colonic inflammation induced by rectal injection of iodoacetoamide (Al-Saghir et al., 2009). The results showed that, similarly to *C. ainetensis* water extract, Sal A significantly reduced inflammatory cytokines and acted as a preventive agent to reduce inflammation.

C. ainetensis water extract and Sal A were also tested against different types of cancers (El-Najjar et al., 2007; Ghantous et al., 2007). *In vitro*, they were both non cytotoxic to normal primary murine keratinocytes while they preferentially inhibited neoplastic benign tumors and squamous cell carcinoma growth in a dose-dependent manner. The selective antiproliferative effects were confirmed in leukemic cells at the metastatically invasive stages as well as in human colon carcinomas. Sal A was also tested in combination with another sesquiterpene lactone, the Iso-seco-tanapartholide (TNP) extracted from *Achillea damascene*, against human colon cancer cell lines (Gali-Muhtasib, unpublished findings). The study demonstrated a synergistic apoptotic effect of both sesquiterpene lactones that failed to induce apoptosis when tested alone at the same low concentrations. Finally *in vivo*, the intraperitoneal water extract injection in Balb/c mice before chemically inducing colon cancer reduced drastically the mean size of aberrant crypt foci which is indicative of the extract's cancer preventive activity.

6. Salograviolide A and inflammation: Mechanisms and targets

Natural products derivatives have contributed over the last 25 years to approximately one fourth of the anti-inflammatory drugs used in the clinic (Newman & Cragg, 2007). In 2008, 18 additional natural product derived drugs were being tested at different clinical stages (Harvey, 2008). Terpenoids including sesquiterpene lactones have also reached clinical trials as potential anti-inflammatory agents. For instance, andrographolide; a labdane diterpenoid derived from the plant *Andrographis paniculata* of the Acanthacaea family, reached phase II clinical trials for rheumatoid arthritis. The sesquiterpene lactone parthenolide that made it to phase I cancer clinical trials, has also reached phase II and III clinical trials for the treatment of allergic contact dermatitis (refer to http://www.clinicaltrials.gov/).

Drugs with anti-inflammatory activities have common targets and modes of action that lead to the downregulation of the signs of inflammation as well as the chemical mediators controlling the mechanisms of inflammation. Elements of the complement system, angiogenic factors, prostaglandins, cytokines such as interleukins and matrix metalloproteinases (MMPs) are some of the most common inflammatory mediators.

Prostaglandins play a role in the modulation of blood flow. They are derived from the arachidonic acid due to the action of two prostaglandins H synthases isoforms known as the cyclooxygenases 1 and 2 (COX-1 and COX-2). COX-1 is constitutively expressed in different tissues while COX-2 is induced by inflammatory stimuli and is therefore thought to be the only isoform involved in propagating the inflammatory response (Larsen & Henson, 1983).

IL-6 secreted by the macrophages releases proteinases and elastases which bind to IL-6 receptor and generate signals implicated in humoral inflammation (Heinrich et al., 2003). IL-1, on the other hand, induces the mobilization of the arachidonic acid and its metabolism into prostaglandins thus contributing to cellular inflammation. It was also shown that IL-1 induces the synthesis of COX-2 through the activation of the nuclear factor Kappa B (NF-κB) transcription factor (Larsen & Henson, 1983). NF-κB is a key modulator of inflammation and is implicated in inflammation-induced tumor formation as well (Karin & Greten, 2005). It is known to promote the expression of target genes of the inflammation response such as interleukins, COX-2, and inducible nitric-oxide synthase (iNOS) (Mazor et al., 2000).

Finally, components of the MMP family have been reported to act in wound healing and embryogenesis (Mainardi et al., 1991). Gelatinase A or MMP-2 (72 KDa) and gelatinase B or MMP-9 (92 KDa) have been identified as pro-inflammatory agents. They enable the digestion of components of the basement membrane; a function that is referred to as gelatinolysis (Birkedal-Hansen et al., 1993).

Sal A and *C. ainetensis* water extract were shown to modulate some of these major players of the inflammatory response. They both inhibit IL-6 expression (Talhouk et al., 2008) and IL-1-induced COX-2 expression by interfering with their synthesis (Al-Saghir et al., 2009). Only the effect of the water extract on the expression levels of the gelatinases A and B was assessed. The results indicate that the water extract decreased the expression of both proteins with preferential inhibition of gelatinase B 9 h post treatment with endotoxin (Talhouk et al., 2008). Similarly, only the effect of Sal A on the NF-κB signaling was investigated. NF-κB is composed of the two subunits p50 and p65 and is only active after translocation of the subunits into the nucleus and their dimerization. In normal conditions, NF-κB is inactive due to its retention in the cytoplasm by the inhibitor of NF-κB (IκB). Pro-inflammatory stimuli such as IL-1 cause the phosphorylation of the IκB by the inhibitor of NFκB- β (IKK). The phosphorylation in return leads to IκB degradation enabling thus the translocation to the cytoplasm and the dimerization of the NF-κB subunits, their binding to target DNA sequences, initiation of transcription and activation of the NF-κB transduction pathway (Baeuerele & Baltimore, 1996).

It was demonstrated that Sal A inhibits the NF-κB activation by two mechanisms. The first involved the stabilization of IκB, since combination treatment of Sal A with IL-1 decreased the degradation of IκB observed in response to treatment with IL-1 alone. The second involved inhibiting NF-κB translocation and binding to DNA, since the incubation of cells with Sal A after IL-1 addition (hence after IκB degradation) still caused a reduction in the activity of NF-κB (Fig. 4) (Al-Saghir et al., 2009).

7. Salograviolide A and cancer: Mechanisms and targets

The mechanism behind the anticancer activity of sesquiterpene lactones has been extensively investigated. For example, parthenolide was shown to induce cell cycle arrest, promote cell differentiation and trigger apoptosis (Pajak et al., 2008). The molecular basis for parthenolide activity in cancer cells include among others, inhibiting NF-κB and stimulating apoptosis by accumulation of reactive oxygen species (ROS) as well as by regulating the levels of anti-apoptotic and pro-apoptotic proteins (Pajak et al., 2008). Interestingly, parthenolide showed a synergistic effect when used in combination with paclitaxel and increased apoptosis in breast cancer cells (Patel et al., 2000).

As mentioned earlier, *C. ainetensis* crude extract and Sal A were tested against skin, colon and blood cancer cell lines and showed selective antineoplastic effects with no cytotoxicity to normal cells. At the cellular level, *C. ainetensis* crude extract induced G_0/G_1 cell cycle arrest in neoplastic epidermal cells while Sal A increased the population in Pre-G_1. In accordance with this finding, the levels of cyclin D1 whose activity is required for the G_1/S transition were reduced (Li et al., 2011). On the other hand, the levels of the tumor suppressors p16 and p21 which are associated with greater susceptibility to chemotherapy and with calcium induced differentiation in keratinocytes, respectively were increased (Hochhauser, 1997; Di Cunto et al., 1998, as cited in Ghantous et al., 2007). Moreover, p21 proteins were differentially regulated: they were upregulated in the presence of the crude extract which was consistent with the observed G_0/G_1 cell cycle arrest, whereas their upregulation in the presence of Sal A was found to be transient. This transient upregulation of p21 has been reported as critical for its role in differentiation (Di Cunto et al., 1998).

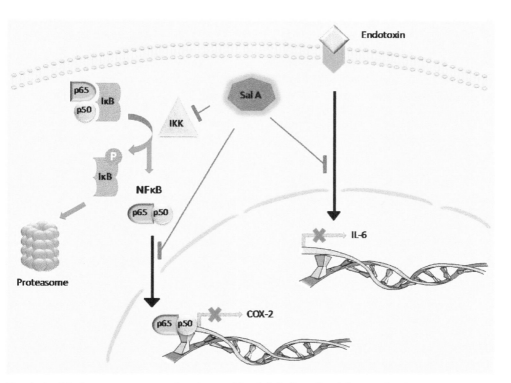

Fig. 4. Anti-inflammatory cascade triggered by Sal A. Details of the mechanism are explained in section 6 above.

In addition to cell cycle modulation, characteristic signs of apoptosis such as the partial and complete condensation of the chromatin were noted in the presence of Sal A. Furthermore, the ratio of the pro-apoptotic protein Bax to the anti-apoptotic protein Bcl-2 was found to be elevated. Bax and Bcl-2 have counteracting roles regarding the mitochondrial membrane permeabilization and thus the high ratio of Bax to Bcl-2 reflects the permeabilization of the mitochondrial membrane to release factors such as cytochrome c and the apoptosis inducing factor that will induce cell death. In conjunction, a considerable amount of ROS accumulated in the cells in the presence of Sal A. In fact, the accumulation of ROS was even shown to precede the growth inhibition and indicated an oxidant role of Sal A in these cells. Finally, the crude extract and Sal A had a contradictory regulatory effect on NF-κB. The crude plant extract decreased in a dose-dependent manner the binding of NF-κB to the DNA without affecting the expression level of IκB, whereas Sal A increased it. It is worth noting that in cancer, the role of NF-κB activation or inhibition is in itself conflicting. NF-κB can be best described as a double edged sword for its activation can promote tumorigenesis (by inducing inflammatory mediators) or promote differentiation and thus inhibit tumorigenesis (Seitz et al., 1998, as cited in Ghantous et al., 2007).

In addition, the crude extract was assessed in human colon cancers and showed both an increase in p21 protein level of expression and in the ratio of Bax to Bcl-2 proteins. In colon cancer, cyclin B1 levels were decreased by the extract, while they were found to be unaffected by neither Sal A nor the extract in skin cancer. Cyclin B1 decrease is important for the exit from mitosis and for the cytokinesis (Takizawa & Morgan, 2000, as cited in El-Najjar et al., 2007). Another protein which was differentially modulated in skin *vs* colon cancer is p53. In colon cancer, the crude extract increased the expression levels of the p53 protein, while the levels were unaffected in skin cancer.

In leukemic cells, similarly to what was shown with the other two types of cancers, the extract induced pre-G_1 cell cycle arrest, increased the levels of p53 and p21 as well as the ratio of Bax to Bcl-2, and decreased cyclin D1 levels. In addition, the secretion of the vascular endothelial growth factor (VEGF) was significantly decreased by Sal A and the crude extract, adding VEGF to the list of targets of Sal A (El-Sabban, unpublished findings). Finally, Sal A was tested in combination with TNP against human colon cancer cell lines (Gali-Muhtasib, unpublished findings). At low concentrations, Sal A and TNP induced G_2/M cell cycle arrest when tested separately. At the same low concentrations, the combination of Sal A and TNP synergistically inhibited tumor growth and triggered apoptosis. ROS, which increased by a factor of 25 upon combination treatment, were found to be responsible for the synergistic-induced cell death. The pretreatment of the colorectal cancer cells with the antioxidant N-acetyl-L-cysteine (NAC), which diminishes the intracellular ROS, reversed the synergistic anti-proliferative effect and protected the cells from apoptosis and therefore confirmed the implication of ROS in the induction of apoptosis. Moreover, p38 kinase, the extracellular signal regulated kinase (ERK) and the c-Jun N-terminal kinase (JNK) of the mitogen-activated protein kinases (MAPK) pathway were found to be phosphorylated and thus induced after the combination treatment. Literature strongly advocates for the MAPK pathway implication in ROS induced cell death (Zhang et al., 2003). Using specific inhibitors of both ERK (usually involved in mitogenic signals and cellular proliferation), and of p38 (associated with stress along with JNK and commonly known as the stress activated protein kinases (Lewis et al., 1998)) abolished the apoptotic synergistic effect of the combination treatment and emphasized the pathway's association to cell death. Further studies with Sal A and TNP suggested a cross-talk between ROS, JNK and Bcl-2 family in the induction of apoptosis. ROS accumulation was found to induce Bax relocalization to the mitochondrial membrane on the one hand and to decrease the ani-apoptotic Bcl-2 expression levels on the other (Gali-Muhtasib, unpublished findings). Bcl-2 decrease was also associated with a maximal JNK activation which suggested that JNK might play a role in further inactivation of Bcl-2. In accordance with our findings several studies have reported the involvement of JNK but not ERK nor p38 in the phosphorylation and inactivation of Bcl-2 (Srivasta et al., 1999).

Taken together these results indicate a promising chemotherapeutic effect for using Sal A alone or in combination against various cancer types.

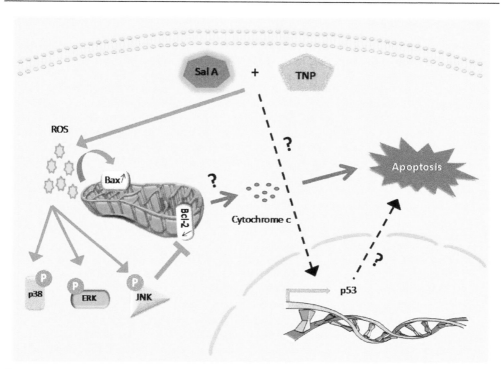

Fig. 5. Anticancer cascade triggered by the combination of Sal A and TNP in colon cancer cells. The combination caused increase in ROS and activation of MAPK molecules, ERK, JNK and p38 leading to apoptosis. It is still unclear whether apoptosis is associated with the modulation of p21, p53, and cyclin B1 proteins or the release of cytochrome c from mitochondria.

8. Conclusion and future direction

Cancer progression is characterized by seven hallmarks: sustaining proliferative signaling, insensitivity to growth suppressors, evading apoptosis, acquisition of replicative immortality, induction of angiogenesis, activation of invasion and metastasis and finally chronic inflammation (Colotta F. Et al., 2009).

In a nutshell, the evidence that has been collected so far by multiple investigators suggests that Sal A is a promising compound for cancer drug discovery for it acts at least on three cancer hallmarks: it upregulates tumor suppressors, triggers apoptosis and downregulates the mediators of inflammation. Its selectivity toward tumor cells and ability to target multiple pathways involved in inflammation and cancer imply that this compound is unlikely to have a single target that is responsible for its biological activities. Although a large body of information supports the role of Sal A against cancer and inflammation, there are yet no studies assessing its toxicology profiles or its absorption, distribution and metabolism in animals and humans. Such studies are warranted to better determine its potential for future applications in the clinical setting whether alone or in combination with standard clinical drugs.

9. Acknowledgement

This work was supported by grants from UNISANTIS and the research was conducted under the direction of the Nature Conservation Center for Sustainable Futures (Ibsar) at the American University of Beirut, Lebanon. Dr. Salma Talhouk and many researchers contributed to the establishment of Ibsar. Plant collection was supervised by Dr. Salma Talhouk and carried out by Mr. Khaled Sleem. Extraction and fractionation of plant extracts were supervised by Dr. Najat Saliba. Inflammation studies on Sal A were supervised by Dr. Fadia Homeidan and Dr. Rabih Talhouk, skin cancer studies by Dr. Nadine Darwiche, colon cancer by Dr. Hala Gali-Muhtasib, leukemia by Dr. Marwan El-Sabban and the microbial studies by Dr. Elie Barbour. The following graduate students have contributed to this work: Ms. Nahed El-Najjar, Mr. Akram Ghantous, Mr. Mohammad Salla, Ms. Saada Dakdouki, Mr. Ahmad Abou Tayyoun, Mr. Wassim El-Jouni, Ms. Melody Saikaly, Mr. Houssam Shaib, Ms. Myriam El-Khoury, Ms. Jamal Al-Saghir and Ms. Noura Abdallah.

10. References

Akkol, EK.; Arif, R.; Ergun, F. & Yesilada, E. (2009). Sesquiterpene lactones with antinociceptive and antipyretic activity from two Centaurea species. *J Ethnopharmacol.* 122, 2 (March 2009), pp. 210-5.

Al-Saghir, J.; Al-Ashi, R.; Salloum, R.; Saliba, NA.; Talhouk, RS. & Homaidan FR. (2009). Anti-inflammatory properties of Salograviolide A purified from Lebanese plant Centaurea ainetensis. *BMC Complement Altern Med.* 9, 36, (September 2009).

Awadallah, A. (1984). *Al'Ilaj Bil Aa'shab Wal Nabatat Al Shafiya* (Arabic). Published by Dar Ikraa, Beirut, Lebanon.

Azaizeh, H., Saad, B., Cooper, E. & Said, O. (2008). Traditional Arabic and Islamic Medicine, a Re-emerging Health Aid. *Evid Based Complement Alternat Med.* 7, 4, (Jun 2008), pp. 419-424.

Bach, SM.; Fortuna, MA.; Attarian, R.; de Trimarco, JT.; Catalán, CA.; Av-Gay, Y. & Bach, H. (2011). Antibacterial and cytotoxic activities of the sesquiterpene lactones cnicin and onopordopicrin. *Nat Prod Commun.* 6, 2, (February 2011), pp. 163-6.

Baeuerle, PA. & Baltimore, D. (1996). NF-kappa B: ten years after. *Cell.* 87, 1, (October 1996), pp. 13-20.

Balunas, MJ. & Kinghorn, AD. (2005). Drug discovery from medicinal plants. *Life Sci.* 78, 5, (December 2005), pp. 431-41. Review.

Barbour, EK.; Al Sharif, M.; Sagherian, VK.; Habre, AN.; Talhouk, RS. & Talhouk, SN. (2004). Screening of selected indigenous plants of Lebanon for antimicrobial activity. *J Ethnopharmacol.* 93, 1, (July 2004), pp. 1-7.

Birkedal-Hansen, H.; Moore, WGI.; Windsor, LJ.; Birkedal-Hansen, B.; DeCarlo, A. & Engler, JA. (1993). Matrix metalloproteinases: A Review. *Crit Rev Oral Biol And Med.* 4, 2, pp. 197-250

Bruno, M.; Rosselli, S.; Maggio, A.; Raccuglia, RA.; Bastow KF., Wu CC & Lee, KH. (2005). Cytotoxic activity of some natural and synthetic sesquiterpene lactones. *Planta Med.*71, 12, (December 2005), pp. 1176-8.

Cheng, CH.; Costall, B.; Hamburger, M.; Hostettmann, K.; Naylor, RJ.; Wang, Y. & Jenner, P. (1992). Toxic effects of solstitialin A 13-acetate and cynaropicrin from Centaurea solstitialis L. (Asteraceae) in cell cultures of foetal rat brain. *Neuropharmacology*.31, 3, (March 1992), pp. 271-7.

Chicca, A.; Tebano, M.; Adinolfi, B.; Ertugrul, K.; Flamini, G. & Nieri, P. (2011). Anti-proliferative activity of aguerin B and a new rare nor-guaianolide lactone isolated from the aerial parts of Centaurea deflexa. *Eur J Med Chem*. (March 2011).

Cho, JY.; Kim, AR.; Jung, JH.; Chun, T.; Rhee, MH. & Yoo, ES. (2004). Cytotoxic and pro-apoptotic activities of cynaropicrin, a sesquiterpene lactone, on the viability of leukocyte cancer cell lines. *Eur J Pharmacol*. 492, 2-3, (May 2004), pp. 85-94.

Clinical trials (2010): http://www.clinicaltrials.gov/ct2/search/browse?brwse=intr_cat_Infl

Colotta, F.; Allavena, P.; Sica, A.; Garlanda, C. & Mantovani, A. (2009). Cancer-related inflammation, the seventh hallmark of cancer: links to genetic instability. *Carcinogenesis*. 30, 7, (July 2009), pp. 1073-81. Review.

Cragg, G.M. (1998). Paclitaxel (Taxol): a success story with valuable lessons for natural product drug discovery and development. *Med Res Rev*.18, 5 (September 1998), pp. 315-31.

Csupor-Löffler, B.; Hajdú, Z.; Réthy, B.; Zupkó, I.; Máthé, I.; Rédei, T.; Falkay, G. & Hohmann, J. (2009). Antiproliferative activity of Hungarian Asteraceae species against human cancer cell lines. Part II. *Phytother Res*. 23, 8, (August 2009), pp. 1109-15.

Daniewski, W.M.; Nowak, G.; Routsi, E.; Rychlewska, U.; Szczepanska, B. & Skibicki, P. (1992). Salogravilide A, A Sesquiterpene From Centaurea Salonitana. *Phytochemistry*. 31, 8, pp. 2891-2893.

Darwiche, N.; El-Banna, S. & Gali-Muhtasib, H. (2007). Cell cycle modulatory and apoptotic effects of plant-derived anticancer drugs in clinical use or development. *Expert Opinion on Drug Discovery*. 2, 3, (March 2007), pp. 361-379.

Djeddi, S.; Karioti, A.; Sokovic, M.; Koukoulitsa, C. & Skaltsa, H. (2008). A novel sesquiterpene lactone from Centaurea pullata: structure elucidation, antimicrobial activity, and prediction of pharmacokinetic properties. *Bioorg Med Chem*. 16, 7, (April, 2008), pp. 3725-31.

Djeddi, S.; Karioti, A.; Sokovic, M.; Stojkovic, D.; Seridi, R. & Skaltsa, H. (2007). Minor sesquiterpene lactones from Centaurea pullata and their antimicrobial activity. *J Nat Prod*. 70, 11, (November 2007), pp. 1796-9.

El-Najjar, N.; Dakdouki, S.; Darwiche, N.; El-Sabban, M.; Saliba, NA. & Gali-Muhtasib, H. (2008). Anti-colon cancer effects of Salograviolide A isolated from Centaurea ainetensis. *Oncol Rep*. 19, 4, (April 2008), pp. 897-904.

Font, M.; Garcia-Jacas, N.; Vilatersana, R.; Roquet, C. & Susanna, A. (2009). Evolution and biogeography of Centaurea section Acrocentron inferred from nuclear and plastid DNA sequence analyses. *Ann Bot*. 103, 6, (April 2009), pp. 985-97.

Fortuna, AM.; de Riscala, EC.; Catalan, CA.; Gedris, TE. & Herz, W. Sesquiterpene lactones from Centaurea tweediei. *Biochem Syst Ecol*. 29, 9, (October 2001), pp. 967-971.

Gali-Muhtasib, H. & Bakkar, N. (2002). Modulating Cell Cycle: Current Applications and Prospects for Future Drug Development. *Current Cancer Drug Targets*. 2, 4, (December 2002), pp. 309-336.

Genta, SB.; Cabrera, WM.; Mercado, MI.; Grau, A.; Catalán, CA. & Sánchez, SS. (2010). Hypoglycemic activity of leaf organic extracts from Smallanthus sonchifolius: Constituents of the most active fractions. *Chem Biol Interact*. 185, 2, (April 2010), pp. 143-52.

Ghantous, A.; Tayyoun, AA;, Lteif, GA.; Saliba, NA.; Gali-Muhtasib, H.; El-Sabban, M. & Darwiche, N. (2008). Purified Salograviolide A Isolated From Centaurea ainetensis Causes Growth Inhibition and Apoptosis in Neoplastic Epidermal Cells. *Int J Oncol*. 32, 4, (April 2008), pp. 841-9.

Ghantous, A.; Gali-Muhtasib, H.; Vuorela, H.; Saliba, NA. & Darwiche, N. (2010). What made sesquiterpene lactones reach cancer clinical trials? *Drug Discov Today*. 15, 15-16, (August 2010), pp. 668-78.

González, AG.; Darias, V.; Alonso, G. & Estévez, E. (1980). The cytostatic activity of the chlorohyssopifolins, chlorinated sesquiterpene lactones from Centaurea. *Planta Med*. 40, 2, (October 1980), pp. 179-84.

Gürbüz, I. & Yesilada, E. Evaluation of the anti-ulcerogenic effect of sesquiterpene lactones from Centaurea solstitialis L. ssp. solstitialis by using various in vivo and biochemical techniques. *J Ethnopharmacol*. 112, 2, (Jun 2007), pp. 284-91.

Harvey, AL. Natural products in drug discovery. (2008). *Drug Discov Today*. 13, 19-20, (October 2008), pp. 894-901. Review.

Heinrich, PC.; Behrmann, I.; Haan, S.; Hermanns, HM.; Müller-Newen, G. & Schaper, F. (2003). Principles of interleukin (IL)-6-type cytokine signaling and its regulation. *Biochem J*. 15, 374(Pt 1), (August 2003), pp. 1-20. Review.

Heywood, V.H.; Harborne, J.B. & Turner, B.L. (1997). The biology and chemistry of the compositae, vols I and II, *Academic press: New York*.

Ibsar: Traditional Knowledge and Biotechnology > plants > Centaurea ainetensis (2010) http://www.ibsar.org/research/Traditional%20Knowledge%20and%20Biotechnol ogy/plants/Centaurea%20ainetensis.htm.

Karin, M. & Greten, FR. (2002). NF-kappaB: linking inflammation and immunity to cancer development and progression. *Nat Rev Immunol*. 5, 10, (October 2005), pp. 749-59. Review.

Koukoulitsa, E.; Skaltsa, H.; Karioti, A.; Demetzos, C. & Dimas, K. (2002). Bioactive sesquiterpene lactones from Centaurea species and their cytotoxic/cytostatic activity against human cell lines in vitro. *Planta Med*. 68, 7, (July 2002), pp. 649-52.

Lakhal, H.; Boudiar, T.; Kabouche, A.; Kabouche, Z.; Touzani R.; & Bruneau, C. (2010). New sesquiterpene lactone and other constituents from Centaurea sulphurea (Asteraceae). *Nat Prod Commun*. 5, 6, (Jun 2010), pp. 849-50.

Larsen, GL. & Henson, PM. (1983). Mediators of inflammation. *Annu Rev Immunol*. 1983, 1, pp. 335-59. Review.

Lewis, T S.; Shapiro, P S. & Ahn, N G. (1998). Signal transduction through MAP kinase cascades. *Advances in Cancer Research*. 1998, 74, pp. 49-139.

Li, J.; Huang, X.; Xie, X.; Wang, J. & Duan, M. (2011). Human telomerase reverse transcriptase regulates cyclin D1 and G1/S phase transition in laryngeal squamous carcinoma. *Acta Otolaryngol*. 131, 5, (May 2011), pp. 546-51.

Lonergan, G.; Routsi, E.; Georgiadis, T.; Agelis, G.; Hondrelis, J.; Matsoukas, J.; Larsen, LK. & Caplan, FR. (1992). Isolation, NMR studies, and biological activities of onopordopicrin from Centaurea sonchifolia. *J Nat Prod.* 55, 2, (February, 1992), pp. 225-8.

Mainardi, CL.; Pourmotabbed, TF. & Hasty, KA. (1991). Inflammation phagocytes and connective tissue degrading metalloproteinases. *Am J Med Sci.* 302, 3, (September 1991), pp. 171-175.

Mazor, R L.; Menendez, I Y.; Ryan, M A.; Fiedler, M A. & Wong, H R. (2000). Sesquiterpene lactones are potent inhibitors of interleukin 8 gene expression in cultured human respiratory epithelium. *Cytokine.* 12, 3, (March 2000), p. 239-45.

McGovern, PE.; Mirzoian, A. & Hall, GR. (2009). Ancient Egyptian herbal wines. *Proc Natl Acad Sci USA.* 106, 18, (May 2009), pp. 7361-6.

Medjroubi, K.; Benayache, F. & Bermejo, J. Sesquiterpene lactones from Centaurea musimomum. (2005). Antiplasmodial and cytotoxic activities. *Fitoterapia.* 76,7-8, (December 2005), pp. 744-6.

Moukarzel K., 1997 Al Tadawi Bil Nabatat Al Tabi'iya, Kitab Tob Cha'bi Mouzawad Bil Souwar Wal Fahares (Arabic) published by Dar Al Hadara, Beirut, Lebanon.

Nehmeh M., 1977. Wild Flowers of Lebanon, National Council for Scientific Research, Beirut, Lebanon.

Newman, DJ. & Cragg, GM. (2007). Natural products as sources of new drugs over the last 25 years. *J Nat Prod.* 70, 3, (March 2007), pp. 461-77. Review.

Nowak, G. (1993). Chromatography of Twentysix Sesquiterpene Lactones from Centaurea bella. *Chromatographia.* 35, 5/6, (March 1993)

Ozçelik, B.; Gürbüz, I.; Karaoglu, T. & Yeşilada, E. (2007). Antiviral and antimicrobial activities of three sesquiterpene lactones from Centaurea solstitialis L. ssp. solstitialis. *Microbiol Res.* 164, 5, (July 2007), p. 545-52.

Pajak, B.; Gajkowska, B. & Orzechowski, A. (2008). Molecular basis of parthenolide-dependent proapoptotic activity in cancer cells. *Folia Histochem Cytobiol.* 46, 2, pp. 129-35. Review.

Patel, N M.; Nozaki, S.; Shortle, N H.; Bhat-Nakshatri, P.; Newton, T R.; Rice, S.; Gelfanov, V.; Boswell, S H.; Goulet, R J.; Sledge, G W. & Nakshatri H. (2000). Paclitaxel sensitivity of breast cancer cells with constitutively active NF-kappaB is enhanced by IkappaBalpha super-repressor and parthenolide Oncogen. 19, 36, (August, 2000), pp. 4159-69.

Rychlewska, U.; Szczepafiska, B.; Daniewski, W.M. & Nowak G. (1992). Crystal structure of salograviolide A, a guaiane-type sesquiterpene lactone. *Journal of Crystallographic and Spectroscopic Research.* 22, 6, (February 1992), pp. 659-663.

Saliba, NA.; Dakdouki, S.; Homeidan, FR.; Kogan, J.; Bouhadir, K.; Talhouk, SN. & Talhouk, RS. (2009). Bio-guided identification of an anti-inflammatory guaianolide from Centaurea ainetensis. *Pharmaceutical Biology.* 47, 8, (August 2009), pp. 701-707.

Saroglou, V.; Karioti, A.; Demetzos, C.; Dimas, K. & Skaltsa, H. (2005). Sesquiterpene lactones from Centaurea spinosa and their antibacterial and cytotoxic activities. *J Nat Prod.* 68, 9, (September 2005), pp. 1404-7.

Solecki, R.S. (1975). Shanidar IV, a Neanderthal flower burial in northern Iraq. *Science.* 190, 4217, (1975), pp. 880–881.

Talhouk RS, El-Jouni W, Baalbaki R, Gali-Muhtasib H, Kogan J & Talhouk SN. Anti-inflammatory bio-activities in water extract of Centaurea ainetensis Journal of *Medicinal Plants Research.* 2, 2, (February 2008), pp. 024-033.

Vajs, V.; Todorović, N.; Ristić, M.; Tesević, V.; Todorović, B.; Janaćković, P.; Marin, P. & Milosavljević, S. (1999). Guaianolides from Centaurea nicolai: antifungal activity. *Phytochemistry.* 52, 3, (October 1999), pp. 383-6.

Webster's Revised Unabridged Dictionary. Published in 1913 by C. & G. Merriam Co. Edited by Noah Porter. United States of America.

Zhang, X.; Shan, P.; Sasidhar, M.; Chupp, G L.; Flavell, R A.; Choi, A M. & Lee, P J. (2003). Reactive oxygen species and extracellular signal-regulated kinase 1/2 mitogen-activated protein kinase mediate hyperoxia-induced cell death in lung epithelium. *American journal of respiratory cell and molecular biology.* 28, 3, (March 2003), pp. 305-315.

Part 2

Inflammation, Immune System and Cancer

3

The Role of Inflammation in Cancer

O'Leary D.P., Neary P.M. and Redmond H.P.
Department of Academic Surgery, Cork University Hospital
Ireland

1. Introduction

Cancer is a pro-inflammatory disease. The link between inflammation and cancer was first noticed over 150 years ago. In 1863, Virchow observed that tumours tend to occur at sites of chronic inflammation (Balkwill, 2001).

Epidemiological studies have recently emerged which support the association between cancer and inflammation. Viruses and bacteria cause chronic inflammation and are significant risk factors in the development of malignancy. Human papilloma viruses, hepatitis B, hepatitis C and helicobacter pylori are well studied examples of this phenomenon which result in cervical cancer, hepatocellular cancer, lympho-proliferative disorders and gastric cancer respectively. Furthermore, increased risk of malignancy is associated with chronic inflammation caused by chemical and physical agents (Gulumian, 1999). In addition to epidemiological data, gene-cluster polymorphisms that lead to increased levels of pro-inflammatory cytokine release are associated with a poorer prognosis and disease severity in cancer patients (Warzocha, 1998; El-Omar, 2000). Moreover, the fact that chronic use of NSAIDs, such as aspirin are shown to reduce the incidence of numerous cancer types including colon, lung and stomach, gives additional supporting evidence for the link between inflammation and cancer (Wang, 2003).

2. NF-κB – A key player

Recent studies have implicated an inflammation-induced protein called nuclear factor kappa B (NF-κB) as a central figure in the link between cancer and inflammation. In 1986, Baltimore et al., originally discovered NF- κB as a factor in the nucleus of B cells that binds to the enhancer of the kappa light chain of immunoglobulin (Sen, 1986). NF- κB activity is considered a hallmark of inflammation. It is shown that NF-κB manipulation can convert inflammation-driven tumour growth into inflammation-induced tumour regression (Luo, 2004). Furthermore, many oncogenes and carcinogens can cause activation of NF-κB, whereas chemicals with chemo-protective properties can interfere with NF-κB activation (Bharti, 2002).

In unstimulated cells, the majority of NF-κB complexes are kept predominantly cytoplasmic and in an inactive form by binding a family of inhibitors known as Inhibitor-κB (IκB). The NF-κB pathway can be activated by numerous stimuli including bacteria, viruses and pro-inflammatory cytokines especially tumour necrosis factor (TNF). Phosphorylation of NF-κB bound I-kappa-B kinases (IκK) on two conserved serine residues within the N-terminal domain of the IκB proteins, which allows for proteasomal degradation and resultant NF-κB liberation. Activation of the NF-κB signalling cascade results in complete degradation of IκB allowing translocation of NF-κB to the nucleus where it induces transcription. The NF-κB family of transcription factors is composed of homodimers and heterodimers derived from 5 subunits - including REL-A(p65), c-REL, REL-B, p50(NF-κB1) and p52 (NF-κB2). When these subunits enter the nucleus, they can mediate transcription of target genes (Hayden, 2004). All family members share a highly conserved Rel homology domain responsible for DNA binding, dimerization domain and interaction with IκBs, the intracellular inhibitor of NF-κB. Cellular stresses including ionising radiation and chemotherapeutic agents can also activate NF-kB. The subsequent release of pro-inflammatory mediators (CSF-1, COX-2, IL-6, IL-1, VEGF, TNF) (Luo, 2004; Marx, 2004) and known anti-apoptotic regulators (BCL-2 and GADD45β) are thought to potentiate tumour growth. In 2004, Karin et al discovered the mechanism that NF-κB contributes to tumourigenesis (Luo, 2004). Prior to this study evidence implicating NF-κB and cancer was mostly circumstantial. Using a murine model of colitis-associated cancer, researchers were able to use genetically altered mice which had the NF-κB activator enzyme IκK knocked out of intestinal epithelial cells and macrophages. In the absence of the IκK gene, neither cell could activate NF-κB. Interestingly, loss of NF-κB activity in both macrophages and epithelial cells individually reduced tumour incidence. They also found that this occurred through two different mechanisms. Tumour incidence decreased by approximately 50% with the loss of NF-κB activity in macrophages through a reduction in growth factors produced by inflammatory cells normally induced by NF-κB activation. Secondly, the loss of NF-κB activity in intestinal epithelial cells resulted in an 80% drop in tumour incidence. The mechanism seen here was different to that seen with the macrophages. Inflammation was not reduced as with the macrophages, instead, apoptosis was no longer inhibited in intestinal cells (Karin, 2004). Pikarsky et al had similar findings in a murine model of inflammation-associated liver cancer where they inhibited NF-κB by adding a gene encoding for IκB, a natural NF-κB inhibitor (Pikarsky, 2004).

The NF-κB family of transcription factors plays a key role in regulation of immune and inflammatory responses including apoptosis and oncogenesis (Baldwin, 2001). NF-κB regulated gene products including those encoding ICAM-1, the extracellular matrix protein tenascin C, vascular endothelial growth factor (VEGF), the chemokine IL-8, the pro-inflammatory enzyme COX2 and matrix metalloprotease 9 (MMP9) are associated with tumour progression and metastasis (Karin, 2002). However NF-κB may also control the expression of apoptosis promoting cytokines such as TNF alpha and FAS ligand (Kasibhatla, 1998).

NF-κB activation is required for endotoxin induced tumour growth. Lou et al showed both tumour nodule numbers and lung weights in the Lipopolysaccharide (LPS) challenged CT26 and CT26 vector groups were significantly higher than the controls (<0.05) (Luo, 2004). This demonstrates that inhibition of NF-κB activity in cancer cells converts the LPS-induced proliferative response to an apoptotic response. LPS was shown to induce NF-κB dependent genes in tumour cells. TNF alpha was shown to mediate LPS induced tumour growth and NF-κB activation. TRAIL mediates LPS induced regression of NF-κB deficient tumours. Overall, NF-κB in CT26 cells is responsible for induction of several anti-apoptotic proteins including Bcl-2 and Bcl-X. Most importantly the inhibition of NF-κB converted the growth promoting effect of LPS mediated by TNF alpha into a cytocidal effect. Trail is a weak inducer of inflammation which is an important characteristic, most likely related to its poor

NF-κB activating ability. In addition to preventing the expression of anti-apoptotic proteins, inhibition of NF-κB also led to increased expression of the Trail receptor DR5. Type I and II interferons (IFN) are efficient inducers of Trail. The authors postulate that IFN based therapy with anti-TNF alpha medications may reduce inflammation associated toxicities, block inflammation induced tumour growth and potentiate Trail dependent tumour killing.

The bcl-2 family of proto-oncogenes are a critical regulator of apoptosis and are frequently deregulated in a wide variety of cancers. They have recently been identified as having an NF-κB binding site in the bcl-2 p2 promoter (Catz, 2001). Thus chemotherapeutic drugs that activate NF-κB can also activate bcl-2 family proteins in various cancer cell lines. Activated NF-κB binds to specific DNA sequences in target genes, designated as kB elements and regulates transcription of over 400 genes involved in immunoregulation, growth, inflammation, carcinogenesis and apoptosis.

Several chemotherapeutic agents including 5-fluorouracil (5-FU) have been reported to induce NF-κB activation in various cell lines (Cusack, 1999). Cytotoxic drugs induce NF-κB with delayed kinetics. This delay is due to the time required to induce nuclear DNA damage and relay the damage signal to the cytoplasmic IκK complex. Treatment with 5-FU can also induce activation of NF-κB in colorectal cancer cells (Wang, 2003). Using RKO human colorectal cell line and two NF-κB signalling deficient RKO mutants, Fukuyama et al demonstrated that 5-FU stimulates NF-κB and RKO cell survival through induction of IκK activity (Fukuyama, 2007). Several studies have shown that inhibition of NF-κB activation results in reversal of chemoresistance (Jones, 2000; Arlt, 2001; Cusack, 2001). It was shown that the inhibition of inducible NF-κB by a NF-κB decoy could induce apoptosis and reduce chemoresistance against 5-FU (Uetsuka, 2003). Inhibition of NF-κB activity reduces chemoresistance to 5-fluorouracil (5-FU) in human stomach cancer. Ionising radiation (IR) has been reported to activate NF-κB in both in vitro and in vivo studies (Rithidech, 2005; Ahmed, 2006). Laszlo et al recently reported that IkB-alpha depletion in the late phase of IR is a result of a combined regulation at both transcription and translation levels (Laszlo, 2008).

3. Toll-like receptors

3.1 Overview

Inflammation is initiated through many cellular transmembrane receptors of which the best characterised are the TLR family. Toll like receptors (TLRs) have been the subject of extensive investigation since their discovery in 1996. The first Toll receptor was discovered in Drosophila and it was revealed that the innate immune system may be activated once the receptor was bound by an extracellular ligand (Belvin, 1996). Subsequent research has revealed a total of 13 mammalian TLRs, 11 of which are expressed in humans. They are involved in the recognition by immune and non-immune cells of stimuli such as lipopolysaccharides (LPS) and dsRNA. They signal through the use of adapter proteins such as TRIF-related adaptor molecule (TRAF) and myeloid differentiation factor 88 (Myd88) (Killeen, 2009). Recognition of pathogen–associated molecular patterns (PAMPS) through TLRs, either alone or in heterodimerization with other TLRs or non-TLRs, triggers signals responsible for activation of the innate and adaptive immune responses. Most TLRs are found in innate immune cells such as polymorphonuclear neutrophils, monocytes/macrophages and dendritic cells where they trigger an immediate response. More recently TLRs have been shown to be expressed in a number of different cancer cells (Cheadle, 2002; Huang, 2008). Recent experimental evidence shows that TLRs display both tumouricidal and tumourigenesis properties (Salaun, 2006; Killeen, 2008). Each TLR recognises a different ligand. All TLRs (except for TLR3) signal through the adapter protein MyD88. MyD88 has been found to play a key role in inflammation induced tumour growth, principally through the innate immune system (Rakoff-Nahoum S, 2007). MyD88 mediates NF-κB activation through the canonical pathway (O'Neill, 2008; Akira, 2006). MyD88 is capable of NF-κB signalling selectively via TLR2 (Fitzgerald, 2003; Horng, 2001). Hence, both TLR2 and TLR4 both of which are expressed on the plasma membrane of cells appear to be involved in NF-κB inflammation-associated tumourigenesis. TLR2 is stimulated by numerous pro-inflammatory stimuli and helps activate the innate immune system.

Several TLRs are responsible for NF-κB activation. TLR4 induces tumour growth through NF-κB activation mediated by TNF-α (Luo, 2004). Interestingly, endotoxin or LPS, which binds specifically to TLR4 in cells is shown to be capable of inducing tumour growth (Pigeon, 1999). Endotoxin is a molecule found in the outer membrane of Gram-negative bacteria and elicits a strong inflammatory response in animals. Hence, it appears that the pro-tumorigenic effects of endotoxin occur through TLR4 mediated NF-κB activation. The focus of recent cancer immunology and medical oncology research has been aimed at activating the immune system in order to inhibit cancer cell growth and induce cancer cell apoptosis. Thus, TLRs offer a unique target for cancer therapy.

3.2 Toll-like receptor-3

TLR3 is a type 1 trans-membrane receptor protein located intracellularly on the endosome of eukaryotic cells. TLR3 has been shown to be an important "danger" signalling receptor that has a dual role in controlling the delicate balance between tolerance and inflammation on one hand and inflammation and disease on the other hand (Vercammen, 2008). TLR3 is composed of an ectodomain (ECD) containing multiple leucine rich repeats (LRRs), a transmembrane region and a cytoplasmic tail containing the Toll interleukin-1 receptor (TIR) domain (Vercammen, 2008). The LRRs form a horse shoe shaped solenoid structure which is capped at one end by a LRR N-terminal (LRR-NT) and at the other end by a LRR C-terminal (LRR-CT) (Bell, 2005). The TLR3 ectodomain (ECD) binds dsRNA. This can only occur in an acidic environment (pH<6.5) reflecting the endosomal location of the receptor. DsRNA binding initiates a signalling pathway that recruits the TIR domain containing adaptor protein (TRIF) to its cytoplasmic domain. TLR3 is the sole TLR to interact directly with TRIF. The TIr domain of TLR3 then binds to TRIF. This indirectly activates several transcription factors including NFκB and IRF3. TRIF knockout mice have shown impaired Interferon-B production in response to a TLR3 ligand which proves that TRIF is essential to the signalling pathway (Takeuchi, 2003). TRIF is an adaptor molecule which is essential for TLR-3 signalling pathways (Yamamoto, 2003). The activity of TRIF allows indirect activation of several transcription factors such as NF-κB and IRF-3.

TLR3 is the critical sensor of the dsRNA. In response to dsRNA stimulation, specific signalling pathways are activated leading to activation of transcription factors such as nuclear factor- κB (NF-κB) and interferon regulatory factor 3 (IRF-3). This response acts as a defence mechanism against a viral insult to the body. The dsRNA itself is produced during viral replication (Jacobs, 1996). Strong or sustained TLR-3 signalling is potentially harmful and in some cases fatal to the host cell. It appears that the mammalian cells have adapted to this using a negative feedback mechanism. PIK3 and RIP-1 binding to TRIF has been shown to inhibit the actions of TRIF signalling (Meylan, 2004). Polyribosinic:polyriboctidic acid (poly I:C) is a stable synthetic dsRNA which acts as an agonist on the TLR3 receptor. It has been the subject of anti-cancer immunotherapy trials for decades. However its activity on the TLR3 receptor as well as RIG-1 and MDA-5 has only been recently identified. It activates the human innate system which subsequently regulates adaptive immunity. Poly I:C is recognised by both endosomal receptor TLR3 and cytosolic receptors including RNA helicases such as RIG-1 melanoma differentiation associated gene 5 (MDA5). TLR3 preferentially recognizes synthetic poly(I:C) rather than a virus derived dsRNA (Okahira, 2005). The important role played by TLR3 in poly I:C recognition was shown in one study which used TLR3 deficient mice. These mice demonstrated reduced responses to poly I:C and produced lower levels of inflammatory cytokines (Alexopoulou, 2001). Poly I:C has several side effects such as nephrotoxicity, coagulopathies and hypersensitivity reactions. In order to reduce this toxicity a modified form of poly I:C known as Poly I:C$_{12U}$ has been produced. This substitutes uridine for cytosine at a ratio of 1:12 and results of a clinical trial of patients with HIV have proven Poly I:C$_{12u}$ to be very safe. Studies using differing lengths of poly I:C showed that longer duplexes are better inducers of TLR3 signalling (Boone, 2004; Okahira, 2005). There are various alternatives to Poly I:C available. Poly I:C$_{12}$U is a mismatched dsRNA helix in which uridine has replaced cytosine. It has a rapid half-life compared to Poly I:C which has opened the door for its use as a clinically useful drug. Poly I:C$_{12}$U is more specific in its binding to TLR3 and this may account for its reduced toxicity and safe use in clinical trials (Mitchell, 2006). No evidence exists of dose limiting organ toxicity including haematological, liver or renal toxicity following intravenous administration to HIV positive patients (Thompson, 1996). Poly I:C mediates a potent adjuvant effect in cells expressing TLR3 and this strongly enhances antigen specific CD8+ T-cell responses, promotes antigen cross presentation by dendritic cells (Cui, 2006; Schulz, 2005) and directly acts on effector CD8+ T and natural killer cells to alter the release of IFN-γ (Tabiasco, 2006). It is the most potent type 1 interferon stimulant that is recognised by TLR3 (Yoneyama, 2004; Matsumoto, 2008).

TLR3 stimulation by dsRNA can cause direct apoptosis and inhibit cell proliferation in various types of cancer cells including colon, breast and melanoma (Taura, 2010; Salaun, 2006, 2007). It is now known that expression and function of TLR3 is dependent on p53 activation (Taura, 2008). Salaun et al recently used poly I:C to treat a breast cancer cell line by triggering apoptosis (Salaun, 2006). They showed that poly I:C can directly cause apoptosis without the involvement of the immune system. They also showed that poly I:C induced apoptosis occurred through the Fas-associated protein death domain-caspase 8 signalling pathway. The extrinsic apoptotic pathway was also shown to be involved by the same group in selected cancer cells (Salaun, 2007). Polyadenylic:polyuridylic acid (poly A:U) is another synthetic double stranded RNA. Poly A:U is unique as it only signals through TLR3. Poly A:U has been used with moderate success to treat breast and gastric cancer as a monotherapy (Laplanche, 2000; Jeung, 2010). Interferons (IFN) are a group of cytokines that can cause antiviral, antiproliferative and apoptotic effects through the Jak/STAT pathway signal transducers (Stark, 2007). In particular, IFN-α, a type I IFN has been shown to induce TLR3 expression and thus significantly enhance tumour cell apoptosis when combined with Poly I:C compared to each treatment alone (Taura 2010). The same study combined IFN-α, Poly I:C and 5-FU which resulted in a significant increase in cancer cell death in a colon cancer cell line. They also showed that by inhibiting the JAK/STAT pathway, induction of TLR3 by INF- α caused a reduced response of TLR3 to INF- α stimulation. Several clinical trials have examined the effect of combining a TLR3 agonist and INF-α with or without a chemotherapeutic agent. Wadler et al combined 5-FU with INF-α and achieved a good response in colon cancer cells however this combination was not effective in clinical trials (Wadler, 1990). Early clinical trials involving a TLR3 agonist as a single adjuvant therapy in colorectal cancer showed mixed results. Lacour et al showed that Poly A:U alone as an adjuvant therapy in colorectal cancer patients who had undergone a resection of the primary tumour was unable to improve the overall survival of patients after five years compared to a placebo (Lacour, 1992). However, when used as a combination therapy there have been very positive results in a clinical trial to demonstrate a positive role for Poly A:U in cancer treatment. After a 14 year median follow-up Laplanche et al reported the results of a trial which combined Poly A:U with loco-regional radiotherapy versus chemotherapy with cyclophosphamide, methotrexate and fluorouracil (CMF) in women with operable breast cancer. They reported that the Poly A:U combination group had a significantly improved disease free survival (p=0.03) and significantly reduced the incidence of metastasis when compared to the CMF group. This trial did not however differentiate the role that Poly A:U and radiotherapy had as single therapies (Laplanche, 2000). Several studies have reported that caspase 3 is up-regulated by TLR3 agonist activity which would suggest a role for caspase 3 in cancer cell apoptosis induced by TLR3 agonists (Salaun, 2006; Khvalevsky, 2007). A recent study by Conforti et al demonstrated the synergistic effects between vaccines, chemotherapy and poly A:U (Conforti, 2010). A vaccine (OVA plus CpG) was administered prior to the combination of oxaliplatin and poly A:U and this significantly reduced tumour growth and prolonged survival. Interestingly these results were not demonstrated in nude and TRIF knockout mice.

3.3 Toll-like receptor-4

TLR4 was first discovered in 1998. Lipopolysaccharide (LPS) is a cell wall protein in gram negative bacteria and works as a ligand for TLR4. The recognition of LPS by TLR4 requires other proteins including LPS binding protein, CD14 and MD2. In resting cells TLR4 is located in the Golgi apparatus. The translocation of TLR4 from the Golgi apparatus to the plasma membrane and the binding of LPS is dependent on MD2 (Nagai, 2002; Shimazu, 1999). TLR4 signals through two pathways: the MyD88-dependant pathway and the MyD88-independant pathway. In the MyD88-dependant pathway, MyD88 binds to the Toll-IL-1 receptor domain of the TLR4 receptor and activates IL-1 receptor associated kinase (IRAK). IRAK in turn phosphorylates TRAF6, which in turn activates a MAP-3-kinase called TAK1, and TAK1 phosphorylates and activates the IκK complex. IκK then liberates NFκB. Killeen et al showed that bacterial endotoxins directly promote tumour cell adhesion and invasion through up-regulation of urokinase plasminogen activator and urokinase plasminogen activator receptor through TLR4 dependant activation of NF_KB (Killeen 2009). TLR4 can also signal through the MyD88-independant pathway to stimulate the production of Interferon-B. Wang et al showed that TLR4/MyD88 over-expression was frequently detected in colo-rectal cancer with liver metastasis and TLR4/MyD88 levels were significantly higher in these patients (Wang, 2010). Although there have been a number of studies investigating the role of TLR4 in colo-rectal cancer, the exact impact of TLR4 signalling in comparison to TLR3 signalling in colon cancer cells has yet to be established.
TLR4 signalling has been shown to promote resistance of cancer cells to apoptosis following introduction of a TLR4 ligand in colon cancer cells (Cianchi, 2010). TLR4 signalling appears to promote the development of colitis associated cancer by mechanisms including enhanced

Cox-2 expression and increased EGFR signalling (Fukata, 2007). Recent experimental studies have shown that TLR4 induced inflammatory factors may cause tumour cell escape from immune surveillance and resistance to chemotherapy and radiotherapy (He, 2007).

One proposed mechanism by which tumour cells resist treatment involves an impairment of the immune response by the inflammatory microenvironment at the tumour site (Coussens, 2002). TLR4 upregulation has been shown to increase the secretion of immunosuppressive cytokines TGF-β, VEGF and pro-angiogenic chemokine IL-8 in human lung cancer cells and induces resistance of human lung cancer cells to TNF-α and TRAIL induced apoptosis (He, 2007). The same study demonstrated secretion of VEGF and IL-8 is p38MAPK dependent and the ERK1/2 and JNK1/2 proteins are not activated. NF-κB activation contributes to apoptosis resistance of human lung cancer cells after LPS stimulation and LPS-induced apoptosis is dependent on NF-κB activation in human lung cancer cells. NF-κB is an anti-apoptotic transcriptional factor induced by cellular components such as LPS, radiation and various chemotherapy drugs.

Contrasting evidence for the role of TLR4 in chemotherapy and radiotherapy resistance was reported by Apetoh et al who demonstrated reduced tumour growth and prolonged survival in immunocompetent wild type mice when treated with chemotherapeutic agents such as oxaliplatin and doxorubicin but this effect was significantly less in TLR4$^{-/-}$ mice and nu/nu mice (Apetoh, 2007). These findings were also demonstrated in TRIF$^{-/-}$ mice which behaved like the wild type mice but Myd88$^{-/-}$ mice behaved like TLR$^{-/-}$ mice. This suggests a certain dependence of tumour treatment resistance on the MyD88 dependent pathway in TLR4 signalling. These results show that when TLR4 itself is knocked out this will lead to a reduction in tumour growth when the tumour is exposed to an appropriate chemotherapeutic agent or radiotherapy. However, when TLR4 is up regulated in the presence of LPS, this results in resistance to chemotherapy and arguably radiotherapy treatment.

Various agents have been suggested as having a role in reversing TLR4 induced tumour apoptotic resistance. Rapamycin is one such agent. Rapamycin is a macrolide antifungal agent and is a potent immunosuppressive medication that is used as an anti-inflammatory and immunosuppressive drug for the treatment of autoimmune diseases such as Systemic lupus erythematosus (SLE) and transplantation rejection (Fernandez, 2006; Hackstein, 2003). In terms of cancer treatment Rapamycin has been shown to display a number of useful anti-cancer cell properties including inhibition of cancer cell proliferation and induction of apoptosis (Hartford, 2007; Zhang, 2007). Rapamycin can also inhibit invasion and metastasis of tumour cells (Abraham, 2007). One study focused on Rapamycins ability to reverse the apoptotic resistance that can occur following TLR4 stimulation with LPS. Sun et al showed that Rapamycin reverses TLR4 ligation induced apoptotic resistance in colon cancer cells (Sun, 2008). Interestingly this same study showed that Rapamycin inhibits anti-apoptotic protein bcl-xL expression and activation of Akt and NF-κB pathways following LPS treatment of cells and this was shown to reverse apoptosis when Akt and NF-κB were inhibited. Paclitaxel has been described as a potential ligand to TLR4 (Asselin, 2001). Kelly et al demonstrated that TLR4 signalling promotes tumour growth and paclitaxel chemo-resistance in ovarian cancer cells (Kelly, 2006). This behaviour was mediated by MyD88 expression.

4. Role of chemokines and cytokines

4.1 Overview

Both TLR3 and TLR4 signalling produce a pro-inflammatory response including chemokines and it has previously been shown that the pro-inflammatory response may contribute to tumorigenesis (Kelly, 2006). Chemokines and cytokines are markers of inflammation which normally recruit leucocytes and aid in blood vessel remodelling. Pathophysiological roles for chemokines include acting as autocrine growth factors, disruption of basement membranes, increasing motility and tumour invasion (Rollins, 2006; Balkwill 2004).

4.2 CXCL-8/IL-8

A recent paper examined the presence of cytokines, chemokines and their receptors in colon cancer using a Taqman Low Density Array with probes for 24 ligands and 17 receptors. This revealed CCL3, CCL4 and CXCL8 levels to be significantly increased in colon cancer samples compared to normal tissue (Erreni, 2009). Further analysis of the levels of CCL3, CCL4 and CXCL8 mRNA expression showed that CCL4 and CCL3 levels were higher in normal and tumour tissue. However, CXCL8 expression was significantly increased in tumour tissue ($p<0.0001$). There was no correlation with tumour stage for all three inflammatory markers. SW620 and HT29 cell lines showed low but detectable levels of CXCL8 which increased with stimulation with TNFα and TGFβ. Interestingly there was high levels of two anti-angiogenic chemokines found in these samples also, CXCL9 and CXCL10 but their receptor was not significantly expressed.

The main function of CXCL8 is the recruitment of neutrophils. These leucocytes have a short life span and have no presence or role in the tumour micro-environment. CXCL8 has however been reported to have a role in the tumour micro-environment by stimulating tumour advancement and invasion by stimulating the process of neoangiogenesis and by activating tumour matrix proteases (Zhu, 2004; Bates, 2004). However, CCL3 and CCL4 are not products of TLR3 and TLR4 signalling, but CXCL8 is produced as a result of signalling by TLR3 and TLR4. Elevated levels of CXCL8 or Interleukin-8 has been associated with increased angiogenesis in normal and transformed tissue adjacent to colon cancer tumours (Fox, 1998; Kuniyasi, 2000). Also, increased CXCL8 protein expression in primary colo-rectal tumours increases the risk of metastasis (Haraguchi, 2002). To date CXCL8 has two known receptors, CXCR1 and CXCR2. These receptors are known broadly as G-protein coupled receptors (GPCR). Recently GPCR antagonists have been developed which can block the biological effects of GPCR signalling. [D-Arg[1,] D-Trp[5,7,9],Leu[11]]SP or substance P antagonist is a potent GPCR antagonist and has been shown to inhibit small cell lung cancer cell proliferation both in vitro and in vivo (Seckl, 1997) and in pancreatic cancer cell proliferation in vitro and in vivo (Guha, 2005). The GPCR ligand/receptor interaction has been shown to result in neuropeptide-induced Ca^{2+} mobilisation which increases intra-cellular Ca^{2+} and this proves useful as a marker of GPCR function (Ryder, 2001). A GPCR antagonist has previously been shown to prevent GPCR agonist induced increase in Ca^{2+}, DNA synthesis and anchorage independent growth in pancreatic cancer cells (Guha, 2005). The role of a GPCR antagonist in colon cancer has yet to be established. IL-8 is produced and has been shown to be produced by tumour cells and the level of its production correlates directly with the metastatic potential of the tumour (Abdollahi, 2003; Bruserud, 2004).

5. Immuno-surveillance

The interaction between cancer cells and the innate and adaptive immune system is complex. As described previously, pro-inflammatory cytokines promote tumour growth; however the immune system has a means of restricting cancer development through immuno-surveillance and immuno-editing. The pro-tumorigenic effect of the inflammatory immune response appears generally to be a consequence of the innate immune system, whereas the adaptive immune system exerts anti-tumorigenic effects (Karin, 2005).

Cancer immunosurveillance is a theory formulated in 1957 by Burnet and Thomas, who proposed that lymphocytes act as sentinels in recognising and eliminating continuously arising transformed cells (Dunn, 2002; Burnet, 1957). Cancer immunosurveillance appears to be an important host protection process that inhibits carcinogenesis and maintains regular cellular homeostasis (Kim 2007). It has been shown that when mice are deficient in genes that encode for cells integral to the adaptive immune response such as T cells, B cells and natural killer T (NKT) cells, tumour incidence and tumour growth are increased (Shankaran, 2001). With the aid of additional studies, natural killer cells and T cells now appear to be the dominant cells involved in tumour immuno-surveillance. Interestingly, interferon-γ (IFN-γ) is produced by both NKT and T cells. Furthermore, IFN-γ is the most influential cytokine released by these cells. Recent studies have now shown that mice deficient in IFN-γ are more susceptible to spontaneous carcinogenesis (Shankaran, 2001).

The mechanism involved in the anticancer protective effect of the immune system is complex. Generally, it is theorised that cells of the immune system recognise the presence of a growing tumour which has undergone stromal remodelling, causing local tissue damage. This is followed by the induction of inflammatory signals which recruits natural killer cells, NKT cells and macrophages to the tumour site. During this phase, the infiltrating lymphocytes such as the natural killer cells and NKT cells are stimulated to produce IFN-γ. Newly synthesised IFN-γ then induces tumour death as well as promoting the production of chemokines which play an important role in promoting tumour death by blocking the formation of new blood vessels.

Similarly, IL-4 is released in large quantities by NKT cells upon activation and is a key regulator in the adaptive immunity. Therapeutic attempts to recruit the immune system to curtail cancer growth have now become a keen area of interest. Although, attempts have met with limited success thus far, this is the basis of vaccine guided anti-cancer therapy which is a rapidly progressing area of research (Dranoff, 2004).

It is clear that elements of the immune system can restrict tumour growth. However, as discussed previously pro-inflammatory cytokine release initiated by the immune system can also promote tumour growth. Therefore, the immune system appears to have the effect of a double edged sword on cancer growth. If we had full understanding and control of these pathways, this could potentially lead to successful cures for cancer.

5.1 Vaccines

Recently vaccines have been developed to take advantage of the role played by the immune system in cancer. The discovery of tumour associated antigens (TAA) expressed by colorectal carcinoma as well as recent advances in tumour immunology are providing new focus to develop biologically targeted immunotherapeutic strategies. It has been reported that immuno-deficient animals as well as humans, e.g. transplant patients, are at greater risk of developing malignancy (Penn, 2000). It has also been reported that cytotoxic T lymphocytes (CTL) and antibodies specific for TAA have been demonstrated in patients with cancers including colorectal cancer (Nagorsen, 2000). Therefore there is an ideal niche in cancer treatment for an active specific immunotherapy. Previously identified or undefined TAAs can be administered to cancer patients in order to cause a systemic immune response which will lead to malignant cell destruction (Rosenberg, 2001).

Despite the huge amount of evidence and theoretical potential of this treatment strategy, the clinical results are limited to date. There is evidence to support the tumouricidal effects of active specific immunotherapy however it appears cancer cells are able to survive the tumouricidal effects as the disease progresses. This phenomenon has become known as 'tumour immune escape'. Several mechanisms have been proposed as to how this phenomenon occurs. One body of evidence shows evidence that cancer genetic instability leads to TAA/HLA downregulation as well as to disruption of the TAA processing/presenting machinery which then allows malignant cells to evade the surveillance of immune sentinels (Seliger, 2001; Yang, 2003). Another proposed mechanism lies in the ability of cancer cells to produce immunosuppressive cytokines e.g. IL-10, and thus counteract the immune system response (Mocellin, 2001; Walker, 1997). The challenge for tumour immunologists currently is to overcome this 'tumour immune escape' and increase the proportion of patients mounting an immune response and increase the rate of responses from the targeted tumour.

The role of macrophages in the development of colorectal cancer is controversial. One study demonstrated that increased numbers of macrophages in all areas of the tumour correlated with an advanced tumour stage (Bailey, 2007). On the other hand Forssell et al showed that the presence of macrophages positively influenced prognosis in colorectal cancer (Forssell, 2007). Another group demonstrated that macrophages have the ability to inhibit or stimulate tumour growth according to their polarisation and state of activation (Mantovani, 2005). This group showed that M1-polarised macrophages activated by IFNγ and bacterial products like LPS display tumouricidal effects whereas M2 macrophages differentiated in the presence of Th2 cytokines, IL-4, IL-13 or IL-10, have the opposite effect. These macrophages favour tumour cell proliferation and stimulate tumour progression and tumour invasion. These studies are crucial in demonstrating the important role that inflammatory mediators such as chemokines and cytokines play in the establishment of the tumour microenvironment. The tumorgenicity of proinflammatory mediators such as interleukin-6 and tumour necrosis factor-α (TNFα) was shown by Coussens et al (Coussens, 2002).

6. Surgery, inflammation and tumourigenesis

At present, the only recognised curative treatment for cancer is surgery. As a result, surgery is the mainstay treatment for tumours. However, surgery is not indicated for all patients with a cancer diagnosis. Surgery is only indicated in these patients if the cancer has not dissipated and spread to distant organs. In fact, surgery in these patients worsens outcome and survival. This begs the question, is surgery tumorigenic? Numerous studies have examined the role of surgery itself on tumour growth. Interestingly, cancer surgery in the presence of micrometastases increases metastatic burden and enhances peri-operative tumour growth (Pigeon, 1999; MS, 1997; Coffey, 2002). The presence of undetected micro-metastases is thought to be largely responsible for these recurrences. Cancer patients often harbour micrometastases which are undetectable at the time of surgery. Surgical intervention in these patients is thought not only to accelerate their progression but also to be responsible for activating dormant micrometastases that may have remained inactive in the absence of surgery. In addition, the extent of the surgery is proportional to the post-operative recurrence rate. This is evidenced by the meta-analyses that show that minimally invasive surgery is more effective than open surgery in improving tumour recurrence, and cancer-related survival (Hensler, 1997), although equally studies exist that do not support this idea (Jayne, 2010). Considering surgery is the only curative treatment of solid tumours, this knowledge has prompted efforts to understand this undesired effect of surgery. It is hoped that this understanding will eventually help develop therapeutic treatments that may attenuate or eliminate this unwelcome consequence of surgery.

6.1 Mechanisms of surgery induced tumourigenesis

Considering what is already known concerning the role of inflammation in tumourigenesis, it is not surprising that surgery is tumorigenic. Surgery confers a traumatic insult to the body which like all traumas induce a potent pro-inflammatory response. Surgery is followed by a biologic period of repair to help restore homeostasis. It induces an early hyper-inflammatory response, which is characterised by pro-inflammatory TNF-α, IL-1 and IL-6 cytokine release (Walker, 1999) and neutrophil activation (Hensler, 1997). Several of these cytokines have been shown to potentiate tumour growth (Coussens, 2004). The massive and continuous IL-6 release subsequently accounts for the up-regulation of major anti-inflammatory mediators, such as PGE_2, IL-10, and TGF-ß (Walker 1999). The magnitude and duration of this hyper-inflammatory response is proportional to the severity of the trauma which may explain how laparoscopic versus open surgery may result in lower tumour recurrence (Colacchio, 1994; Baigrie, 1992). Following surgery, angiogenesis is also stimulated as the body initiates a period of healing and biological repair. Pro-angiogenic substances such as VEGF become elevated post-operatively. Moreover, anti-angiogenic substances such as endostatin and angiostatin are not detectable in the serum shortly after tumour excision (Li, 2001; Holmgren 1995; O'Reilly, 1994). This incites the formation of capillaries and new blood vessels not only to the areas of tissue insult but also to all parts of the body including areas of residual metastatic disease which promotes tumour growth.

Furthermore, surgery also influences immune system function. Immuno-suppression is a feature of the post-operative stress response and is also associated with anaesthesia, blood transfusion and the release of acute-phase proteins (Lee, 1977). The immune system appears to be an important regulator in identifying and eliminating any abnormal cells with cancerous potential. Hence, any disruption of immune function as a result of surgery can also lead to potentiating tumour growth. Interestingly, this immuno-suppression is greater dependent on the extent of surgery (Da Costa, 1998; Da Costa, 1999). The immunosuppressive effects of surgery can last anywhere from between 4 to 14 days depending on the size of surgical trauma induced but peaks day three post-operatively in most cases. Likewise, this may explain why laparoscopic versus open surgery in colon cancer patients confers a greater survival advantage, although the evidence supporting this is not equivocal.

Endotoxaemia also occurs following surgery involving bowel manipulation. Endotoxin, a potent inflammatory mediator, is a component on the wall of Gram negative bacteria often found in the lumen of the gastrointestinal system. Upon manipulation, endotoxin or LPS translocates across the intestinal lumen and enters the circulation. Endotoxaemia further potentiates the hyper-inflammatory response following surgery such as colorectal cancer resection. One study examined the effect of endotoxin administration on a murine breast cancer model (Pigeon, 1999). Interestingly, they found enhanced metastatic growth in the endotoxin treated group compared to controls. In a later study the same group found that endotoxin-induced metastatic growth was associated with increased angiogenesis, vascular permeability and tumour cell invasion and migration (Harmey, 2002). Therefore, this is another potential mechanism of surgically induced tumour growth especially in regard to colorectal cancer operations. In addition, the actual manipulation of the tumour during surgery results in the dissemination of tumour cells into the circulation. These tumour cells can potentially seed in distant sites throughout the body facilitating metastatic spread. Surgeons will make efforts to minimise tumour manipulation intra-operatively to minimise this potential.

Peri-operative tumour growth appears to significantly impact on tumour recurrence following "curative" surgery. Following a deeper understanding of this mechanism, therapeutic efforts are now being sought. Peri-operative immunomodulators such as IL-2, known to abrogate the immune changes that follow excisional cancer surgery, are being investigated as potential peri-operative treatments showing promising initial results (Den Otter, 1996). Even current chemotherapeutic regimes known to induce cell death in rapidly dividing cells have been given immediately post-operatively resulting in increased long-term survival. However, most of these treatments are limited by their toxicities as tissue and wound healing are essential in the immediate post-operative period.

7. Conclusion

Overall, our understanding of the relationship between inflammation and cancer has improved greatly since Virchow first made his observation over 150 years ago. The unravelling of signalling pathways shared by cancer and inflammation will provide the focus for future cancer treatment strategies.

8. References

Abdollahi T, Robertson NM, Abdollahi A, Litwack G. 2003. Identification of interleukin 8 as an inhibitor of tumor necrosis factor-related apoptosis-inducing ligand-induced apoptosis in the ovarian carcinoma cell line OVCAR3. Cancer Res. 63, 4521–4526.

Abraham RT, Gibbons JJ. The mammalian target of rapamycin signaling pathway: twists and turns in the road to cancer therapy. Clin Cancer Res 2007;13:3109–14.

Ahmed KM, Dong S, Fan M, Li JJ. Nuclear factor-kappaB p65 inhibits mitogen activated protein kinase signaling pathway in radioresistant breast cancer cells. Mol. Cancer Res. 4 (2006) 945–955

Akira S, Uematsu S, Takeuchi O. Pathogen recognition and innate immunity. Cell 2006;124(4):783-801.

Alexopoulou, L., A. C. Holt, R. Medzhitov, and R. A. Flavell. 2001. Recognition of double-stranded RNA and activation of NF-kB by Toll-like receptor 3. Nature 413:732–738.

Apetoh L, Ghiringhelli F, Tesniere A. Toll-like receptor 4-dependent contribution of the immune system to anticancer chemotherapy and radiotherapy. Nature Medicine. 2007;13(9):1050–1059.

Arlt A, Vorndamm J, Breitenbroich M, Folsch UR, Kalthoff H, Schmidt WE, Schafer H. Inhibition of NF-kappaB sensitizes human pancreatic carcinoma cells to apoptosis induced by etoposide (VP16) or doxorubicin, Oncogene 20 (2001) 859–868.

Asselin E, Mills GB, Tsang BK. XIAP regulates Akt activity and caspase-3-dependent cleavage during cisplatin-induced apoptosis in human ovarian epithelial cancer cells. Cancer Res 2001;61:1862–8.

Baigrie R, Lamont P, Kwiatkowski D, Dallman M, Morris P. Systemic cytokine response after major surgery. British Journal of Surgery 1992;79(8): 757–760.

Bailey C, Negus R, Morris A, Ziprin P, Goldin R et al. Chemokine expression is associated with the accumulation of tumour associated macrophages (TAMs) and progression in human colorectal cancer, Clin. Exp. Metastasis 24 (2007), pp. 121–130

Baldwin, A.S., Jr. (2001). Series introduction: The transcription factor NF-B and human disease. J. Clin. Invest. 107, 3–6.

Balkwill F, Mantovani A. Inflammation and cancer: back to Virchow? The Lancet 2001;357(9255): 539-545.

Balkwill F. Cancer and the Chemokine Network. Nature Reviews, Cancer 2004;4:540–50.

Bates RC, DeLeo MJ, Arthur M. The epithelial–mesenchymal transition of colon carcinoma involves expression of IL-8 and CXCR-1-mediated chemotaxis. Mercurio Experimental Cell Research 299 (2004) 315– 324.

Baud V, Karin M. Is NF-kappaB a good target for cancer therapy? Hopes and pitfalls, Nat. Rev. Drug Discov. 8 (2009) 33–40

Bell JK. Proc. Natl. Acad. Sci. U.S.A. 102, 10976 (2005).

Belvin MP, Anderson KV. A CONSERVED SIGNALING PATHWAY: The Drosophila Toll-Dorsal Pathway. Annual Review Cell Dev. Biol. 1996. 12:393–416

Bharti AC AB. Chemopreventive agents induce suppression of nuclear factor-kappaB leading to chemosensitization. Ann N Y Acad Sci 2002;973(Nov): 392-395.

Böhm B, Schwenk W, Hucke H, Stock W. Does methodic long-term follow-up affect survival after curative resection of colorectal carcinoma? Diseases of the Colon & Rectum 1993;36(3): 280-286.

Boone DL, Turer EE, Lee EG, Ahmad RC, Wheeler MT et al. 2004. The ubiquitin-modifying enzyme A20 is required for termination of Toll-like receptor responses. Nat. Immunol.5:1052–1060.

Braumann C, Winkler G, Rogalla P, Menenakos C, Jacobi C. Prevention of disease progression in a patient with a gastric cancer-re-recurrence. Outcome after intravenous treatment with the novel antineoplastic agent taurolidine. Report of a case. World Journal of Surgical Oncology 2006;4(1): 34.

Bruserud O, Ryningen A, Wergeland L, Glenjen NI, Gjertsen BT. 2004. Osteoblasts increase proliferation and release of pro-angiogenic interleukin 8 by native human acute myelogenous leukemia blasts. Haematologica 89, 391–402.

Burnet F. Cancer-A biological approach. 37. Med J 1957;1: 779-841.

Catz SD, Johnson JL, Transcriptional regulation of bcl-2 by nuclear factor kappa B and its significance in prostate cancer, Oncogene 20 (2001) 7342–7351.

Cheadle EJ, Jackson AM. (2002) Bugs as drugs for cancer. Immunology 107:10–19

Coffey J, Doyle M, O'Mahony L. Probiotics confer protection against perioperative metastatic tumour growth. Ann Surg Oncol 2002;9: 93.

Colacchio T, Yeager M, Hildebrandt L. Perioperative immunomodulation in cancer surgery. American journal of surgery 1994;167(1): 174

Conforti R, Ma Y, Morel Y, Paturel C, Terme M, Viaud S, Ryffel B, Ferrantini M, Uppaluri R, Schreiber R, Combadière C, Chaput N, André F, Kroemer G, Zitvogel L. Opposing effects of toll-like receptor (TLR3) signaling in tumors can be therapeutically uncoupled to optimize the anticancer efficacy of TLR3 ligands. Cancer Res. 2010 Jan 15;70(2):490-500.

Coussens L. Inflammation and cancer. Toxicologic Pathology 2004;32(6): 732-734.

Coussens LM, Werb Z. Inflammation and cancer. Nature 2002; 420: 860–66.

Cui Z, Qiu F. Synthetic double-stranded RNA poly(I:C) as a potent peptide vaccine adjuvant: therapeutic activity against human cervical cancer in a rodent model. Cancer Immunol Immunother 2006;55: 1267–79.

Cusack JC, Liu R, Baldwin AS. NF- kappa B and chemoresistance: potentiation of cancer drugs via inhibition of NF- kappa B, Drug Resist. Updat. 2 (1999) 271–273

Cusack JC, Liu R, Houston M, Abendroth K, Elliott PJ, Adams J, Baldwin AS. Enhanced chemosensitivity to CPT-11 with proteasome inhibitor PS-341: implications for systemic nuclear factor-kappaB inhibition, Cancer Res. 61(2001) 3535–3540.

Da Costa M, Redmond H, Bouchier-Hayes D. The effect of laparotomy and laparoscopy on the establishment of spontaneous tumor metastases. The Journal of Urology 1999;162(2): 633-634.

Da Costa M, Redmond H, Finnegan N, Flynn M, Bouchier-Hayes D. Laparotomy and laparoscopy differentially accelerate experimental flank tumour growth. British Journal of Surgery 1998;85(10).

Den Otter W, De Groot J, Bernsen M, Heintz A, Maas R, Jan Hordijk G, Hill F, Klein W, Ruitenberg E, Rutten V. Optimal regimes for local IL-2 tumour therapy. International Journal of Cancer 1996;66(3).

Dranoff G. Cytokines in cancer pathogenesis and cancer therapy. Nature Reviews Cancer 2004;4(1): 11-22.

Dunn G, Bruce A, Ikeda H, Old L, Schreiber R. Cancer immunoediting: from immunosurveillance to tumor escape. Nature immunology 2002;3(11): 991-998.

Erreni M, Bianchi P, Laghi L, Mirolo M, Fabbri M et al. Expression of Chemokines and Chemokine Receptors in Human Colon Cancer Methods in Enzymology, Volume 460, 2009, Pages 105-121.

Fernandez D, Bonilla E, Mirza N, Niland B, Perl A. Rapamycin reduces disease activity and normalizes T cell activation-induced calcium fluxing in patients with systemic lupus erythematosus. Arthritis Rheum 2006;54:2983–8.

Fitzgerald KA, McWhirter SM, Faia KL, Rowe DC, Latz E, Golenbock DT, Coyle AJ, Liao SM, Maniatis T. IKKε and TBK1 are essential components of the IRF3 signaling pathway. Nature immunology 2003;4(5): 491-496.

Forssell J, Oberg A, Henriksson ML, Stenling R, Jung A, Palmqvist R. High macrophage infiltration along the tumor front correlates with improved survival in colon cancer, Clin. Cancer Res. 13 (2007), pp. 1472–1479

Fox SH, Whalen GF, Sanders MM, Burleson JA, Jennings K, Kurtzman S, Kreutzer D. Angiogenesis in normal tissue adjacent to colon cancer. Journal of Surgical Oncology 1998;69:230–4.

Fukata M, Chen A, Vamadevan AS, Cohen J, Breglio K, Krishnareddy S, Hsu D, Xu R, Harpaz N, Dannenberg AJ, Subbaramaiah K, Cooper HS, Itzkowitz SH, Abreu MT (2007) Toll-like receptor-4 promotes the development of colitis-associated colorectal tumors. Gastroenterology 133: 1869–1881.

Fukuyama R, Ng KP, Cicek M, Kelleher C, Niculaita R, Casey G, Sizemore N. Role of IKK and oscillatory NFkappaB kinetics in MMP-9 gene expression and chemoresistance to 5-fluorouracil in RKO colorectal cancer cells, Mol. Carcinog. 46 (2007) 402–413.

Guha S, Eibl G, Kisfalvi K, Fan R, Burdick M. Broad-Spectrum G Protein–Coupled Receptor Antagonist, [D-Arg1,D-Trp5,7,9,Leu11]SP: A Dual Inhibitor of Growth and Angiogenesis in Pancreatic Cancer. Cancer Res April 1, 2005 65; 2738.

Gulumian M. The role of oxidative stress in diseases caused by mineral dusts and fibres: current status and future of prophylaxis and treatment. Molecular and cellular biochemistry 1999;196(1): 69-77.

Hackstein H, Taner T, Zahorchak AF, Morelli AE, Logar AJ, Gessner A, et al. Rapamycin inhibits IL-4-induced dendritic cell maturation in vitro and dendritic cell mobilization and function in vivo. Blood 2003;101:4457–63.

Haraguchi M, Komuta K, Akashi A, Matsuzzaki S, Furui J, Kanematsu T. Elevated IL-8 levels in the drainage vein of resectable Duke's C colorectal cancer indicate high risk for developing hepatic metastasis. Oncology Reports 2002;9:159–65.

Harmey J, Bucana C, Lu W, Byrne A, McDonnell S, Lynch C, Bouchier-Hayes D, Dong Z. Lipopolysaccharide-induced metastatic growth is associated with increased angiogenesis, vascular permeability and tumor cell invasion. International Journal of Cancer 2002;101(5): 415-422.

Hartford CM, Ratain MJ. Rapamycin: something old, something new, sometimes borrowed and now renewed. Clin Pharmacol Ther 2007;82:381–8.

Hayden MS, Ghosh S. Signaling to NF- B. Genes & development 2004;18(18): 2195-2224.

He W, Liu Q, et al. (2007). TLR4 signaling promotes immune escape of human lung cancer cells by inducing immunosuppressive cytokines and apoptosis resistance. Molecular immunology 44(11): 2850-2859.

Hensler T, Hecker H, Heeg K, Heidecke C, Bartels H, Barthlen W, Wagner H, Siewert J, Holzmann B. Distinct mechanisms of immunosuppression as a consequence of major surgery. Infection and immunity 1997;65(6): 2283.

Holmgren L, O'Reilly M, Folkman J. Dormancy of micrometastases: balanced proliferation and apoptosis in the presence of angiogenesis suppression. Nature Medicine 1995;1(2): 149-153.

Horng T, Barton GM, Medzhitov R. TIRAP: an adapter molecule in the Toll signaling pathway. Nature immunology 2001;2(9): 835-841.

Huang B, Zhao J, Li H, He KL, Chen Y, Chen SH, et al. Toll-like receptors on tumor cells facilitate evasion of immune surveillance. Cancer Res 2005;65:5009–14.

Huang B, Zhao J, Unkeless JC, Feng ZH, Xiong H. (2008) TLR signalling by tumor and immune cells: a double-edged sword. Oncogene 27:218–224.

Jacobi C, Peter F, Wenger F, Ordemann J, Müller J. New therapeutic strategies to avoid intra- and extraperitoneal metastases during laparoscopy: results of a tumor model in the rat. Dig Surg 1999;16: 393-399.

Jacobi C, Sabat R, Ordemann J, Wenger F, Volk H, Müller J. Peritoneal instillation of taurolidine and heparin for preventing intraperitoneal tumor growth and trocar metastases in laparoscopic operations in the rat model. Langenbecks Archiv für Chirurgie 1997;382(4 Suppl 1): S31.

Jacobs BL, Langland JO. When two strands are better than one: the mediators and modulators of the cellular responses to double stranded RNA. Virology 1996 219:339-349.

Jayne D, Thorpe H, Copeland J, Quirke P, Brown J, Guillou P. Five year follow up of the Medical Research Council CLASICC trial of laparoscopically assisted versus open surgery for colorectal cancer. Br J Surg. 2010 Nov;97(11):1638-45.

Jeung HC, Moon YW, Rha SY, et al. Phase III trial of adjuvant 5-fluorouracil and Adriamycin versus 5-fluorouracil, Adriamycin, and Optimizing Poly(A:U) Anticancer Therapy. Cancer Res; 70(2) January 15, 2010 499.

Jones DR, Broad RM, Madrid LV, Baldwin AS, Mayo MW. Inhibition of NFkappaB sensitises non-small cell lung cancer cells to chemotherapy-induced apoptosis, Ann. Thorac. Surg. 70 (2000) 930–936 discussion 936–937.

Karin M, Greten F. NF- B: linking inflammation and immunity to cancer development and progression. Nature Reviews Immunology 2005;5(10): 749-759.

Karin M, Lin A. (2002). NF-B at the crossroads of life and death. Nat. Immunol. 3, 221-27 227.

Kasibhatla, S., Brunner, T., Genestier, L., Echeverri, F., Mahboubi, A., Green, D.R. (1998). DNA damaging agents induce expression of Fas and subsequent apoptosis in T lymphocytes via the activation of NF-kB and AP-1. Mol. Cell 1, 543–551.

Kelly MG, Alvero AB, Chen R, et al. TLR-4 signaling promotes tumor growth and paclitaxel chemoresistance in ovarian cancer. Cancer Res 2006;66:3859–68.

Khvalevsky E, Rivkin L, Rachmilewitz J, Galun E, Giladi H. TLR3 signaling in a hepatoma cell line is skewed towards apoptosis. J Cell Biochem 2007;100: 1301–12.

Killeen SD, Wang JH, Andrews EJ, Redmond HP (2008) Exploitation of the Toll-like receptor system in cancer: a doubled-edged sword? Br J Cancer 95: 247–252.

Killeen SD, Wang JH, Andrews EJ, Redmond HP. Bacterial endotoxin enhances colorectal cancer cell adhesion and invasion through TLR-4 and NF-kB-dependent activation of the urokinase plasminogen activator system. British Journal of Cancer (2009) 100, 1589 – 1602.

Kim R, Emi M, Tanabe K. Cancer immunoediting from immune surveillance to immune escape. Immunology 2007;121(1):1.

Knight B, Skellern G, Smail G, Browne M, Pfirrmann R. NMR studies and GC analysis of the antibacterial agent taurolidine. Journal of Pharmaceutical Sciences 1983;72(6): 705-707.

Kuniyasu H, Yasui W, Shinohara H, Yano S, Ellis LM, Wilson MR, Bucana CD, Rikita T, Tahara, E, Fidler I. Induction of angiogenesis by hyperplastic colonic mucosa adjacent to colon cancer. American Journal of Pathology 2000;157:1523–35.

Lacour J, Laplanche A, Malafosse M, Gallot D, Julien M et al. Polyadenylic-polyuridylic acid as an adjuvant in resectable colorectal carcinoma: a 6 1/2 year follow-up analysis of a multicentric double blind randomized trial. Eur J Surg Oncol. 1992 Dec;18(6):599-604.

Laplanche A, Alzieu L, Delozier T, Berlie J, Veyret C, Fargeot P, Luboinski M, Lacour J. Polyadenylic–polyuridylic acid plus locoregional radiotherapy versus chemotherapy with CMF in operable breast cancer: a 14 year follow-up analysis of a randomized trial of the F´ed´eration Nationale des Centres de Lutte Contre le Cancer (FNCLCC). Breast Cancer Research and Treatment 64: 189–191, 2000.

Laszlo CF, Wu S. Mechanism of UV-induced IkappaBalpha-independent activation of NF-kappaB, Photochem. Photobiol. 84 (2008) 1564–1568

Lee SJ, Lim KT. UDN glycoprotein regulates activities of manganese-superoxide dismutase, activator protein-1, and nuclear factor-kappaB stimulated by reactive oxygen radicals in lipopolysaccharide-stimulated HCT-116 cells. Cancer Lett 2007;254:274–87.

Lee Y. Effect of anesthesia and surgery on immunity. Journal of Surgical Oncology 1977;9(5).

Li T, Kaneda Y, Ueda K, Hamano K, Zempo N, Esato K. The influence of tumour resection on angiostatin levels and tumour growth—an experimental study in tumour-bearing mice. European Journal of Cancer 2001;37(17): 2283-2288.

Little D, Regan M, BOUCHIER-HAYES D. Perioperative immune modulation. Surgery 1993;114(1): 87-91.

Luo JL, Maeda S, Hsu LC, Yagita H, Karin M. Inhibition of NF- B in cancer cells converts inflammation-induced tumor growth mediated by TNF to TRAIL-mediated tumor regression. Cancer Cell 2004;6(3): 297-305.

Mantovani A. Cancer: Inflammation by remote control, Nature 435 (2005), pp. 752–753.

Marx J. Cancer research: Inflammation and cancer: The link grows stronger. In; 2004. p. 966-968.

Matsumoto M, Seya T. TLR3: Interferon induction by double-stranded RNA including poly(I:C). Adv Drug Deliv Rev 2008; 60:805-12.

Meylan, E., K. Burns, K. Hofmann, V. Blancheteau, F. Martinon, M. Kelliher, and J. Tschopp. 2004. RIP1 is an essential mediator of Toll-like receptor 3-induced NF-_B activation. Nat. Immunol. 5:503–507.

Mitchell W. 2006. Review of Ampligen clinical trials in chronic fatigue syndrome. J. Clin. Virol. 37:S113.

Mocellin S, Wang E, Marincola FM. Cytokines and immune response in the tumor microenvironment. J Immunother 2001;24:392–407

MS O, Boehm T, Shing Y, Fukai N, Vasios G, Lane W, Flynn E, Birkhead J, Olsen B, Folkman J. Endostatin: an endogenous inhibitor of angiogenesis and tumor growth. Cell 1997;88(2): 277-285.

Nagai Y, Akashi S, Nagafuku M, Ogata M, Iwakura Y, Akira S, Kitamura T, Kosugi A et al. Essential role of MD-2 in LPS responsiveness and TLR4 distribution. Nat Immunol 3 (2002), pp. 667–672.

Nagorsen D, Keilholz U, Rivoltini L. Schmittel A, Letsch A, Asemissen AM, Berger G, Buhr HJ, Theil E, Scheibenbogen C. Natural T-cell response against MHC class I epitopes of epithelial cell adhesion molecule, her-2/neu, and carcinoembryonic antigen in patients with colorectal cancer. Cancer Res 2000;60:4850–4854.

Okahira S, Nishikawa F, Nishikawa S, Akazawa T, Seya T, Matsumoto M. 2005. Interferon-beta induction through Toll-like receptor 3 depends on double-stranded RNA structure. DNA Cell Biol. 24:614–623.

O'Neill LAJ. The interleukin-1 receptor/Toll-like receptor superfamily: 10 years of progress. Immunological Reviews 2008;226(1):10.

O'Reilly M, Holmgren L, Shing Y, Chen C, Rosenthal R, Moses M, Lane W, Cao Y, Sage E, Folkman J. Angiostatin: a novel angiogenesis inhibitor that mediates the suppression of metastases by a Lewis lung carcinoma. Cell 1994;79(2): 315-328.

Penn I. Post-transplant malignancy: the role of immunosuppression. Drug Saf 2000;23:101–113.

Pidgeon G, Harmey J, Kay E, Da Costa M, Redmond H, Bouchier-Hayes D. The role of endotoxin/lipopolysaccharide in surgically induced tumour growth in a murine model of metastatic disease. British journal of cancer 1999;81(8): 1311-1317.

Pikarsky E, Porat RM, Stein I, Abramovitch R, Amit S, Kasem S, Gutkovich-Pyest E, Urieli-Shoval S, Galun E, Ben-Neriah Y. NF- B functions as a tumour promoter in inflammation-associated cancer. Nature 2004;431(7007): 461-466.

Rakoff-Nahoum S, Medzhitov R. Regulation of spontaneous intestinal tumorigenesis through the adaptor protein MyD88. Science 2007;317(5834):124.

Reith H. Therapy of peritonitis today. Surgical management and adjuvant therapy strategies. Langenbecks Archiv für Chirurgie 1997;382(4 Suppl 1): S14.

Rithidech KN, Tungjai M, Arbab E, Simon SR. Activation of NF-kappaB in bone marrow cells of BALB/cJ mice following exposure in vivo to low doses of (137)Cs gamma-rays, Radiat. Environ. Biophys. 44 (2005) 139–143.

Rollins B. Inflammatory chemokines in cancer growth and progression. European Journal of Cancer. 2006;42:760–7.

Rosenberg SA. Progress in human tumour immunology and immunotherapy. Nature 2001;411:380–384.

Ryder NM, Guha S, Hines OJ, Reber HA, Rozengurt E. G protein-coupled receptor signaling in human ductal pancreatic cancer cells: neurotensin responsiveness and mitogenic stimulation. J Cell Physiol 2001; 186: 53–64.

Salaun B, Coste I, Rissoan MC, Lebecque SJ, Renno T. TLR3 can directly trigger apoptosis in human cancer cells. J Immunol 2006; 176: 4894–901.

Salaun B, Lebecque S, Matikainen S, Rimoldi D, Romero P. Toll-like receptor 3 expressed by melanoma cells as a target for therapy? Clin Cancer Res 2007;13: 4565–74.

Schulz O, Diebold SS, Chen M, et al. Toll-like receptor 3 promotes cross-priming to virus-infected cells. Nature 2005;433:887–92.

Seckl MJ, Higgins T, Widmer F, Rozengurt E. [DArg1,D-Trp5,7,9,Leu11]substance P: a novel potent inhibitor of signal transduction and growth in vitro and in vivo in small cell lung cancer cells. Cancer Res 1997;57;51–4

Seliger B, Wollscheid U, Momburg F, Blankenstein T, Huber C. Characterization of the major histocompatibility complex class I deficiencies in B16 melanoma cells. Cancer Res 2001;61:1095–1099

Sen R, Baltimore D. Inducibility of kappa immunoglobulin enhancer-binding protein Nf-kappa B by a posttranslational mechanism. Cell 1986;47(6): 921-928.

Shankaran V, Ikeda H, Bruce A, White J, Swanson P, Old L, Schreiber R. IFN and lymphocytes prevent primary tumour development and shape tumour immunogenicity. Nature 2001;410(6832): 1107-1111.

Shimazu R, Akashi S, Ogata H, Nagai Y, Fukudome K, Miyake K, Kimoto M. MD-2, a molecule that confers lipopolysaccharide responsiveness on Toll-like receptor 4. J Exp Med 189 (1999), pp. 1777–1782.

Stark GR. How cells respond to interferons revisited: from early history to current complexity. Cytokine Growth Factor Rev 2007; 18: 419–23.

Sun Q, Zheng Y, Liu Q, Cao X. International Immunopharmacology 8 (2008) 1854–1858.

Tabiasco J, Devevre E, Rufer N, et al. Human effector CD8+ T lymphocytes express TLR3 as a functional coreceptor. J Immunol 2006;177:8708–13.

Takeuchi, M. Sugiyama, M. Okabe, K. Takeda, and S. Akira. 2003. Role of adaptor TRIF in the MyD88-independent Toll-like receptor signaling pathway. Science 301:640–643.

Taura M, Eguma A, Suico MA et al. p53 regulates Toll-like receptor 3 expression and function in human epithelial cell lines. Mol Cell Biol 2008; 28: 6557–67.

Taura M, Fukuda R, Suico MA, Eguma A, Koga T et al. TLR3 induction by anticancer drugs potentiates poly I:C-induced tumor cell apoptosis. Cancer Sci | July 2010 | vol. 101 | no. 7 | 1615

Thompson KA, Strayer DR, Salvato, PD, Thompson CE, Klimas N, Molavi A et al. Results of a double blinded placebo controlled study of the double stranded RNA drug poly1:polyC12U in the treatment of HIV infection. Eur J Clin Microbiol Infect Dis 1996;15(7):580-7.

Uetsuka H, Haisa M, Kimura M, Gunduz M, Kaneda Y et al. Inhibition of inducible NF-kappaB activity reduces chemoresistance to 5-fluorouracil in human stomach cancer cell line, Exp. Cell Res. 289 (2003) 27–35.

Vercammen E, Staal J, Beyaert R. Sensing of Viral Infection and Activation of Innate Immunity by Toll-Like Receptor 3. CLINICAL MICROBIOLOGY REVIEWS, Jan. 2008, p. 13–25 Vol. 21, No. 1.

Wadler S, Schwartz EL. Antineoplastic activity of the combination of interferon and cytotoxic agents against experimental and human malignancies: a review. Cancer Res 1990; 50: 3473–86.

Walker C, Bruce D, Heys S, Gough D, Binnie N, Eremin O. Minimal modulation of lymphocyte and natural killer cell subsets following minimal access surgery. American journal of surgery 1999;177(1): 48.

Walker PR, Saas P, Dietrich PY. Role of Fas ligand (CD95L) in immune escape: the tumor cell strikes back. J Immunol 1997;158:4521–4524

Wang EL, Qian ZR, Nakasono M, Tanahashi T, Yoshimoto K, Bando Y et al. High expression of Toll-like receptor 4/myeloid differentiation factor 88 signals correlates with poor prognosis in colorectal cancer. British Journal of Cancer (2010) 102, 908 – 915.

Wang L, Liu Q, Sun Q, Zhang C, Chen T, Cao X. TLR4 signaling in cancer cells promotes chemoattraction of immature dendritic cells via autocrine CCL20. Biochem Biophys Res Commun 2008;366:857–61.

Wang WH, Huang JQ, Zheng GF, Lam SK, Karlberg J, Wong BCY. Non-steroidal anti-inflammatory drug use and the risk of gastric cancer: a systematic review and meta-analysis. jnci 2003;95(23): 1784-1791.

Warzocha K, Ribeiro P, Bienvenu J, Roy P, Charlot C, Rigal D, Coiffier B, Salles G. Genetic polymorphisms in the tumor necrosis factor locus influence non-Hodgkin's lymphoma outcome. Blood 1998;91(10): 3574.

Wiemann B, Starnes CO. Coley's toxins, tumor necrosis factor and cancer research: a historical perspective. Pharmacol Ther. 1994;64(3):529-64.

Yakovlev VA, Barani IJ, Rabender CS, Black SM, Leach JK et al. Tyrosine nitration of IkappaBalpha: a novel mechanism for NF-kappaB activation. Biochemistry 46 (2007) 11671–11683.

Yamamoto M, Sato S, Hemmi H, Hoshino K, Kaisho T, Sanjo H, Takeuchi O, Sugiyama M, Okabe M, Takeda K, Akira S. Role of adaptor TRIF in the MyD88-independent toll-like receptor signaling pathway. Science. 2003 Aug 1;301(5633):640-3.

Yang T, McNally BA, Ferrone S, Liu Y, Zheng P. A single-nucleotide deletion leads to rapid degradation of TAP-1 mRNA in a melanoma cell line. J Biol Chem 2003;278:15291–15296

Yoneyama M, Kikuchi M, Natsukawa T, Shinobu N, Imaizumi T, Miyagishi M, et al. The RNA helicase RIG-I has an essential function in double-stranded RNA-induced innate antiviral responses. Nat Immunol 2004; 5:730-7.

Zhang JF, Liu JJ, Lu MQ, Cai CJ, Yang Y, Li H, et al. Rapamycin inhibits cell growth by induction of apoptosis on hepatocellular carcinoma cells in vitro. Transpl Immunol 2007;17:162–8.

Zhu YM, Webster SJ, Flower D, Woll PJ. Interleukin-8/CXCL8 is a growth factor for human lung cancer cells. British Journal of Cancer (2004) 91, 1970 – 1976.

Transcription Regulation and Epigenetic Control of Expression of Natural Killer Cell Receptors and Their Ligands

Zhixia Zhou, Cai Zhang, Jian Zhang and Zhigang Tian
Institute of Immunopharmacology & Immunotherapy,
School of Pharmaceutical Sciences, Shandong University
China

1. Introduction

Throughout the life of an individual organism, a successful host defense relies on the coordination of innate and adaptive immunity (McQueen and Parham, 2002). Natural killer (NK) cells are characteristic cytolytic cells that are integral components of innate immunity and play a major role both in the direct destruction of infected or transformed cells and in the production of cytokines and chemokines that mediate inflammatory responses and exert a regulatory effect on the adaptive immune responses (McQueen and Parham, 2002; Moretta et al., 2006). Cells become susceptible to NK cell-mediated killing following downregulation of cell surface MHC class I expression after virus infection, which ultimately leads to escape from the MHC-restricted adaptive immune system; a phenomenon also seen in metastasized tumor cells. MHC class I-specific NK receptors (NKR) have acquired the ability to detect immune escape variants and in rodents and primates can be grouped into two distinct classes of MHC class I-specific receptor families based on protein structure: the C-type lectin superfamily (Cl-SF) and the immunoglobulin superfamily (Ig-SF). Humans possess a large family of killer cell immunoglobulin-like receptors (KIR) that belong to the Ig superfamily, whereas mice express lectin-like Ly49 receptors that are now not present in humans, except for a single nonfunctional gene fragment (Lanier, 1998, 2001; Vilches and Parham, 2002; Takei et al., 2001). A third family of NKR, the lectin-like CD94/NKG2 heterodimers, are structurally and functionally conserved between rodents and primates and interact with their ligands: nonclassical MHC class I molecules and some specific ligands that are differentially expressed in different tissues in response to different stresses (McQueen and Parham, 2002; Moretta et al., 2006; Raulet et al., 2001; Uhrberg et al., 1997; Valiante et al., 1997). The actions of NK cells, therefore, are thought to be mediated by the complex interactions between inhibitory and activating signals sent by cell-surface receptors following ligation (Lanier, 2005; Ravetch and Lanier, 2000).

Malignant cells in tumor growth frequently demonstrate alterations in MHC class I expression that play a major role in their ability to escape immune recognition and killing (Dunn et al., 2002; Campoli et al., 2005). NK cells enhance their cytotoxic function and immune regulation by using their stimulatory and inhibitory receptors to maintain the constant balance in the immune system (Chang and Ferrone, 2006). There are major questions, however, regarding the molecular mechanisms that govern the shape of the NK-cell receptors and MHC class I molecules or other ligands that exhibit an exceptionally high degree of genetic polymorphism in a clonally distributed fashion. Studies, therefore, that focus on the molecular mechanisms that govern the expression of NK-cell receptors and their ligands may provide improved strategies of active-specific immunotherapy for the treatment of cancer, infection and other diseases (Campoli and Ferrone, 2008; Krukowski et al., 2011; Gao et al., 2009). Some stimulators, including viruses, tumor cells and heat shock, could promote the expression of NK-cell receptors and their ligands via activation of certain transcription factors that are capable of regulating activity of NKG2 promoters. Epigenetic mechanisms, including DNA methylation and histone posttranslational modification, are also critical for expression of NK-cell receptors and their ligands, and may control the clonal distribution of some NK-cell receptors. These effects may influence the performance of NK-cell functions. In this review, we will discuss the recent advances in transcriptional regulation and epigenetic control of the expression of NK-cell receptors and their ligands (and of KIR and NKG2 receptor families in particular).

2. Regulation of gene expression – An introduction in the transcriptional level

Mechanisms that underlie the control of gene expression, which drives the processes of gene morphogenesis and distribution, are complex. Transcription regulation at every step of the process is subject to dynamic regulation in the cell (Beckett, 2009; Pan et al., 2010). This regulation includes structural changes in the chromatin to make a particular gene accessible for transcription, transcription of DNA into RNA, splicing of RNA into mRNA, editing and other covalent modifications of the mRNA, translation of mRNA into protein, and, finally, posttranslational modification of the protein into its mature functional form. Information on molecular details of each of these regulatory steps is becoming increasingly available (Fry and Peterson, 2002; Mitchell and Tjian, 1989).

2.1 Transcriptional factor regulation

Regulation at the transcriptional level is a critical mechanism of controlling gene expression. Transcription is controlled by trans-acting factors that regulate spatiotemporal gene expression by associating with cis-acting elements such as promoters, enhancers, and other regulatory regions. Transcription factors perform this function either alone or with other proteins in a complex and by promoting or blocking the transcription of genetic information from DNA to RNA (Mitchell and Tjian, 1989; Alexander and Beggs, 2010; Brivanlou and Darnell, 2002; Karin, 1990). A defining feature of transcription factors is that they contain one or more DNA-binding domains (DBDs), which attach to specific DNA sequences adjacent to the genes that they regulate. In eukaryotes, an important class of transcription factors, called general transcription factors (GTFs), is necessary for transcription to occur. Many of these GTFs do not actually bind to DNA but are parts of the large transcription preinitiation complex that interact directly with RNA polymerase. The most common GTFs are transcription factor II members (TFIIA/B/D/E/F and TFIIH). There are also some nonclassical transcription factors that play crucial roles in gene regulation, including coactivators, chromatin remodelers, histone acetylases, deacetylases, kinases, and methylases, which lack DNA-binding domains (Brivanlou and Darnell, 2002; Karin, 1990; Dowell, 2010; van Nimwegen, 2003).

2.2 Epigenetic control

Transcription is also controlled by epigenetic regulation that is defined as gene-regulation activity that does not involve changes in the underlying DNA code and includes DNA methylation and a variety of histone protein posttranslational modifications (Feng et al., 2010; Furumatsu and Ozaki, 2010). DNA methylation usually occurs in CpG islands, CG-rich regions that are "upstream" of the promoter region. The letter "p" here signifies that C and G are connected by a phosphodiester bond. In humans, DNA methylation is carried out by a group of enzymes called DNA methyltransferases. These enzymes not only determine DNA methylation patterns during early development, but are also responsible for copying these patterns to the strands generated from DNA replication. DNA methylation can alter condensed chromatin structure by influencing histone–DNA and histone–histone contact. Methylation of the promoter and 5′ region of the gene and methylation of histone are associated with transcriptional silencing (Bird, 2002; Bird and Wolffe, 1999; Law and Jacobsen, 2010).

Acetylation and methylation of histones are the most general and important histone modifications associated with transcriptional activation. Histone acetylation is catalysed by histone acetyl transferases (HATs), whereas the reverse reaction is performed by histone deacetylases (HDACs) (Furumatsu and Ozaki, 2010). HATs and HDACs are classified into many families that are often conserved throughout evolution from yeast to humans. Histone H3 is primarily acetylated at several lysine residues, Lys9, 14, 18, 23, 27 and 56, whereas histone H4 is acetylated at Lys5, 8, 12 and 16 (Su et al., 2004). Interestingly, methylation is often modified at lysine and arginine residues in histones H3 and H4. It has been suggested that these modifications constitute a "histone code"; the "code" hypothesis speculates that this modification pattern is read by proteins that recognize distinct modifications specifically and then regulate chromatin dynamics and genome function (Wang et al., 2004; Kisliouk et al., 2010). Whether these modifications form a true code is still under discussion. The processes of histone modification and DNA methylation can both influence each other. Moreover, DNA methylation and suppressive histone modifications may prevent transcription, even when transcription factors are abundant. In turn, transcription factors may cause alterations in DNA methylation and histone modifications (Furumatsu and Ozaki, 2010; Fernandez-Morera et al., 2010; Strahl and Allis, 2000). Molecular details of the transcriptional regulators involved in expression of many NK-cell receptors and their ligands are becoming increasingly available, especially for the NKG2 and KIR receptor families and their ligands.

3. Transcription factor regulation and epigenetic control of the expression of NK-cell receptors and their ligands

3.1 NKG2 receptor family

In humans, the NKG2 receptor family comprises seven members called NKG2A, NKG2B, NKG2C, NKG2D, NKG2E, NKG2F and NKG2H; NKG2A/B and NKG2E/H pairs are splice variants of the same gene (Brostjan et al., 2000; Glienke et al., 1998). All members of the NKG2 family, except NKG2D, share substantial sequence homology, are closely linked, and of the same transcriptional orientation; they contain conserved sequences at the transcriptional start site and at other transcription factor-binding sites, such as the TCF-1 (testosterone conversion factor-1) and GATA-1 (GATA-binding factor 1) sites. These members of the NKG2 family form disulfide-linked heterodimers with CD94. Each member of the NKG2 family, however, has a unique repeat Alu sequence that functions as a gene promoter. Alu repeats are the putative binding sites for several transcription factors: activator protein-1/3 (AP-1/3), cAMP response element binding/activating transcription factors (CREB/ATF), CCAAT/enhancer binding protein (C/EBP), transcription factor-1 (Sp1), nuclear factor-1/CCAAT transcription factor (NF-1/CTF) and lymphocyte-specific DNA-binding protein-1 (LyF-1), and may contribute to differences in gene regulation among family members (Brostjan et al., 2000; Glienke et al., 1998). The CD94 protein associates with different NKG2 isoforms to form heterodimeric receptors that function either to inhibit or to trigger cytotoxicity of NK cells, depending on the NKG2 isoform. Functionally, therefore, CD94/NKG2 heterodimers are divided into activating (NKG2C, NKG2E/H) or inhibitory (NKG2A/B) isotypes (Glienke et al., 1998). It has also been shown that several cytokines, including interleukin (IL)-12 (Derre et al., 2002), transforming growth factor (TGF)-β (Bertone et al., 1999), IL-15 (Mingari et al., 1998) and IL-10 (Romero et al., 2001), are capable of inducing expression of CD94/NKG2 in human NK or T cells, in which IL-15 and TGF-β can upregulate CD94/NKG2A, but not other CD94/NKG2 receptors (Wilhelm et al., 2003). NKG2D is a special activating receptor that is not covalently associated with CD94. NKG2D is downmodulated by TGF-β, but markedly upregulated by IL-15, interferon (IFN)-α and IL-12 stimulation in primary NK cells (Dasgupta et al., 2005). IFN-α can stimulate the expression of NKG2D, but inhibits the expression of the inhibitory receptor NKG2A, and therefore alters the balance of stimulatory and inhibitory receptors in favor of activation, leading to NK-cell-mediated cytotoxicity. IFN-γ addition exerts the opposite effect (Zhang et al., 2005).

CD94 is a C-type lectin and is required for the dimerization of the CD94/NKG2 family of receptors, which are expressed on NK cells and T-cell subsets. The CD94 and NKG2 genes are located in the center of the NK-gene complex between the NKRP1 and PRB3 loci in the region containing the STS markers D12S77 and D12S1093. All six genes are closely linked and are situated 100 to 200 kb proximal to the D12S77 STS marker (Sobanov et al., 1999). The CD94 gene is placed in the opposite orientation relative to the NKG2 gene family members (which all have the same transcriptional orientation). CD94 gene expression is regulated by distal and proximal promoters that transcribe unique initial exons specific for each promoter. Both promoters contain elements with IFN-γ-activated and E26 transformation-specific (ETS)-binding sites (called GAS and EBS respectively). The two promoters differentially regulate expression of the CD94 gene in response to treatment with IL-2 or IL-15 (Lieto et al., 2003).

3.2 Ligands of NKG2D-MIC

The two types of NKG2D ligands are MHC class I chain-related proteins (MICA and MICB) and UL16-binding proteins (ULBP) (Sutherland et al., 2001; Bauer et al., 1999). MICA and MICB are located in the MHC complex within the 6q21.3 chromosomal region. The ULBP family contains 10 genes, of which five are expressed (ULBP1–5). ULBPs are located outside the MHC gene complex, in the 6q24.2–25.3 region (Samarakoon et al., 2009). These molecules exhibit highly restricted expression in healthy tissues but are widely expressed on epithelial tumors. In hematological malignancies they are upregulated in nontumor and tumor cells by genotoxic stress (Kim et al., 2006; Venkataraman et al., 2007). Aligned cosmid-derived regions 1.5 kb upstream of the translation start codon (ATG) in MICA and MICB share approximately 90% sequence identity. The 5'-end flanking regions of MICA and

MICB contain putative heat shock elements (HSE) that are prototypic transcription inducer sites in heat shock protein-70 (HSP70) genes and that bind activated trimeric heat shock factor protein-1 (HSF1). Cytomegalovirus (CMV) infection results in up to a 10-fold increase in cell surface MIC expression and is associated with induced HSP70 expression. TATA-like elements and Sp1 consensus sites, as with HSE, are located unusually far "upstream" from MIC gene, but can also moderately or profoundly affect stress-induced and proliferation-associated induction. The common integrating conjugative element (ICE), however, appears to be a negative regulator of MICB, but not of MICA. It is an important to note, although the sequences of MICA and MICB promoters are very similar, the baseline transcriptional activity of MICA is higher than that of MICB and they have different regulatory mechanisms for expression. Most MICA transcripts start downstream of the conserved AP-1 TATA-like motif, a region that lacks a recognizable RNA start site. In contrast, most MICB transcripts initiate further upstream, proximal to the HSE–Sp1–ICE elements (Venkataraman et al., 2007). Nuclear factor kappa-light-chain-enhancer of activated B cells (NF-κB) regulates MICA expression on activated T lymphocytes and on HeLa tumor cells by binding to a specific sequence in the long intron 1 region of the MICA gene (Molinero et al., 2004). Histone deacetylase inhibitor (HDAC-I) and sodium valproate (VPA) induced transcription of MICA and MICB in hepatocellular carcinoma cells, leading to increased cell surface, soluble and total MIC protein expression (Armeanu et al., 2005). Similar results have been obtained using histone deacetylase inhibitors FR901228 and SAHA (Skov et al., 2005). In our laboratory, we found that VPA can increase the expression of HSP70 and Sp1 and increase the binding of transcription factors Sp1 and HSF1 to the MICA/B promoter. This activation leads to the upregulation of MICA/B in HeLa and HepG2 tumor cells (Zhang et al., 2009).

3.3 Ligands of NKG2D-ULBPs

All expressed ULBPs (ULBP1–5) have good conservation of the coding sequence, but the 5'-end flanking regions of these genes have little homology. This situation suggests that ULBPs are regulated specifically in response to different stimuli or pathogens (Lopez-Soto et al., 2006). Mechanisms that regulate the expression of ULBP1 have been described previously. In the core region of the ULBP1 promoter, there are many binding sites for transcription factors, including a canonical TATA box, three GC boxes, one overlapping sequence GC(4)/AP-2, two cytokinin response element (CRE)-like sequences (CRE1 and CRE2) (Zeng et al., 1997; Wajapeyee and Somasundaram, 2003), and one NF-κB site. Transcription of ULBP1 depends strictly on binding of Sp1 and Sp3 to a CRE1 site located in the ULBP1 minimal promoter. The mutation or deletion of this Sp1/Sp3 binding site abolished ULBP1 transcription; Sp3 is the main transcription factor that regulates ULBP1 through the CRE1 site. AP-2α, however, repressed the expression of ULBP1 by binding to the GC(4)/AP-2α site and interfering with the binding of Sp3 and Sp1 to the ULBP1 promoter (Lopez-Soto et al., 2006). It has been shown that heat shock and ionizing radiation treatment can induce the expression of ULBP1/2/3 in human cancer cell lines; HSP 70 is induced by heat shock but not by ionizing radiation (Kim et al., 2006). Human cytomegalovirus (HCMV) can also induce the expression of ULBP1/2/3 proteins that are predominantly localized in the endoplasmic reticulum of infected fibroblasts together with UL16 (Rolle et al., 2003). There is interplay, however, between virus and host cells depending on the viral dose. At low viral dose, ULBP1 or ULBP2 surface expression is completely inhibited compared with ULBP3, while at a higher viral doses cell surface expression of ULBP1 and ULBP2 is delayed (Rolle et al., 2003). Whether this phenomenon is mediated through the ULBP promoter or through transcription factors needs to be investigated further.

Epigenetic modulations are also likely to play a large part in the observed alteration in ULBP expression. Current observations imply that loss of DNA methylation (deficient in DNA methyltransferase cells) is correlated with increased ULBP2 mRNA levels. It has been shown that both demethylation of the ULPB2 promoter, necessary for increased protein levels, and the RAS/MEK signaling pathway, shown to control DNA methylation (Lund et al., 2006), are necessary for maximal protein expression (Sers et al., 2009). In addition, the HDAC inhibitor trichostatin A (TSA) is reported to upregulate ULBP1–3 expression in tumor cells; Sp3 was found to be crucial for activation of the ULBP1 promoter by TSA. One report showed that HDAC3 is recruited to the ULBP1 promoter and acts as a repressor of ULBP expression in epithelial cancer cells. TSA treatment interfered with this interaction and caused the complete release of HDAC3 from the ULBP1–3 promoters (Lopez-Soto et al., 2009).

3.4 KIR receptor family and their ligands

The KIR family is of particular interest because individual members bind to specific subgroups of HLA allele products, such as HLA-A, HLA-B, HLA-C, and HLA-G, although most KIRs show 90–95% amino acid identity. The high level of homology can facilitate exchange of exons between different KIR loci, by some form of crossing over or gene conversion (Wilson et al., 2000). One study found that due to the polymorphism of KIR genes, two KIR haplotypes segregated at roughly equal frequency in a largely Caucasian population. Group A haplotypes contained seven KIR genes and had KIR2DS4 as the only activating receptor. Group B haplotypes had a greater diversity of KIR genes, had more activating receptors, and were characterized by the KIR2DL2, KIR2DS1, KIR2DS2, KIR2DS3, and KIR2DS5 genes (Uhrberg et al., 1997). KIR can also be further subdivided into inhibitory receptors that carry an inhibitory signal motif within their cytoplasmic domain (KIR2DL and KIR3DL) and into stimulatory receptors (KIR2DS and KIR3DS) that lack this motif. Most of the inhibitory KIRs are specific for the products of HLA class I genes like such as HLA-A/-B and HLA-C (Bellon et al., 1999; Colonna et al., 1993; Dohring et al., 1996). The ligand specificities of many stimulatory KIR are uncertain and might include non-HLA class I ligands. KIR2DL4, however, combines structural and functional features of both stimulatory and inhibitory KIR and is reported to bind to the nonclassical class I protein HLA-G (Chan et al., 2003; Martin et al., 2000; Trompeter et al., 2005; Santourlidis et al., 2002). The expression of KIR appears to be largely independent of each other and the impact of the requirement for inhibition by self class I molecules on the shape of the KIR repertoire is rather subtle.

3.4.1 Transcriptional factors regulation of KIR

Different groups of 2–9 KIR genes are expressed in NK clones, but the sequences of the KIR promoters are homogeneous in their 5'-untranslated regions (5' UTR), except for that of KIR2DL4 (Valiante et al., 1997; Wilson et al., 2000). The sequences of KIR genes comprise a continuous loop that extends seamlessly from gene to gene. The repeat of the loop is broken only by a region 14 kb upstream of the KIR2DL4 locus, which displays some unique features and is characterized by L1 repeats. The sequence upstream of KIR2DL4 may be significant because this gene is unique in this group in being expressed in 100% of NK clones (Valiante et al., 1997; Wilson et al., 2000; Martin et al., 2000). Moreover, KIR2DL4 is the only KIR gene that lacks the repeat region in intron 1. All KIR genes lack typical promoter features such as TATA and CAAT boxes, so many transcription factor binding sites have been predicted to be present in the upstream regions of KIR, including sites for transcription factors CREB, SP1, ETS, AP-1 and AP-4 (Chan et al., 2003; Santourlidis et al., 2002). None of these elements alone, however, is required for or significantly increases promoter activity, except for a CREB site located outside the core promoter region. To date, the basic KIR promoter appears to either require undefined transcription factors or alternatively only interacts with the basic transcription machinery of RNA polymerase II (Trompeter et al., 2005). It has been suggested previously that a binding site for the transcription factor AML/Runx (Runt Homology Domain Transcription Factors) at –100 bp can be essential for KIR expression (Vilches et al., 2000). However, a further study suggested that AML has a general inhibitory influence on KIR expression in mature NK cells and that AML exerts its repressor function by binding directly to the promoter of the different KIR genes (Trompeter et al., 2005). Recently, it was reported that the transcription factor c-Myc upregulated KIR gene transcription through direct binding to an upstream distal promoter element in peripheral blood NK cells, and that IL-15 promoted this effect (Cichocki et al., 2009). It was suggested that the role of the traditional transcription factors in KIR gene expression is different from that in other genes.

3.4.2 Histone modifications of KIR

It was found that histone H3 and H4 proteins are substantially acetylated at the Lys9 and Lys14 positions and H4 acetylation at the 5th, 8th, 12th, and 16th positions in both KIR3DL1+ and KIR3DL1– NK cells (Chan et al., 2005). The level of KIR3DL1-associated histone acetylation and methylation was higher in KIR3DL1+ NK cells than in KIR3DL1– NK cells; however, histone H3 methylation at Lys4 (H3K4) is only 2.6-fold higher in KIR3DL1+ NK cells than that in KIR3DL1– NK cells, although the histone H3K4 methylation levels correlated well with the KIR3DL1 promoter to lead to upregulation of KIR3DL1 gene expression, named KIR3DL1-associated histone H3K4 methylation. These findings indicate that histone acetylation and trimethylated modifications, but not histone H3 methylation, are preferentially associated with the transcribed allele in NK cells with monoallelic KIR expression (Santourlidis et al., 2002; Chan et al., 2005).

KIR expression is increased on T cells with increasing age, and can contribute to age-related diseases (van Bergen et al., 2004). In these cells, the KIR2DL4 promoter is partially demethylated, and dimethylated H3L4 is increased; all other histone modifications are characteristic of an inactive promoter. In comparison, NK cells have a fully demethylated KIR2DL4 promoter and have the full spectrum of histone modifications indicative of active transcription with H3 and H4 acetylation. These findings suggest that an increased T-cell ability to express KIR2DL4 with age is conferred by a selective increase in H3L4 dimethylation and limited DNA demethylation (van Bergen et al., 2004; Li et al., 2008).

3.4.3 DNA demethylation of KIR

Methylation status of CpG islands in NK cells correlates with transcriptional activity of KIR genes. The overall structure of the CpG islands is similar in all expressed KIR, with complete conservation of four CpG dinucleotides upstream of the transcriptional start site, with the exception of KIR2DL4, which shows a highly divergent profile with lower CpG density. In addition, CpG islands with <70% of methylated CpGs are exclusively found in the expressed KIR2DL3, whereas CpG islands of nonexpressed KIR2DL3 and KIR3DL2 are consistently methylated at 70–100% of CpG dinucleotides (Santourlidis et al., 2002). Analysis of the methylation status at individual CpG sites demonstrated that differential methylation of expressed versus nonexpressed KIR is not restricted to specific CpGs, but is consistently found throughout the CpG islands. That is to say, the methylated CpG islands are associated with transcriptionally silent KIR and unmethylated CpG islands with expressed KIR genes (Chan et al., 2003; Santourlidis et al., 2002).

In addition, exposure to a DNA methyltransferase inhibitor, 5-aza-2'-deoxycytidine (5azaC), effectively induced the whole range of KIR expression in NK cells (Gao et al., 2009; Chan et al., 2003; Santourlidis et al., 2002; Chan et al., 2005), but not in other cells of lymphoid or nonlymphoid origin. A weak induction of KIR3DL2 following treatment with 5aza-dC was observed in a T-cell line (Li et al., 2008; Santourlidis et al., 2008). These results suggested that repression of KIR gene transcription is dependent on DNA methylation only in NK cells and T cells, and that allele-specific KIR3DL1 gene expression is not only correlated with promoter but also with 5'-gene DNA hypomethylation. Further studies showed that methylation influenced KIR expression both in immature NK cells and in mature NK cells, because KIR promoter-associated CpG islands are indeed DNA-methylated at an early developmental stage (Li et al., 2008; Liu et al., 2009).

3.4.4 A two-step model of epigenetic regulation of KIR

Recent studies suggested that CpG methylation is functionally linked to histone deacetylation, which, in turn, leads to the formation of condensed, transcriptionally repressive chromatin (Bird, 2002; Bird and Wolffe, 1999). Altering the state of histone acetylation using the deacetylase inhibitor TSA did not change transcriptional activity of either expressed or silent KIR genes. Additionally, combined treatment of 5aza-dC and TSA did not lead to a synergistic effect compared with 5aza-dC alone. In particularly, the expression of KIR2DL4, which is expressed by all human NK clones, was not affected by either demethylating or histone-acetylating treatment. This finding indicated that KIR genes in NK cells might have already acquired a state of transcriptionally competent chromatin. Methylation of KIR CpG islands appears to be the priority epigenetic modification required for silencing of specific KIR genes (Santourlidis et al., 2002). In a further study, this point was addressed. Hematopoietic progenitor cell KIR genes exhibited the major hallmarks of epigenetic repression: dense DNA methylation; inaccessibility of chromatin; and a repressive histone signature, characterized by strong H3K9 dimethylation and reduced H4K8 acetylation. In contrast, KIR genes in NK cells showed active histone signatures characterized by absence of H3K9 dimethylation and presence of H4K8 acetylation. In KIR-competent lineages, active histone signatures were also observed in silenced KIR genes and, in this study, were found in combination with dense DNA methylation of the promoter and nearby regions. The study suggested a two-step model of epigenetic regulation in which lineage-specific acquisition of euchromatic histone is a prerequisite for subsequent gene-specific DNA demethylation and expression of KIR genes (Santourlidis et al., 2008).

3.4.5 HLA-ligand of KIR

Recently, epigenetic alterations were shown to play a role in HLA changes associated with malignant transformation of cells (Campoli and Ferrone, 2008). HLA-G, initially discovered on the fetal–maternal interface, plays a key role in the maintenance of immune tolerance by inhibition of NK cells via the receptor KIR2DL4 (Hofmeister and Weiss, 2003); it is expressed in some surgically removed melanoma lesions, but there is little expression in established cell lines. Treatment of a HLA-G-negative melanoma cell line with 5azaC restored HLA-G expression; similarly 5azaC activated HLA-G expression in human leukemia cell lines, even in malignant hematopoietic cells isolated from patients with acute myeloid leukemia (AML) and chronic lymphocytic leukemia (B-CLL) (Polakova et al., 2009a; Polakova et al., 2009b). Further research found that HLA-G was silenced as a result of CpG hypermethylation within a 5' regulatory region upstream of the start codon (Moreau et al., 2003; Yan et al., 2005). These results determined that regulation of HLA-G expression also involved epigenetic mechanisms, such as DNA methylation. There was no significant difference in HLA-G expression, however, detected in tumor and normal ovarian surface epithelial cells (OSE) samples, although HLA-G expression was significantly increased after treatment with 5azaC. There was no correlation between methylation and HLA-G gene expression in ovarian tumor samples and OSE, which suggested that changes in methylation may be necessary, but not sufficient, for HLA-G expression in ovarian cancer (Menendez et al., 2008).

In addition, the expression of HLA-A, HLA-B and HLA-C, specific ligands for inhibitory KIR (KIR3DL2, KIR3DL1, and KIR2DL1/3) was lost or downregulated in human gastric cancer, where the percentage of promoter methylation was higher than in adjacent nontumor tissues (Ye et al., 2010). In esophageal squamous cell carcinoma lesions, it was also shown that hypermethylation in the gene promoter regions of the HLA-A, HLA-B and HLA-C, and altered chromatin structure of the HLA class I heavy chain gene promoters have both been implicated as a major mechanism for transcriptional inactivation of HLA genes (Nie et al., 2001). Furthermore, the MAPK (mitogen-activated protein kinases) and DNA methyltransferases were shown to downregulate HLA-A expression (Sers et al., 2009). These findings suggest an association between promoter hypermethylation and the downregulated expression of HLA class I molecules.

4. Regulation expression of NK cell receptors and their ligands as potential therapeutics for cancer

The mechanisms of regulation the gene expression, which requires signalling cascades for transducing and integrating regulatory cues to determine which genes are expressed, are obligatory for tumorigenesis, tumor progression and metastasis (Bhalla, 2005; Samarakoon et al., 2009; Stein et al., 2010). Transcriptional gene regulations, particularly in transcriptional factors and epigenetic level, affect several aspects of tumor cell biology, including cell growth, proliferation, phenotype, differentiation, DNA repair, and cell death. NK cells are the major effector lymphocytes of innate immune system that defend against many forms of viral infections and tumor growth without prior sensitizations, by the interaction of inhibitory and activating receptors with corresponding ligands on the target cells. This raises the strong possibility that regulation expression of NK cell receptors on NK cells and their ligands on tumor cells may be an effective treatment strategy for malignant tumors. This treatment strategy, as mentioned above, including activation and suppression of the transcription factors and promoter activity, modification the DNA methylation in the underlying DNA code, and rearrangement the acetylation and methylation of protein in histone posttranslational level, leads to the induced or suppressed expression of NK cells receptors and their ligands (Fig. 1), so that the NK cell-mediated immunotherapy can be carried out fully to cure malignancies. So the regulation expression of NK cell receptors and their ligands provides a strategy for targeting gene expression in tumor cells, and may be with minimal offtarget consequences (Villar-Garea and Esteller, 2004; Bhalla, 2005; Szyf, 2005, Stein et al., 2010).

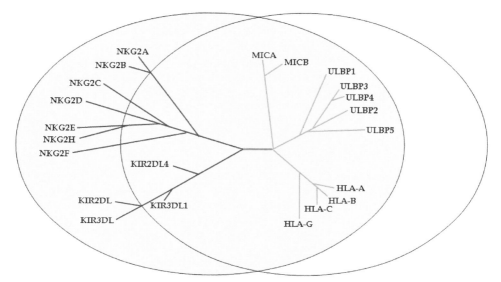

Fig. 1. Transcription regulation and epigenetic control of KIR and NKG2 receptors and their ligands. A dendrogram representing the relatedness of different KIR and NKG2 receptors (blue) and their ligands (green) to each other, and the extent of the sequence relatedness between two genes is shown by the distance of the lines (Raulet, 2003). The left oval shows the gene regulation in transcription factor level, while the right oval shows the gene regulation in epigenetic level, and the overlapping part shows the co-regulation.

5. Concluding remarks

NK cells not only are important players of innate effecter responses, but also participate in the initiation and development of antigen-specific responses through secretion of immunoregulatory cytokines (such as IFN-γ, tumor necrosis factor-α (TNF-α) and granulocyte–macrophage colony-stimulating factor (GM–CSF)) and through cell-to-cell contact (Biron et al., 1999). Regulation of the expression of NK-cell receptors and their ligands refers to the control of the amount, the timing of appearance, and the functional products of these genes, leading to the flexibility of NK cells or other immune cells to adapt to a variable environment, external signals, and damages to target cells (Wu et al., 2005). In particular, the modification of NK-cell receptors and their ligands is a potential therapeutic implication for cancer treatment. Although the regulation mechanism of expression of NK-cell receptors and related ligands has acquired important progress at the transcription level, the regulatory mechanisms of a number of crucial receptors and ligands, for example signaling lymphocytic activating molecule (SLAM)-related receptors (CD150, 2B4, Ly-9,

CD84, and NTB-A) (Sidorenko and Clark, 2003; Engel et al., 2003; Morra et al., 2001), are not well understood. More research is needed into other regulated stages of gene expression, such as posttranscriptional modification, RNA transport, translation, and mRNA degradation. Investigation of the regulatory mechanisms of NK-cell receptors and their ligands might aid in the design of therapy against cancer, infection, inflammation, or autoimmune diseases.

6. Acknowledgment

This work was supported by grants from the Natural Science Foundation of China (No. 90713033), the National 973 Basic Science Program of China (No. 2007CB815800) and the Important National Science & Technology Specific Projects of China (No. 2008ZX10002-008).

7. References

Armeanu, S., Bitzer, M., Lauer, U. M., Venturelli, S., Pathil, A., Krusch, M., Kaiser, S., Jobst, J., Smirnow, I., Wagner, A., Steinle, A. & Salih, H. R. (2005). Natural killer cell-mediated lysis of hepatoma cells via specific induction of NKG2D ligands by the histone deacetylase inhibitor sodium valproate. *Cancer Res*, Vol.65, No.14, pp. 6321-6329, ISSN 1538-7445

Alexander, R. & Beggs, J. D. (2010). Cross-talk in transcription, splicing and chromatin: who makes the first call? *Biochem Soc Trans*, Vol.38, No.5, pp. 1251-1256, ISSN 0300-5127

Bauer, S., Groh, V., Wu, J., Steinle, A., Phillips, J. H., Lanier, L. L. & Spies, T. (1999). Activation of NK cells and T cells by NKG2D, a receptor for stress-inducible MICA. *Science*, Vol. 285, No.5428, pp. 727-729, ISSN 1095-9203

Bellon, T., Heredia, A. B., Llano, M., Minguela, A., Rodriguez, A., Lopez-Botet, M. & Aparicio, P. (1999). Triggering of effector functions on a CD8+ T cell clone upon the aggregation of an activatory CD94/kp39 heterodimer. *J Immunol*, Vol.162, No.7, pp. 3996-4002, ISSN 0732-0582

Bertone, S., Schiavetti, F., Bellomo, R., Vitale, C., Ponte, M., Moretta, L. & Mingari, M. C. (1999). Transforming growth factor-beta-induced expression of CD94/NKG2A inhibitory receptors in human T lymphocytes. *Eur J Immunol*, Vol.29, No.1, pp. 23-29, ISSN 0014-2980

Bird, A. P. & Wolffe, A. P. (1999). Methylation-induced repression--belts, braces, and chromatin. *Cell* , Vol.99, No.5, pp. 451-454, ISSN 0092-8674

Biron, C. A., Nguyen, K. B., Pien, G. C., Cousens, L. P. & Salazar-Mather, T. P. (1999). Natural killer cells in antiviral defense: function and regulation by innate cytokines. *Annu Rev Immunol*, Vol.17, pp. 189-220, ISSN 0732-0582

Brostjan, C., Sobanov, Y., Glienke, J., Hayer, S., Lehrach, H., Francis, F. & Hofer, E. (2000). The NKG2 natural killer cell receptor family: comparative analysis of promoter sequences. *Genes Immun*, Vol.6, No.8, pp. 504-508, ISSN 1466-4879

Brivanlou, A. H. & Darnell, J. E., Jr. (2002). Signal transduction and the control of gene expression. *Science*, Vol.295, No.5556, pp. 813-818, ISSN 0036-8075

Bird, A. (2002). DNA methylation patterns and epigenetic memory. *Genes Dev*, Vol.16, No.1, pp. 6-21, ISSN 1549-5477

Bhalla, K. N. (2005). Epigenetic and chromatin modifiers as targeted therapy of hematologic malignancies. *J Clin Oncol*, Vol.23, No.17, pp. 3971-3993, ISSN 0732-183X

Beckett, D. (2009). Regulating transcription regulators via allostery and flexibility. Proc Natl Acad Sci U S A , Vol.106, No.52, pp. 22035-22036, ISSN 0027-8424 Campoli, M., Ferrone, S., Zea, A. H., Rodriguez, P. C. & Ochoa, A. C. (2005). Mechanisms of tumor evasion. *Cancer Treat Res*, Vol.123, pp. 61-88, ISSN 0927-3042

Colonna, M., Borsellino, G., Falco, M., Ferrara, G. B. & Strominger, J. L. (1993). HLA-C is the inhibitory ligand that determines dominant resistance to lysis by NK1- and NK2-specific natural killer cells. *Proc Natl Acad Sci U S A* , Vol.90, No.24, pp. 12000-12004, ISSN 0027-8424

Chan, H. W., Kurago, Z. B., Stewart, C. A., Wilson, M. J., Martin, M. P., Mace, B. E., Carrington, M., Trowsdale, J. & Lutz, C. T. (2003). DNA methylation maintains allele-specific KIR gene expression in human natural killer cells. *J Exp Med*, Vol.197, No.2, pp. 245-255, ISSN 0022-1007

Chan, H. W., Miller, J. S., Moore, M. B. & Lutz, C. T. (2005). Epigenetic control of highly homologous killer Ig-like receptor gene alleles. *J Immunol*, Vol.175, No.9, pp. 5966-5974, ISSN 0022-1767

Chang, C. C. & Ferrone, S. (2006). NK cell activating ligands on human malignant cells: molecular and functional defects and potential clinical relevance. *Semin Cancer Biol*, Vol.16, No.3, pp. 359-393, ISSN 1044-579X

Campoli, M. & Ferrone, S. (2008). HLA antigen changes in malignant cells: epigenetic mechanisms and biologic significance. *Oncogene,* Vol.27, No.45, pp. 5869-5885, ISSN 0950-9232

Cichocki, F., Hanson, R. J., Lenvik, T., Pitt, M., McCullar, V., Li, H., Anderson, S. K. & Miller, J. S. (2009). The transcription factor c-Myc enhances KIR gene transcription through direct binding to an upstream distal promoter element. *Blood*, Vol.113, No.14, pp. 3245-3253, ISSN 0006-4971

Dohring, C., Scheidegger, D., Samaridis, J., Cella, M. & Colonna, M. (1996). A human killer inhibitory receptor specific for HLA-A1,2. *J Immunol*, Vol.156, No.9, pp. 3098-3101, ISSN 0022-1767

Derre, L., Corvaisier, M., Pandolfino, M. C., Diez, E., Jotereau, F. & Gervois, N. (2002). Expression of CD94/NKG2-A on human T lymphocytes is induced by IL-12: implications for adoptive immunotherapy. *J Immunol*, Vol.168, No.10, pp. 4864-4870, ISSN 0022-1767

Dunn, G. P., Bruce, A. T., Ikeda, H., Old, L. J. & Schreiber, R. D. (2002). Cancer immunoediting: from immunosurveillance to tumor escape. *Nat Immunol*, Vol.3, No.11, pp. 991-998, ISSN 1529-2908

Dasgupta, S., Bhattacharya-Chatterjee, M., O'Malley, B. W., Jr. & Chatterjee, S. K. (2005). Inhibition of NK cell activity through TGF-beta 1 by down-regulation of NKG2D in a murine model of head and neck cancer. *J Immunol*, Vol.175, No.8, pp. 5541-5550, ISSN 0022-1767

Dowell, R. D. (2010). Transcription factor binding variation in the evolution of gene regulation. *Trends Genet*, Vol.26, No.11, pp. 468-475, ISSN 0168-9525

Engel, P., Eck, M. J. & Terhorst, C. (2003). The SAP and SLAM families in immune responses and X-linked lymphoproliferative disease. *Nat Rev Immunol*, Vol.3, No.10, pp. 813-821, ISSN 0732-0582

Fry, C. J. & Peterson, C. L. (2002). Transcription. Unlocking the gates to gene expression. *Science*, Vol.295, No.5561, pp. 1847-1848, ISSN 0036-8075

Feng, S., Jacobsen, S. E. & Reik, W. (2010). Epigenetic reprogramming in plant and animal development.*Science*, Vol. 330, No. 6004, pp. 622-627, ISSN 0036-8075

Fernandez-Morera, J. L., Calvanese, V., Rodriguez-Rodero, S., Menendez-Torre, E. & Fraga, M. F. (2010). Epigenetic regulation of the immune system in health and disease. *Tissue Antigens*, Vol.76, No.6, pp. 431-439, ISSN 0001-2815

Furumatsu, T. & Ozaki, T. (2010). Epigenetic regulation in chondrogenesis. *Acta Med Okayama*, Vol. 64, No.3, pp. 155-161, ISSN 0386-300X

Glienke, J., Sobanov, Y., Brostjan, C., Steffens, C., Nguyen, C., Lehrach, H., Hofer, E. & Francis, F. (1998). The genomic organization of NKG2C, E, F, and D receptor genes in the human natural killer gene complex. *Immunogenetics*, Vol.48, No.3, pp. 163-173, ISSN 0093-7711

Gao, X. N., Lin, J., Wang, L. L. & Yu, L. (2009). Demethylating treatment suppresses natural killer cell cytolytic activity. *Mol Immunol*, Vol.46, No.10, pp. 2064-2070, ISSN 1672-7681

Hofmeister, V. & Weiss, E. H. (2003). HLA-G modulates immune responses by diverse receptor interactions. Semin Cancer Biol , Vol.13, No.5, pp. 317-323, ISSN 1044-579X

Karin, M. (1990). Too many transcription factors: positive and negative interactions. *New Biol*, Vol.2, No.2, pp. 126-131, ISSN 0090-0028

Kim, J. Y., Son, Y. O., Park, S. W., Bae, J. H., Chung, J. S., Kim, H. H., Chung, B. S., Kim, S. H. & Kang, C. D. (2006). Increase of NKG2D ligands and sensitivity to NK cell-mediated cytotoxicity of tumor cells by heat shock and ionizing radiation. *Exp Mol Med*, Vol.38, No.5, pp. 474-484, ISSN 1226-3613

Kisliouk, T., Ziv, M. & Meiri, N. (2010). Epigenetic control of translation regulation: alterations in histone H3 lysine 9 post-translation modifications are correlated with the expression of the translation initiation factor 2B (Eif2b5) during thermal control establishment. *Dev Neurobiol*, Vol.70, No.2, pp. 100-113, ISSN 1064-0517

Krukowski, K., Eddy, J., Kosik, K. L., Konley, T., Janusek, L. W. & Mathews, H. L. (2011). Glucocorticoid dysregulation of natural killer cell function through epigenetic modification. *Brain Behav Immun*, Vol.25, No.2, pp. 239-249, ISSN 0889-1591

Lanier, L. L. (1998). NK cell receptors. Annu Rev Immunol, Vol.16, No.3, pp. 359-393, ISSN 0732-0582

Lanier, L. L. (2001). On guard--activating NK cell receptors. *Nat Immunol*, Vol.2, No.1, pp. 23-27, ISSN 1529-2908

Lieto, L. D., Borrego, F., You, C. H. & Coligan, J. E. (2003). Human CD94 gene expression: dual promoters differing in responsiveness to IL-2 or IL-15. *J Immunol*, Vol.171, No.3, pp. 5277-5286, ISSN 0022-1767

Lanier, L. L. (2005). "NK cell recognition. *Annu Rev Immunol*, Vol.23, pp. 225-274, ISSN 0732-0582

Lopez-Soto, A., Quinones-Lombrana, A., Lopez-Arbesu, R., Lopez-Larrea, C. & Gonzalez, S. (2006). Transcriptional regulation of ULBP1, a human ligand of the NKG2D receptor.*J Biol Chem*, Vol.281, No.41, pp. 30419-30430, ISSN 0021-9258

Lund, P., Weisshaupt, K., Mikeska, T., Jammas, D., Chen, X., Kuban, R. J., Ungethum, U., Krapfenbauer, U., Herzel, H. P., Schafer, R., Walter, J. & Sers, C. (2006). Oncogenic HRAS suppresses clusterin expression through promoter hypermethylation. *Oncogene*, Vol.25, No.35, pp.4890-4903, ISSN 0950-9232

Li, G., Weyand, C. M. & Goronzy, J. J. (2008). Epigenetic mechanisms of age-dependent KIR2DL4 expression in T cells. *J Leukoc Biol*, Vol.84, No.3, pp. 824-834, ISSN 0741-5400

Liu, Y., Kuick, R., Hanash, S. & Richardson, B. (2009). DNA methylation inhibition increases T cell KIR expression through effects on both promoter methylation and transcription factors. *Clin Immunol*, Vol.130, No.2, pp. 213-224, ISSN 1521-6616

Lopez-Soto, A., Folgueras, A. R., Seto, E. & Gonzalez, S. (2009). HDAC3 represses the expression of NKG2D ligands ULBPs in epithelial tumour cells: potential implications for the immunosurveillance of cancer. *Oncogene*, Vol. 28, No.25, pp. 2370-2382, ISSN 0950-9232

Law, J. A. & Jacobsen, S. E. (2010). Establishing, maintaining and modifying DNA methylation patterns in plants and animals. *Nat Rev Genet*, Vol.11, No.3, pp. 204-220, ISSN 1471-0056

Mitchell, P. J. & Tjian, R. (1989). Transcriptional regulation in mammalian cells by sequence-specific DNA binding proteins.*Science*, Vol.245, No.4916, pp. 371-378, ISSN 0036-8075

Mingari, M. C., Ponte, M., Bertone, S., Schiavetti, F., Vitale, C., Bellomo, R., Moretta, A. & Moretta, L. (1998). HLA class I-specific inhibitory receptors in human T lymphocytes: interleukin 15-induced expression of CD94/NKG2A in superantigen- or alloantigen-activated CD8+ T cells. *Proc Natl Acad Sci U S A*, Vol.95, No.3, pp. 1172-1177, ISSN 0027-8424

Martin, A. M., Freitas, E. M., Witt, C. S. & Christiansen, F. T. (2000). The genomic organization and evolution of the natural killer immunoglobulin-like receptor (KIR) gene cluster. *Immunogenetics*, Vol.51, No. 4-5, pp. 268-280, ISSN 0093-7711

Morra, M., Howie, D., Grande, M. S., Sayos, J., Wang, N., Wu, C., Engel, P. & Terhorst, C. (2001). X-linked lymphoproliferative disease: a progressive immunodeficiency. *Annu Rev Immunol*, Vol.119, pp. 657-682, ISSN 0732-0582

McQueen, K. L. & Parham, P. (2002). Variable receptors controlling activation and inhibition of NK cells. *Curr Opin Immunol*, Vol.14, No.5, pp. 615-621, ISSN 0952-7915

Moreau, P., Mouillot, G., Rousseau, P., Marcou, C., Dausset, J. & Carosella, E. D. (2003). HLA-G gene repression is reversed by demethylation. *Proc Natl Acad Sci U S A*, Vol.100, No.3, pp. 1191-1196, ISSN 0027-8424

Molinero, L. L., Fuertes, M. B., Girart, M. V., Fainboim, L., Rabinovich, G. A., Costas, M. A. & Zwirner, N. W. (2004). NF-kappa B regulates expression of the MHC class I-related chain A gene in activated T lymphocytes. *J Immunol*, Vol.173, No.9, pp. 5583-5590, ISSN0022-1767

Moretta, L., Bottino, C., Pende, D., Castriconi, R., Mingari, M. C. & Moretta, A. (2006). Surface NK receptors and their ligands on tumor cells. *Semin Immunol*, Vol.18, No.3, pp. 151-158, ISSN 1044-5323

Menendez, L., Walker, L. D., Matyunina, L. V., Totten, K. A., Benigno, B. B. & McDonald, J. F. (2008). Epigenetic changes within the promoter region of the HLA-G gene in ovarian tumors. *Mol Cancer*, Vol.7, pp. 43, ISSN 1476-4598

Nie, Y., Yang, G., Song, Y., Zhao, X., So, C., Liao, J., Wang, L. D. & Yang, C. S. (2001). DNA hypermethylation is a mechanism for loss of expression of the HLA class I genes in human esophageal squamous cell carcinomas. *Carcinogenesis*, Vol.22, No.10, pp. 1615-1623, ISSN 0143-3334

Polakova, K., Bandzuchova, E., Sabty, F. A., Mistrik, M., Demitrovicova, L. & Russ, G. (2009a). Activation of HLA-G expression by 5-aza-2 - deoxycytidine in malignant hematopoetic cells isolated from leukemia patients. *Neoplasma*, Vol.56, No.6, pp. 514-520, ISSN 0028- 2685

Polakova, K., Bandzuchova, E., Kuba, D. & Russ, G. (2009b). Demethylating agent 5-aza-2'-deoxycytidine activates HLA-G expression in human leukemia cell lines. *Leuk Res*, Vol.33, No.4, pp. 518-524, ISSN 0145-2126

Pan, Y., Tsai, C. J., Ma, B. & Nussinov, R. (2010). Mechanisms of transcription factor selectivity.*Trends Genet*, Vol.26, No.2, pp. 75-83, ISSN 0168-9525

Raulet, D. H., Vance, R. E. & McMahon, C. W. (2001). Regulation of the natural killer cell receptor repertoire. *Annu Rev Immunol*, Vol.19, pp.291-330, ISSN 0732-0582

Romero, P., Ortega, C., Palma, A., Molina, I. J., Pena, J. & Santamaria, M. (2001). Expression of CD94 and NKG2 molecules on human CD4(+) T cells in response to CD3-mediated stimulation. *J Leukoc Biol*, Vol.70, No.2, pp. 219-224, ISSN 0741-5400

Ravetch, J. V. & Lanier, L. L. (2000). Immune inhibitory receptors. *Science*, Vol.290, No.5489, pp. 84-89, ISSN 0036-8075

Raulet, D. H. (2003). Roles of the NKG2D immunoreceptor and its ligands. *Annu Rev Immunol*, Vol.3, No.10, pp.781-790, ISSN 0732-0582

Rolle, A., Mousavi-Jazi, M., Eriksson, M., Odeberg, J., Soderberg-Naucler, C., Cosman, D., Karre, K. & Cerboni, C. (2003). Effects of human cytomegalovirus infection on ligands for the activating NKG2D receptor of NK cells: up-regulation of UL16-binding protein (ULBP)1 and ULBP2 is counteracted by the viral UL16 protein. *J Immunol*, Vol.171, No.2, pp. 902-908, ISSN 0022-1767

Sobanov, Y., Glienke, J., Brostjan, C., Lehrach, H., Francis, F. & Hofer, E. (1999). Linkage of the NKG2 and CD94 receptor genes to D12S77 in the human natural killer gene complex. *Immunogenetics*, Vol.49, No.2, pp. 99-105, ISSN 1744-313X

Strahl, B. D. & Allis, C. D. (2000). The language of covalent histone modifications. *Nature*, Vol. 403, No. 6765, pp. 41-45, ISSN 0028-0836

Sutherland, C. L., Chalupny, N. J. & Cosman, D. (2001). The UL16-binding proteins, a novel family of MHC class I-related ligands for NKG2D, activate natural killer cell functions. *Immunol Rev*, Vol.181, No.3, pp. 185-192, ISSN 0105-2896

Santourlidis, S., Trompeter, H. I., Weinhold, S., Eisermann, B., Meyer, K. L., Wernet, P. & Uhrberg, M. (2002). Crucial role of DNA methylation in determination of clonally distributed killer cell Ig-like receptor expression patterns in NK cells. *J Immunol,* Vol.169, No.8, pp. 4253-4261, ISSN 0022-1767

Sidorenko, S. P. & Clark, E. A. (2003). The dual-function CD150 receptor subfamily: the viral attraction. *Nat Immunol,* Vol.4, No.1, pp. 19-24, ISSN 1529-2908

Su, R. C., Brown, K. E., Saaber, S., Fisher, A. G., Merkenschlager, M. & Smale, S. T. (2004). Dynamic assembly of silent chromatin during thymocyte maturation." *Nat Genet,* Vol.36, No.5, pp. 502-506, ISSN 1061-4036

Skov, S., Pedersen, M. T., Andresen, L., Straten, P. T., Woetmann, A. & Odum, N. (2005). Cancer cells become susceptible to natural killer cell killing after exposure to histone deacetylase inhibitors due to glycogen synthase kinase-3-dependent expression of MHC class I-related chain A and B. *Cancer Res,* Vol.65, No.23, pp. 11136-11145, ISSN 1538-7445

Szyf, M. (2005). DNA methylation and demethylation as targets for anticancer therapy. *Biochemistry (Mosc) ,* Vol.70, No.5, pp. 533-549, ISSN 0006-2979

Santourlidis, S., Graffmann, N., Christ, J. & Uhrberg, M. (2008). Lineage-specific transition of histone signatures in the killer cell Ig-like receptor locus from hematopoietic progenitor to NK cells. *J Immunol,* Vol.180, No.1, pp. 418-425, ISSN0022-1767

Samarakoon, A., Chu, H. & Malarkannan, S. (2009). Murine NKG2D ligands: "double, double toil and trouble". *Mol Immunol,* Vol.46, No.6, pp. 1011-1019, ISSN 1672-7681

Sers, C., Kuner, R., Falk, C. S., Lund, P., Sueltmann, H., Braun, M., Buness, A., Ruschhaupt, M., Conrad, J., Mang-Fatehi, S., Stelniec, I., Krapfenbauer, U., Poustka, A. & Schafer, R. (2009). Down-regulation of HLA Class I and NKG2D ligands through a concerted action of MAPK and DNA methyltransferases in colorectal cancer cells." *Int J Cancer,* Vol.125, No.7, pp. 1626-1639, ISSN 1097-0215

Stein, G. S., Stein, J. L., Van Wijnen, A. J., Lian, J. B., Montecino, M., Croce, C. M., Choi, J. Y., Ali, S. A., Pande, S., Hassan, M. Q., Zaidi, S. K. and Young, D. W. (2010). Transcription factor-mediated epigenetic regulation of cell growth and phenotype for biological control and cancer. *Adv Enzyme Regul,* Vol.50, No.1, pp. 160-167, ISSN 0065-2571

Takei, F., McQueen, K. L., Maeda, M., Wilhelm, B. T., Lohwasser, S., Lian, R. H. & Mager, D. L. (2001). Ly49 and CD94/NKG2: developmentally regulated expression and evolution. *Immunol Rev,* Vol.181, , pp. 90-103, ISSN 0105-2896

Trompeter, H. I., Gomez-Lozano, N., Santourlidis, S., Eisermann, B., Wernet, P., Vilches, C. & Uhrberg, M. (2005). Three structurally and functionally divergent kinds of promoters regulate expression of clonally distributed killer cell Ig-like receptors (KIR), of KIR2DL4, and of KIR3DL3. *J Immunol,* Vol.174, No.7, pp. 4135-4143, ISSN 0022-1767

Uhrberg, M., Valiante, N. M., Shum, B. P., Shilling, H. G., Lienert-Weidenbach, K., Corliss, B., Tyan, D., Lanier, L. L. & Parham, P. (1997). Human diversity in killer cell inhibitory receptor genes. *Immunity,* Vol.7, No.6, pp. 753-763, ISSN1074-7613

Valiante, N. M., Lienert, K., Shilling, H. G., Smits, B. J. & Parham, P. (1997). Killer cell receptors: keeping pace with MHC class I evolution. *Immunol Rev*, Vol.155, pp. 155-164, ISSN 0105-2896

Vilches, C., Gardiner, C. M. & Parham, P. (2000). Gene structure and promoter variation of expressed and nonexpressed variants of the KIR2DL5 gene. *J Immunol*, Vol.165, No.11, pp. 6416-6421, ISSN 0022-1767

Vilches, C. & Parham, P. (2002). KIR: diverse, rapidly evolving receptors of innate and adaptive immunity. *Annu Rev Immunol*, Vol.20, pp. 217-251, ISSN 0732-0582

van Nimwegen, E. (2003). Scaling laws in the functional content of genomes. *Trends Genet* , Vol.19, No.9, pp. 479-484, ISSN 0168-9525

van Bergen, J., Thompson, A., van der Slik, A., Ottenhoff, T. H., Gussekloo, J. & Koning, F. (2004). Phenotypic and functional characterization of CD4 T cells expressing killer Ig-like receptors. *J Immunol*, Vol.173, No.11, pp. 6719-6726, ISSN 0022-1767

Villar-Garea, A. & Esteller, M. (2004). Histone deacetylase inhibitors: understanding a new wave of anticancer agents. *Int J Cancer*, Vol.112, No.2, pp. 171-178, ISSN 1097-0215

Venkataraman, G. M., Suciu, D., Groh, V., Boss, J. M. & Spies, T. (2007). Promoter region architecture and transcriptional regulation of the genes for the MHC class I-related chain A and B ligands of NKG2D. *J Immunol*, Vol.178, No.2, pp. 961-969, ISSN 0022-1767

Wilson, M. J., Torkar, M., Haude, A., Milne, S., Jones, T., Sheer, D., Beck, S. & Trowsdale, J. (2000). Plasticity in the organization and sequences of human KIR/ILT gene families. *Proc Natl Acad Sci U S A*, Vol.97, No.9, pp. 4778-4783, ISSN 0027-8424

Wajapeyee, N. & Somasundaram, K. (2003). Cell cycle arrest and apoptosis induction by activator protein 2alpha (AP-2alpha) and the role of p53 and p21WAF1/CIP1 in AP-2alpha-mediated growth inhibition. *J Biol Chem*, Vol.278, No.52, pp. 52093-52101, ISSN 0021-9258

Wilhelm, B. T., Landry, J. R., Takei, F. & Mager, D. L. (2003). Transcriptional control of murine CD94 gene: differential usage of dual promoters by lymphoid cell types. *J Immunol*, Vol.171, No.8, pp. 4219-4226, ISSN 0022-1767

Wang, Y., Fischle, W., Cheung, W., Jacobs, S., Khorasanizadeh, S. & Allis, C. D. (2004). Beyond the double helix: writing and reading the histone code. *Novartis Found Symp*, Vol.259, pp. 3-17, ISSN 1528-2511

Wu, P., Wei, H., Zhang, C., Zhang, J. & Tian, Z. (2005). Regulation of NK cell activation by stimulatory and inhibitory receptors in tumor escape from innate immunity. *Front Biosci*, Vol.10, pp. 3132-3142, ISSN 1093-9946

Yan, W. H., Lin, A. F., Chang, C. C. & Ferrone, S. (2005). Induction of HLA-G expression in a melanoma cell line OCM-1A following the treatment with 5-aza-2'-deoxycytidine. *Cell Res*, Vol.15, No.7, pp. 523-531, ISSN 1001-0602

Ye, Q., Shen, Y., Wang, X., Yang, J., Miao, F., Shen, C. & Zhang, J. (2010). Hypermethylation of HLA class I gene is associated with HLA class I down-regulation in human gastric cancer. *Tissue Antigens*, Vol.75, No.1, pp. 30-39, ISSN 0001-2815

Zeng, Y. X., Somasundaram, K. & el-Deiry, W. S. (1997). AP2 inhibits cancer cell growth and activates p21WAF1/CIP1 expression. *Nat Genet*, Vol.15, No.1, pp. 78-82, ISSN 1061-4036

Zhang, C., Zhang, J., Sun, R., Feng, J., Wei, H. & Tian, Z. (2005). Opposing effect of IFNgamma and IFNalpha on expression of NKG2 receptors: negative regulation of IFNgamma on NK cells. *Int Immunopharmacol*, Vol.5, No.6, pp. 1057-1067, ISSN 1567- 5769

Zhang, C., Wang, Y., Zhou, Z., Zhang, J. & Tian, Z. (2009). Sodium butyrate upregulates expression of NKG2D ligand MICA/B in HeLa and HepG2 cell lines and increases their susceptibility to NK lysis. *Cancer Immunol Immunother*, Vol.58, No.8, pp. 1275-1285, ISSN 0340-7004

5

CD277 an Immune Regulator of T Cell Function and Tumor Cell Recognition

Jose Francisco Zambrano-Zaragoza[1,2] et al.[*]
[1]INSERM, UMR 891, CRCM, Institut Paoli-Calmettes,
Universite Medierranée, Marseille, France
[2]Universidad Autónoma de Nayarit,
Ciencias Químico Biológicas y Farmacéuticas, Tepic Nayarit,
Mexico

1. Introduction

Molecules involved in tumor cell recognition are potentially important targets in cancer therapeutics. Therefore, research on the identification of tumor cell antigens as well as, immune-regulatory molecules is essential. The study of new co-stimulatory molecules has attracted special interest due to, their role in activation and/or inhibition of effector function of immune cells. In this chapter, we focused on the study of CD277 and its putative counter-receptor, and their possible role in activation or inhibition of immune cells and recognition of cancer cells.

CD277 has been involved in immune cells regulation, because of its role in activating or inhibiting effector, cytokine secretion and cytotoxic functions, depending on the activating conditions of these cells. Moreover, the fact that the stimulation of tumor cell lines with anti-CD277 leave to a better recognition and killing by γδ and αβ T cells lead us to postulate that these molecules is involved also in tumor recognition. We will discuss different aspects of CD277 and its counter-receptor in this chapter.

Classically, the immune response has been divided into innate and adaptive immunity, with distinct properties. The innate immune response uses a small number of receptors that detect a limited set of conserved antigens. Induction of the adaptive immune response involves antigen presenting cells (APC) and T cells (Borghesi & Milcarek, 2007). The interaction between the T cell and the APC is the pivotal step that controls a series of events, including T cell activation, cell division and effector differentiation (Zhu & Chen, 2009). However, recognition of the processed antigenic peptide coupled to Major

[*] Nassima Messal[1], Sonia Pastor[1], Emmanuel Scotet[3], Marc Bonneville[3], Danièle Saverino[4],
Marcello Bagnasco[5], Crystelle Harly[3], Yves Guillaume[1], Jacques Nunes[1], Pierre Pontarotti[6],
Marc Lopez[1] and Daniel Olive[1]
[1]INSERM, UMR 891, CRCM, Institut Paoli-Calmettes, Universite Medierranée, Marseille, France
[2]Universidad Autónoma de Nayarit, Ciencias Químico Biológicas y Farmacéuticas,Tepic Nayarit, Mexico
[3]Centre de Recherche en Cancerologie de Nantes Angers, IRT UN, INSERM UMR 892, Nantes France
[4]Department of Experimental Medicine-Section Human Anatomy, University of Genova, Italy
[5]Medical and Radio metabolic Therapy Unit, Department of Internal Medicine, University of Genova, Italy
[6]Université Aix Marseille 1, UMR 6632 Marseille, France

Histocompatilibity Complex (MHC) class I or II molecules on APC is not enough to activate T cells, they require an antigen independent second signal involving the B7 family molecules. The lack of this co-stimulatory signal induces anergy (Ledbetter et al., 1990).

CD28 and the related molecule CTLA-4, together with their natural ligands CD80 and CD86 are the classical co-stimulatory molecules (Ward, 1996). CD28 is constitutively expressed on T cells and is involved in their activation through signal transduction. CTLA-4, which delivers a strong inhibitory signal, is expressed on the T cell surface after engagement of TCR. CD80 and CD86 belong to the B7 co-signalling receptors family, they are cell surface glycoproteins that are essential to modulate and tune the T cell receptor (TCR)-mediated activation of T lymphocytes (Moretta & Bottino, 2004). Other members of this family are PD1 and their ligands PDL-1 and PDL-2 with inhibitory properties on T cell activation and ICOS and ICOSL, involved in T cell activation (Moretta & Bottino, 2004; Rietz & Chen, 2004). Members of the related B7 family belong to the immunoglobulins superfamily (IgSF). They have two Ig extracellular domains and show similarity to the variable (V) and the constant (C) domains of Ig. Previous studies have shown that IgV-like domains of B7.1 and B7.2 share similarity with myelin oligodendrocyte glycoprotein (MOG), chicken blood group system protein (BG) and butyrophillin (BT). Thus, these five proteins depict a subfamily in the IgSF. MOG is expressed only in the central nervous system (CNS) as a component of the myelin sheath and is involved as autoantigen in the pathogenesis of multiple sclerosis; BG proteins are only expressed in chicken and are associated with immunological functions acting as strong adjuvants when used in co-immunization with other proteins and; BT is a glycoprotein that forms a major component of milk fat globule membrane and is expressed in mammary gland at the end of pregnancy and during lactation but its function remains unknown. Whereas MOG and BG have only one extracellular IgV-like domain, BT has a B7-"like" structure with an IgV-like and an IgC-like domain (Henry et al., 1999). Furthermore, BT has an intracellular domain of 166 amino acids named B30.2 and is presumably involved in the regulation of intracellular superoxide concentrations (Henry et al., 1997).

Interestingly, the human bt and mog genes map to the distal part of the MHC class I region and six additional BT members were identified in this region. The six genes could be divided in two groups called BT2 and BT3 and are named using three different nomenclatures. Within these groups, there are BT2.1 (also called BTF1or BTN2A1], BT2.2 (also called BTF2 or BTN2A2], BT2.3 (also called BTF1 or BTN2A1], BT3.1 (also called BTF5 or BTN3A1], BT3.2 (also called BTF4 or BTN3A2], BT3.3 (also called BTF3 or BTN3A3]. The degree of identity between members of BT2 and BT3 groups is around 50 %, while identity is around 95% within the same sub-family. Among these molecules BT3.1 or CD277 has a wide tissue distribution and its ligands are expressed on T cells suggesting that it could play a role in immune functions (Compte et al., 2004). Other members of this family have also been identified on chromosome 6 (BTNL2) or other chromosomes.

Expasy site annotates 15 butyrophilin-like genes in humans including BT and MOG. Butyrophilin proteins typically have a signal peptide, an IgV-like and IgC-like domain, and a transmembrane and cytoplasmic domain. In addition, they often possess a heptad repeat which is a 7-aa sequence encoded by a single exon. Many butyrophilin molecules also contain a 166 aa B30.2 domain in the cytoplasmic region also found in tripartite motif (TRIM) proteins and stonutoxin. The precise function of the B30.2 domain in butyrophilin remains unclear. The B30.2 domain is also present in the C terminal part of various types of proteins which N-terminal globular domain may either contain Ig fold (butyrophilin), a

RING finger domain or a leucine zipper. It has been recently found that the protein TRIM5 interacts with HIV via its B30.2 domain. Xanthine oxidase interacts with B30.2 and may indirectly regulate nitric oxid production.

In pathological settings, proteins possessing B30.2 domain have been reported in over exuberant inflammatory responses such as Familial Mediterranean Fever (FMF) which is caused by mutation in the B30.2 domain of pyrin/marenostrin. In addition, mutations within this domain in the MID1 protein are also associated to the Opitz syndrome.

Because the IgV-like domains of B7.1 and B7.2 are more similar to the IgV-like domain of butyrophilin than to any other sequence, Linsley et al. proposed that B7 and butyrophilin molecules might have evolved from a common ancestral gene to compose a subfamily within the Ig superfamily. It is unclear whether B7 and butyrophilin molecules share common functions in regulating immune responses (Linsley *et al.*, 1994).

CD277 is thought to be involved in immune response because their expression can be modulated by pro-inflammatory cytokines such as TNF-α and IFN-γ (Compte *et al.*, 2004). Stimulation of BTN3 molecules results in phosphorylation BTN3A3 molecules leading to the attenuation of proliferation and cytokine secretion in CD4+ and CD8+ T cells in a CD4+CD25+ independent manner, demonstrating the agonistic properties of BTN3 to mediate negative-signal transduction (Yamashiro *et al.*, 2010).

In order to expand our knowledge about the CD277 and their role in tumor cell recognition, we analyzed different aspects of stimulation of leukaemia cell lines and some strategies to be used in the identification of the CD277 counter-receptor.

2. CD277: Its role in immune regulation and tumor cell recognition

The CD277 molecule is expressed on αβ, γδ T cells, B and NK lymphocytes, monocytes, dendritic cells and hematopoietic precursors as identified by mRNA expression and flow cytometry. Moreover, the CD277 surface expression is constitutive on endothelial cells and it is increased by pro-inflammatory cytokines such as TNF-α and IFN-γ, suggesting that these molecules might be involved in the early events of tissue damage and inflammation (Compte *et al.*, 2004). Even though there are some reports regarding the effects of CD277 on immune cells, little is known about the functions of the CD277 counter-receptor in leukaemia and tumor cells. Here, we report our findings on functional properties of this counter-receptor and propose some strategies to determine the identity of this molecule.

2.1 Engagement of CD277 regulates αβ T cells functions

Two different monoclonal antibodies (mAb) recognizing CD277 have been reported, 1) BT3.1, obtained from mice immunized with the extracellular domain of BTN3A1 (Compte *et al.*, 2004) and, 2) 232-5, obtained from mice immunized with the extracellular domain of BTN3A3 (Yamashiro *et al.*, 2010). In both cases, no differences in the recognition of the different isoforms of CD277 have been found. Therefore, these antibodies were used for the study of the immunomodulatory functions of CD277 on T cells. Yamashiro *et al.*, have evaluated the proliferation of CD4+ and CD8+ T cells populations in PBMC stimulated with anti-CD3 and anti-CD277 mAb. Interestingly, they found that the proliferation of both CD4+ and CD8+ T cells were suppressed by 232-5 but not by BT3.1 mAb. Moreover, IFN-γ and IL-4 production in CD4 T cells and IFN-γ in CD8+ T cells were down-regulated by 232-5 but not by BT3.1 mAb. Additionally, they report that this effect requires the cross-link of CD277 in the cell surface because the observed effects with the 232-5 mAb were lost when the Fab fragment was used (Yamashiro *et al.*, 2010).

These result suggest the negative effect of CD277 on T cell activation, but considering that the affinity of the BT3.1 mAb is lower than those observed with the 232-5 mAb and that the BT3.1 mAb did not show any effect on the T cell population analyzed it is possible that different effects could be attributed to CD277 on αβ T cells. Using another mAb (20.1) we found that CD277 engagement enhanced the CD3 or CD3/CD28 co-stimulation at the proliferation and cytokine production levels. The effect of this mAb was associated with an increased intracellular signalling (Messal et al., submitted).

On the other hand, T cells expressing γδ TCRs have emerged as an important component of the immune repertoire and are included as component of the innate immune response (Nedellec et al., 2010; Saenz et al., 2010). In humans, the γδ T cells are also located in peripheral organs and peripheral blood. Circulating γδ T cells express a TCR comprising mainly Vδ2 and Vγ9 and cells with this phenotype represent 2% of mononuclear cells. These Vγ9Vδ2 T cells are activated by TCR stimulation with small non peptidic phosphorylated compounds also referred as phosphoantigens (Tanaka et al., 1995). Unlike the conventional T cells, their activation does not require activating co-signals provided by CD28 - CD80 and CD86 interaction. However, their activation can be regulated by NKR (Das et al., 2001; Halary et al., 1997) and TLR (Deetz et al., 2006; Wesch et al., 2006). Moreover, engagement of NKG2D can activate them, without TCR stimulation (Rincon-Orozco et al., 2005). Thus, considering the role of γδ T cells in the anti-tumoral immune response (Tokuyama et al., 2008) it is important to analyze the effects of CD277 on the functions of γδ T cells as well.

2.2 CD277 and dendritic cells
We have reported that CD277 is expressed on the surface of resting and activated monocytes and monocyte-derived dendritic cells (iDC). The effect of CD277 on monocytes and iDC was analyzed in freshly isolated monocytes and monocyte-derived dendritic cells stimulated with anti-CD19 or anti-CD277 (anti-BT3.1). We found that upon stimulation for 24 h, anti-CD277 triggered the activation of monocytes, measured by up-regulation of the expression of CD86 on the cell surface as compared to cells treated with isotype-matched control. No effect was observed when control antibody (anti-CD19) or soluble anti-CD277 were used, indicating that cross-linking is required for the cellular activation observed (Simone et al., 2010). Further, these results demonstrate that receptors for the Fc fragment of immunoglobulins (FcRs) dependent signalling are not responsible for cell activation.

On the other hand, a wide variety of receptors regulate the activity of cells of the myeloid lineage. We have also analyzed the effects of CD277 as co-receptor in proinflammatory responses triggering by pathogenic stimuli by stimulating monocytes and iDC with anti-CD277 in presence of different doses of Toll-like receptors (TLR) ligands (LPS and R-848). We observed that secretion of proinflammatory cytokines (IL8/CXCL8, IL-1β and IL-12/p70) are increased in monocytes cultured with both anti-CD277 and TLR ligands compared with individual stimuli. Parallel experiments performed with iDC shown that cytokine secretion is similar to those observed with monocytes (Simone et al., 2010).

These data suggest a possible role of CD277 as activation receptor on monocytes and dendritic cells. The need of cross-linking to obtain a biological effect on both monocytes and iDC is consistent with their possible agonist nature.

These data suggest a possible role of CD277 molecules as activation receptors on monocytes and dendritic cells. In addition, the need of cross-linking to obtain a biological effect on both monocytes and iDC is consistent with their possible agonist nature.

2.3 CD277 and tumor recognition

The effect of CD277 stimulation on αβ T cells and monocytes and iDC described above, suggests the regulatory role of CD277, by activating or inhibiting the effector functions of immune cells. Moreover, the presence of the putative CD277 counter-receptor in the immune environment may play a critical role in defining where and when CD277 is engaged. We have reported that leukaemia cell lines and solid tumor cells lines such as HeLa and MCF-7, Raji, C91, HUT78 and JA16 (Compte *et al.*, 2004) express both CD277 and the CD277 counter-receptor. In addition, we have recently found (Harly et al., in preparation) that Raji cells stimulated with anti-CD277 are better recognized and killed by Vγ9Vδ2 T cells. We postulated that the effect of CD277 stimulation on Raji cells would stand at the level of regulation of the antigen stimulation of Vγ9Vδ2 T cells and/or over-expression of the counter-receptor for CD277, thus, we investigated the effect of CD277 stimulation on the expression of CD277 counter-receptor in Raji cells. We used these cells because they express low levels of CD277 counter-receptor on the cell surface, therefore its regulation can be followed up by flow cytometry using the CD277-Fc fusion protein.

To analyze the expression of CD277 on different cell lines after treatment with anti-CD277, anti-CD80 or the Fab portion of anti-CD277 monoclonal antibodies, Raji, C91, TF1 or HUT78 cells were plated onto 96 round bottom wells (10^6 cells/well) and incubated with or without these antibodies at different concentrations (from 10 to 0.078125 μg/mL) for 2 hours. Then cells were extensively washed on PBS-FCS and incubated with or without 15 μg/mL of CD277-Fc fusion protein (Compte *et al.*, 2004) for 30 minutes at 4°C. After incubation, cells were washed twice on PBS-2% FCS and stained with 1/100 goat-anti-human-Fc-PE for 15 min at room temperature. After wash, the cells were fixed with PBS - 1% formaldehyde and acquisition was done in a LSRII (BD bioscience). Data were analyzed with flow-jo software.

We found that the expression of CD277 counter-receptor is weak on non-stimulated Raji cells (Figure 1). However, the stimulation of Raji cells with anti-CD277 antibodies enhances the expression of CD277 counter-receptor compared to non-stimulated or stimulated with anti-CD80 antibodies controls (Figure 1A, B and C). These data suggest that up-regulation in the expression of CD277 counter-receptor is due to the CD277 engagement, because Raji cells stimulated with anti-CD80 express the counter-receptor at similar levels as non-stimulated cells non-stimulated (Figure 1B).

This effect was also observed on different cell lines such as C91, HUT78 and TF1. Although different basal levels of CD277 counter-receptor expression was found in these cells, in all cases stimulation with anti-CD277 antibodies lead to a higher expression of the counter-receptor on the cell surface (Figure 2). Additionally, stimulation with the Fab portion of the anti-CD277 has no effect on the expression of the counter-receptor; therefore it is necessary to cross-link CD277 on the cell surface to have the stimulatory effect observed (Figure 3). Moreover, the effect observed was dose-dependent, as shown in Figure 4.

2.4 Stimulation by CD277 and the regulation of the expression of CD277

We know that the expression of CD277 on immune cells is constitutive and that it is increased by proinflammatory cytokines such as IFN-γ and TNF-α (Compte *et al.*, 2004), however, little is known regarding the effect of CD277 stimulation on its own expression.

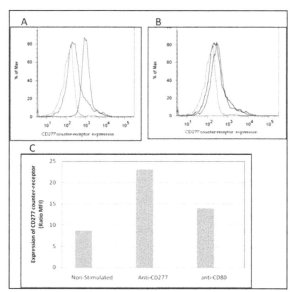

Fig. 1. Effect of CD277 stimulation in the CD277 counter-receptor expression on Raji cells. A) CD277 counter receptor expression in Raji cells after stimulation with anti-CD277 antibodies: Orange, basal fluorescence; green, expression of CD277 counter-receptor in non-stimulated and; blue, expression of CD277 counter-receptor in cells stimulated with anti-CD277 antibodies. B) CD277 counter-receptor expression in Raji cells after stimulation with anti CD80 antibodies(control): Orange, basal fluorescence , green, expression of CD277 counter-receptor in non-stimulated and; Blue, expression of CD277 counter-receptor in cells stimulated with anti-CD80 antibodies. C) MFI ratio was calculated by dividing the fluorescence intensity of cells in different conditions by the fluorescence intensity of the isotype control.

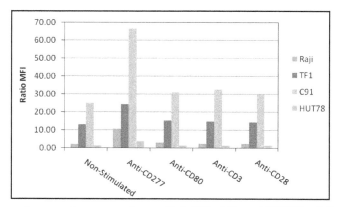

Fig. 2. CD277 counter-receptor expression on Raji, TF1, C91 and HUT78 cell lines stimulated by CD277. Each bar represents the mean fluorescence of triplicates divided by mean fluorescence of the isotype control.

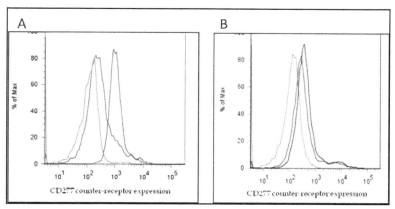

Fig. 3. Effect of CD277 cross-link on the CD277 counter-receptor expression in Raji cells. Orange, basal fluorescence; green, expression of CD277 counter-receptor in non-stimulated and Raji cells and; blue, expression in Raji cells stimulated with (A) anti-CD277 antibodies or (B) Fab of anti-CD277 antibodies.

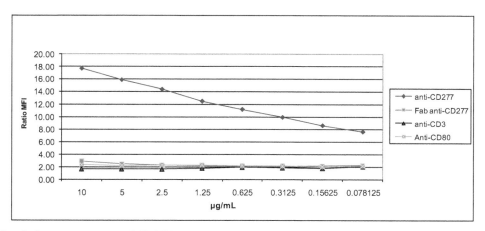

Fig. 4. Over-expression of CD277 counter-receptor in Raji cells is dose-dependent. Raji cells were tested with increasing concentrations of the anti-CD277, the Fab portion of the anti-CD277, anti-CD3 or anti-CD80 monoclonal antibodies and expression of CD277 counter-receptor was followed by flow cytometry.

To test this hypothesis, Raji cells (10×10^6) were cultured in RPMI 1640 + 10% FCS and stimulated with 10 μg/mL of either anti-CD277 or anti-CD80 monoclonal antibodies for 0, 2, 4, 6 or 24 hours at 37°C in a 5% CO_2 atmosphere. RNA was extracted with trizol® and RT-PCR using Taqman assays (Applied Biosystems) for CD277 isoforms (BTN3A1, BTN3A2, BTN3A3), and GAPDH, as endogenous housekeeping gene, was done. Expression of the CD277 isoforms was calculated as follows:

$$\Delta CT_{stimulated} = CT_{Probe} - CT_{GAPDH}$$

$$\Delta\Delta CT = \Delta CT_{stimulated} - \Delta CT_{time = 0}$$

Where CT_{Probe} is the CT for the CD277 isoforms, obtained from Raji cells stimulated with either anti-CD277 or anti-CD80, and $\Delta CT_{time = 0}$ is the ΔCT value for the CD277 isoforms at time = 0 hours (control).

The relative quantity (RQ) expression by using the formula:

$$RQ = 2^{-\Delta\Delta CT}$$

We found that the expression of BTN3A1 and BTN3A3 molecules but not BTN3A2, at 2, 4 and 6 hours is higher in Raji cells stimulated with anti-CD277 monoclonal antibodies and that this effect is lost after 24 hours (Figure 5). Taken together, our data suggest multiple functions of CD277: Promotion of the expression of CD277 counter-receptor and up-regulation of the expression of the CD277 molecules itself.

Although the CD277 monoclonal antibodies tested cannot differentiate between BTN3A1, BTN3A2 and BTN3A3 isoforms, we know that differences in the intracellular region of BTN3 molecules stand mainly with BTN3A2 which lacks the B30.2 domain. Therefore, since our data point out that signal transduction due to CD277 can be mediated by BTN3A1 and BTN3A3 isoforms, it seems likely that the B30.2 domain is involved this effect.

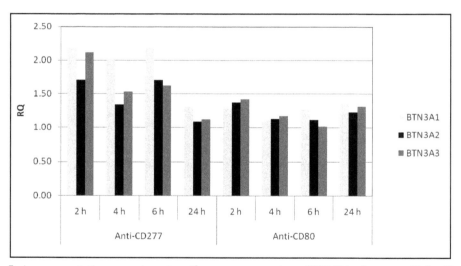

Fig. 5. A representative experiment on the gene expression of BTN3 isoforms on Raji cells stimulated by CD277. BTN3A1, A2 and A3 are the reported isoforms for CD277. The RQ was calculated as described. A RQ value higher than 2.0 was considered as indicative of gene over expression.

2.5 Effect of cytokines on the expression of CD277 counter receptor

It has been reported that cells stimulated by CD277 secrete inflammatory cytokines such as IFN-γ and TNF-α (Cubillos-Ruiz et al., 2010; Yamashiro et al., 2010) and that these cytokines may influence the expression of CD277. However, little is known about the modulation of the expression of the CD277 counter-receptor by these proinflammatory cytokines.

To further investigate the regulatory effects of inflammatory signals on the expression of CD277, C91 cells (50,000 cels/well) were treated with IFN-γ (5, 50, 500 and 5000 ng/mL), TNF-α (0.4, 4, 40 and 400 ng/mL), TGF-β (0.02. 0.2 and 2 ng/mL) and IL-22 (1, 10, 100 and 1000 ng/mL) for 24 hours at 37°C in a 5% CO_2 atmosphere. Following washes with PBS-FCS, the cells were incubated with or without (control) 15 µg/mL of CD277-Fc fusion protein for 30 minutes at 4°C. After incubation, the cells were washed twice on PBS-2% FCS and stained with 1/100 goat-anti-human-Fc-PE for 15 min at room temperature. After wash, cells were fixed on PBS- 1% formaldehyde and expression of CD277 was assessed by flow cytometry (LSRII, BD bioscience). Analysis was done with flow-jo software. Our results show that stimulation with IFN-γ, TNF-α, TGF-β or IL-22 has no effect on the expression of CD277 counter-receptor in C91 cells (Figure 6).

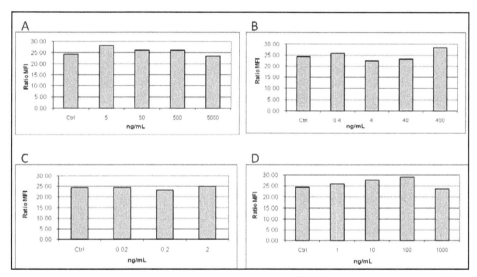

Fig. 6. A representative experiment on the expression of CD277 counter-receptor in C91 cells stimulated with different concentrations of (A) IFN-γ (B) TNF-α (C) TGFβ and (D) IL-22 for 24 hours. Cells were stained with CD277-Fc fusion protein and analyzed by flow cytometry.

2.6 Strategies for CD277 counter receptor identification
The identity of CD277 counter-receptor is one of the main challenges in the near future, for a better understanding of the mechanisms involved in immune cell regulation and tumor cell recognition.

2.6.1 Methods to determine the CD277-counter receptor identity
In spite of the weak expression of the counter-receptor in different cell lines (Compte *et al.*, 2004), C91 cells were selected because of the expression profile is higher than in other cell lines such as Raji, TF1, HUT78 or JA16. In order to obtain a cell population with a stable expression of the CD277 counter-receptor, C91 cells were stained with the CD277-Fc fusion protein as described above. The positive population was identified by comparing to unstained control and the 1% most positive population was selected and purified using a

FacsAria (BD Bioscience). These cells were then cultured in RPMI 1640 supplemented with 10% FCS and antibiotics. Expression of CD277 counter-receptor was followed by flow cytometry to corroborate that its surface expression was stable.

The cells obtained, were used in two different approaches to determine the identity of the CD277 counter-receptor. First, the use of cross-linking assays with Bis (sulfosuccinimidyl) suberate (BS3) a homobifunctional, water-soluble, non-cleavable and membrane impermeable crosslinker and;   second, a classical co-immunoprecipitation assay from post-nuclear membranes.

In the first approach, C91T3.3 cells were incubated with 30 μg/mL of the CD277-Fc fusion protein and then the interaction was covalently stabilized by using 3 mM of BS3. After crosslink a standard co-immunoprecipitation protocol was carried out using anti-CD277 monoclonal antibodies and protein G. A 4-12% polyacrilamide gel electrophoresis-sodium dodecyl sulfate (PAGE-SDS) and western-blot were then used to detect the CD277-Fc crosslinked, bands were then cut from the PAGE-SDS gel and sent to be identified by MALDI (Matrix-Assisted Laser Desorption/Ionization)-TOF in a mass-spectrometry assay.

The second strategy to determine the identity of CD277 counter-receptor involves a procedure to obtain the postnuclear membranes. This procedure leads us to enrich the membrane proteins and eliminate the nuclear contaminants that can interfere with the interaction between CD277 and its counter-receptor. In this approach, the C91T3.3 cells were treated with 3 mM imidazole for cell membrane lysis but not the nuclear membrane. After centrifugation, membranes were recovered and used in a classical co-immunoprecipitation assay with CD277-Fc and CTLA4-Fc as a control. A 4-12% PAGE-SDS was carried out to cut the putative counter-receptors for CD277-Fc and CTLA4-Fc, compared with a control without recombinant proteins. Bands that are in the assay but not in the controls were selected to be identified by MALDI-TOF.

2.6.2 Experimental results

The procedure to enhance the expression of CD277 counter-receptor was done twice and cells obtained were named C91T and C91T2. The expression of CD277 counter-receptor in C91T2 was higher than it was in C91T (Figure 8). A third assay to enrich the cell population expressing CD277 counter-receptor by this method was not possible, because the expression after the procedure was not stable.

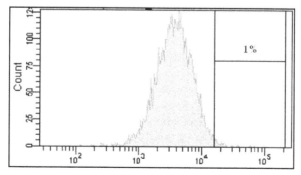

Fig. 7. Population selected from C91, C91T, or C91T2 cells. Flow cytometry was carried out to enhance the stable expression of the CD277 counter-receptor.

From C91T2 cells stained with the CD277-Fc fusion protein we proceeded to clone from the 1% most positive cells (Figure 7). Cloned cells were followed to measure the CD277 counter-receptor expression and the most positive clone obtained was selected and named C91T3.3. As shown in figure 8, increasing expression levels of CD277 counter-receptor were reached with enrichment each step. However, after C91T3.3 no more clones with stable expression of CD277 counter-receptor were obtained. Thus, the highest stable expression of CD277 counter-receptor was that obtained in C91T3.3 cells.

In the first approach to identify the CD277-counter receptor, our preliminary results shown only the homo-polymerization of CD277-Fc by the crosslinking agent BS3 and its detection by mass spectrometry (MALDI-TOF) led us to postulate that this approach is appropriate to determine the identity of CD277 counter-receptor. Nonetheless, the use of additional controls such as CTLA4-Fc is needed to further validate the results. Moreover, as can be seen in our results, it is possible that these homo-polymers mask the potential CD277-Fc - CD277 counter-receptor heterodimerization. Therefore they should be eliminated as collateral products of the reaction in order to select the appropriate band to be analyzed.

Representative 4-12% PAGE-SDS and western-blot analysis are shown in figure 9. The selected bands were analyzed by MALDI-TOF, but only the polymerization of CD277-Fc fusion protein was identified.

The use of the appropriated controls, negative and positive, is essential to validate the results. As a positive control, we used CTLA4-Fc fusion protein in C91 cells (positive by flow cytometry). However, the determination of the identity of CD277 counter-receptor is in process.

In both approaches used (crosslink and co-immunoprecipitation with post-nuclear membranes) the CD80/86 molecules were used to validate these methods. We hypothesized that if detecting CD80/86 was possible, this methodological approach would be useful for the CD277 counter-receptor identification. However, we were not able to detect CD80/86 by any of the strategies tested. Thus, even though this kind of approach has been used in similar circumstances, like the identification of the B7_H6 counter-receptor (Brandt et al., 2009), technical modifications are needed in order to have the validated conditions for the detection of the CD277 counter-receptor.

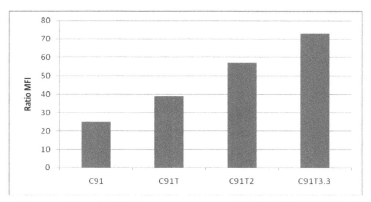

Fig. 8. Enhanced expression of CD277 counter-receptor in C91, C91T, C91T2 and C91T3.3 cells after cell sorting and cloning. Expression was followed-up using CD277-Fc fusion protein by flow cytometry.

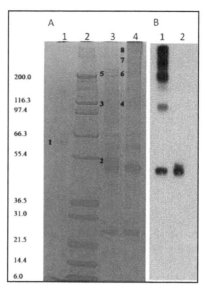

Fig. 9. A typical PAGE-SDS and western-blot analysis for the identification of CD277 counter-receptor. A) 1.- control BSA 2.- molecular weight markers, 3.- assay without BS3 and 4.- with BS3. B) Western-blot line 1 with BS3, line 2 without BS3 and line 3 molecular weight markers. Numbers indicate the selected band to be analyzed by MALDI-TOF.

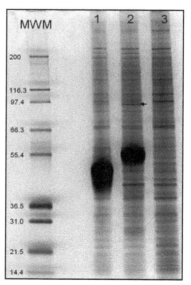

Fig. 10. A typical PAGE-SDS used in co-immunoprecipitation assays using the post-nuclear membranes. 1) Using CTLA4-Fc 2) Using CD277-Fc and 3) control without recombinant proteins. The arrow shows the band to be analyzed.

2.6.3 Monoclonal antibodies against the CD277 counter receptor

The production and use of monoclonal antibodies is another attractive strategy to enhance our knowledge of CD277 counter-receptor. However, the identity of the receptor or a recombinant counter-receptor is not available yet. Thus, we decided to obtain monoclonal antibodies to recognize this counter-receptor using cells expressing it as the immunogenic stimulus. With this rationale we immunized rats with C91T3.3 cells, which as described above, enhanced expression of the CD277 counter-receptor. Spleen cells from these immunized rats were used for the production of hybridomas following standard protocols. Important to note is the fact that when using this type of approach, the screening systems are crucial to identify the relevant hybridomas to be clone and antibodies to be purified.

Considering that the rat immune system will produce antibodies against many of the cell surface proteins of C91T3.3, a first screening was done using the CD277 counter-receptor expressing human erythroleukaemic cell line TF1. Hybridomas secreting antibodies against TF1 cells were selected for a second screening. In addition, since Raji cells stimulated with anti-CD277 mAbs show enhanced expression of the CD277 counter-receptor, these cells were used for a second screening of the clones selected in the first one. This second screening was done in parallel with an inhibitory test using C91T3.3 cells and the CD277-Fc.. With this system, hybridomas secreting antibodies against the Raji cells and with inhibitory activity on C91T3.3 were selected for cloning.

In figure 11 a representative figure is shown. The basal fluorescence of Raji cells is shown (11A). The percentage of positive non-stimulated Raji cells is shown in red and it is compared to the amount of positive stimulated Raji cells (blue) (11B). This supernatant was a potentially useful, thus it was tested for inhibitory activity on C91T3.3 cells (Figure 12). We can see that effectively the antibodies in this supernatant have an inhibitory effect on the CD277-Fc binding. Interestingly, we found that some supernatants enhance the CD277-Fc binding on C91T3.3. These clones were selected too, because they could recognize some accessory molecules for the counter-receptor.

We selected a total of 6 clones with inhibitory activity on C91T3.3 cells. We also obtained one clone whose supernatant has the ability to enhance the CD277-Fc binding on C91T3.3 cells. The identification of the proteins recognized by these antibodies is in progress.

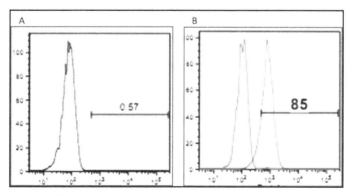

Fig. 11. Representative flow cytometry pattern of a selected clone. A) Basal fluorescence and B) fluorescence of supernatant tested on Raji non stimulated (red) and stimulated with anti-CD277 (blue). The percentage of positive cells is indicated in each pattern.

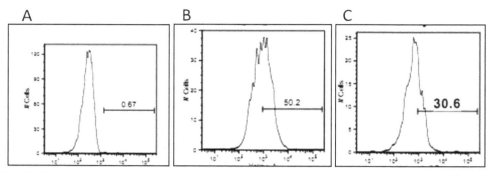

Fig. 12. Representative flow cytometry pattern of a selected clone tested on C91T3.3 cells. A) Basal fluorescence; B) Normal binding of CD277-Fc fusion protein; and C) Inhibitory test showing a reduction in the CD277-Fc binding. The percentage of positive cells is indicated in each pattern.

2.7 Perspectives on the potential use of CD277 and its counter-receptor in cancer therapy

The wide variety of function of CD277 described in this chapter shown the future potential of the use of mAbs anti-CD277 to regulate the immune response against tumor cells. The fact that stimulation of different cells by CD277 lead to the secretion of different cytokines, activation of different signalling pathways, enhance the proliferation of T cells, can be useful to modulate the immune response against tumor cells. Moreover, our results showing that Raji cells stimulated by CD277 are better killed by γδ T cells are potentially useful for cancer therapy.

However, it is necessary to elucidate the mechanisms by which these molecules act and to identify the counter-receptor for CD277. The use of mAbs should be a tool to elucidate the mechanisms, but to be used no to mark the tumor cells, but to modulate the response that lead to kill them.

In the near future, regulation of the expression or activity of molecules such as CD277 or its counter-receptor can be useful for enhance the anti-tumoral immune response, however it is necessary the molecular and fully functional characterization of these molecules, and the mechanisms involved in the observed functions, to be used as modulators of immune response in cancer.

3. Conclusion

Immune responses can be regulated by CD277 in different ways. CD277 affects different immune cells in various ways including inhibition of proliferation, regulation of cytokine secretion in CD4+ and CD8+ T cells, as well as activating monocytes and iDC. Moreover, CD277 promotes the expression of its counter-receptor and this effect may be important for recognition of leukaemia and solid tumor cells.

Proteomics and production and use of monoclonal antibodies are two different approaches we have tested to determine the identity of the CD277 counter-receptor.. However, although functional analysis of CD277 and its counter-receptor has demonstrated a biological effect, it is necessary to identify the counter-receptor and elucidate the signalling pathways involved in the observed response.

4. Acknowledgment

This work was supported by Institut National du Cancer, Institut Paoli Calmettes, Institut National de la Santé et de la Recherche Médicale. J. F Z-Z was a Post-doctoral fellow from Universidad Autónoma de Nayarit.

5. References

Borghesi, L. & Milcarek, C. (2007). Innate versus adaptive immunity: a paradigm past its prime? *Cancer Res* 67(9): 3989-3993.

Brandt, C. S., Baratin, M., Yi, E. C., Kennedy, J., Gao, Z., Fox, B., Haldeman, B., Ostrander, C. D., Kaifu, T., Chabannon, C., Moretta, A., West, R., Xu, W., Vivier, E. & Levin, S. D. (2009). The B7 family member B7-H6 is a tumor cell ligand for the activating natural killer cell receptor NKp30 in humans. *J Exp Med* 206(7): 1495-1503.

Compte, E., Pontarotti, P., Collette, Y., Lopez, M. & Olive, D. (2004). Frontline: Characterization of BT3 molecules belonging to the B7 family expressed on immune cells. *Eur J Immunol* 34(8): 2089-2099.

Cubillos-Ruiz, J. R., Martinez, D., Scarlett, U. K., Rutkowski, M. R., Nesbeth, Y. C., Camposeco-Jacobs, A. L. & Conejo-Garcia, J. R. (2010). cd277 is a Negative Co-stimulatory Molecule Universally Expressed by Ovarian Cancer Microenvironmental Cells. *Oncotarget* 1(5): 329-338.

Das, H., Groh, V., Kuijl, C., Sugita, M., Morita, C. T., Spies, T. & Bukowski, J. F. (2001). MICA engagement by human Vgamma2Vdelta2 T cells enhances their antigen-dependent effector function. *Immunity* 15(1): 83-93.

Deetz, C. O., Hebbeler, A. M., Propp, N. A., Cairo, C., Tikhonov, I. & Pauza, C. D. (2006). Gamma interferon secretion by human Vgamma2Vdelta2 T cells after stimulation with antibody against the T-cell receptor plus the Toll-Like receptor 2 agonist Pam3Cys. *Infect Immun* 74(8): 4505-4511.

Halary, F., Peyrat, M. A., Champagne, E., Lopez-Botet, M., Moretta, A., Moretta, L., Vie, H., Fournie, J. J. & Bonneville, M. (1997). Control of self-reactive cytotoxic T lymphocytes expressing gamma delta T cell receptors by natural killer inhibitory receptors. *Eur J Immunol* 27(11): 2812-2821.

Henry, J., Miller, M. M. & Pontarotti, P. (1999). Structure and evolution of the extended B7 family. *Immunol Today* 20(6): 285-288.

Henry, J., Ribouchon, M., Depetris, D., Mattei, M., Offer, C., Tazi-Ahnini, R. & Pontarotti, P. (1997). Cloning, structural analysis, and mapping of the B30 and B7 multigenic families to the major histocompatibility complex (MHC) and other chromosomal regions. *Immunogenetics* 46(5): 383-395.

Ledbetter, J. A., Imboden, J. B., Schieven, G. L., Grosmaire, L. S., Rabinovitch, P. S., Lindsten, T., Thompson, C. B. & June, C. H. (1990). CD28 ligation in T-cell activation: evidence for two signal transduction pathways. *Blood* 75(7): 1531-1539.

Linsley, P. S., Peach, R., Gladstone, P. & Bajorath, J. (1994). Extending the B7 (CD80) gene family. *Protein Sci* 3(8): 1341-1343.

Moretta, A. & Bottino, C. (2004). Commentary: Regulated equilibrium between opposite signals: a general paradigm for T cell function? *Eur J Immunol* 34(8): 2084-2088.

Nedellec, S., Bonneville, M. & Scotet, E. (2010). Human V gamma 9V delta 2 T cells: From signals to functions. *Seminars in Immunology* 22(4): 199-206.

Rietz, C. & Chen, L. (2004). New B7 family members with positive and negative costimulatory function. *Am J Transplant* 4(1): 8-14.

Rincon-Orozco, B., Kunzmann, V., Wrobel, P., Kabelitz, D., Steinle, A. & Herrmann, T. (2005). Activation of V gamma 9V delta 2 T cells by NKG2D. *J Immunol* 175(4): 2144-2151.

Saenz, S. A., Noti, M. & Artis, D. (2010). Innate immune cell populations function as initiators and effectors in Th2 cytokine responses. *Trends Immunol* 31(11): 407-413.

Simone, R., Barbarat, B., Rabellino, A., Icardi, G., Bagnasco, M., Pesce, G., Olive, D. & Saverino, D. (2010). Ligation of the BT3 molecules, members of the B7 family, enhance the proinflammatory responses of human monocytes and monocyte-derived dendritic cells. *Molecular Immunology* 48(1-3): 109-118.

Tanaka, Y., Morita, C. T., Nieves, E., Brenner, M. B. & Bloom, B. R. (1995). Natural and synthetic non-peptide antigens recognized by human gamma delta T cells. *Nature* 375(6527): 155-158.

Tokuyama, H., Hagi, T., Mattarollo, S. R., Morley, J., Wang, Q., Fai-So, H., Moriyasu, F., Nieda, M. & Nicol, A. J. (2008). V gamma 9 V delta 2 T cell cytotoxicity against tumor cells is enhanced by monoclonal antibody drugs--rituximab and trastuzumab. *Int J Cancer* 122(11): 2526-2534.

Ward, S. G. (1996). CD28: a signalling perspective. *Biochem J* 318 (Pt 2): 361-377.

Wesch, D., Beetz, S., Oberg, H. H., Marget, M., Krengel, K. & Kabelitz, D. (2006). Direct costimulatory effect of TLR3 ligand poly(I:C) on human gamma delta T lymphocytes. *J Immunol* 176(3): 1348-1354.

Yamashiro, H., Yoshizaki, S., Tadaki, T., Egawa, K. & Seo, N. (2010). Stimulation of human butyrophilin 3 molecules results in negative regulation of cellular immunity. *Journal of Leukocyte Biology* 88(4): 757-767.

Zhu, Y. & Chen, L. (2009). Turning the tide of lymphocyte costimulation. *J Immunol* 182(5): 2557-2558.

Part 3

Cancer Diagnostic Technologies

6

Prospective Applications
of Microwaves in Medicine

Jaroslav Vorlíček, Barbora Vrbova and Jan Vrba
Czech Technical University
Czech Republic

1. Introduction

Research of interactions between Electromagnetic (EM) Field and biological systems is of growing interests elsewhere. In this area of research very important activity are studies of prospective medical applications of microwaves (i.e. a possibility to use microwave energy and/or microwave technique and technology for treatment purposes) are a quite new and a very rapidly developing field. Microwave thermotherapy is being used in medicine for the cancer treatment and for some other diseases since early eighties. Most common methods used for treatment of cancer are radiotherapy and chemotherapy. These therapeutic methods have many undesirable effects, such as usage of ionizing radiation. Another method used for treatment of cancer is hyperthermia. This method is based on the principle of destruction of malignant cells by artificially increased temperature in the temperature range between 41 and 45 °C fails self-protective mechanism of malignant cells. In contrast with chemotherapy and radiotherapy, hyperthermia is not limited by the number of doses of radiation.

2. Prospective applications of microwaves in medicine

In the following text we would like to outline scope and new trends in medical applications of microwaves. We can divide these results and new trends into two major groups:
- clinical results and trends,
- technical results and trends.

2.1 Clinical results and trends
Applications of microwaves in medicine is a quite a new field of a high interest in the world (since early 80's). It is necessary to mention one of the most important trends in the research of medical applications of microwaves, i.e. the thermal effects of EM field (since early 80's a microwave thermotherapy is used for cancer treatment, Benign Prostate Hyperplasia (BPH) treatment and for some other areas of medicine; it can be used in combination with other complementary treatment methods also.
To give a basic overview, we can divide medical applications of microwaves in following three basic groups according to purpose, how are microwaves used:
- Microwave energy and/or technique used for the **treatment of patients** (with the use of either thermal or non-thermal effects – sometimes both of these types of effects can play its role).

- Microwave energy and/or technique used for **diagnostics of diseases** (e.g. by aid of permittivity measurements, attenuation measurements and very prospective in the near future can be a microwave tomography).
- Microwave energy and/or technique used as a **part of a treatment or diagnostic system** (e.g.linear accelerator).

As is given above, until now medical applications of microwaves are above all represented by the treatment methods based on thermal effect – i.e. we can speak about the Microwave thermotherapy, which can be further divided into three different modalities distinguished according to the goal temperature level or interval:

- diathermia: heating up to 41 C   (applications in physiotherapy)
- hyperthermia: heating into the interval of 41-45 C (applications in oncology)
- thermodestruction / thermoablation: over 45 C   (applications in urology)

First three of the following list of thermotherapeutical applications are just largely used in many countries around the world, last three instead are in this moment in the phase of very promising projects:

- Oncology   - cancer treatment.
- Physiotherapy   - treatment of rheumatic diseases.
- Urology   - BPH treatment.
- Cardiology   - heart stimulations.
- Surgery   - growing implants.
- Ophthalmology   - retina corrections.

E.g. in cancer treatment is thermotherapy usually used in the combination with some of other modalities used in the clinical oncology (e.g. radiotherapy, chemotherapy, immunotherapy or chirurgical treatment). It is used in USA, Japan and in many countries in European Union (EU), including the Czech Republic, from early 80s. Up to now local microwave hyperthermia for cancer treatment and thermotherapy of BPH are the most important applications of microwaves in medicine. In the Czech Republic we have treated more than 500 patients. Results of our treatments are given the following table:

Complete response of the tumor	52.4 %
Partial response of the tumor	31.7 %
Without response	15.9 %

Table 1. Clinical results of cancer treatment by radiothermotherapy

Successful treatment thus has been indicated in the case of 84 % of patients. This corresponds very well to the results published in EU and USA. Actual scientific information about microwave thermotherapy and its new developments is possible to get from „International Journal of Hyperthermia" issued by European Society for Hyperthermia Oncology (ESHO) together with North American Hyperthermia Society (NAHS) and Asian Society of Hyperthermia Oncology (ASHO). On the following series of photographs (Fig. 1) there is example of the typical 4 phases of the treatment of one of our patients obtained by radio-thermo-therapy (i.e. combination of microwave hyperthermia with significantly reduced doses of radiotherapy).

Very interesting results for the near future can give us the research of microwave medical applications based on so called non-thermal effects. In the literature it is possible just now to identify research projects on:

- to reduce pain feeling (analogically to analgesics),
- to increase of reaction capabilities of a human being,
- to examine the teaching capabilities, etc.

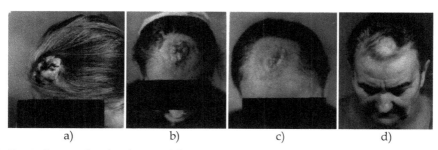

a)   b)   c)   d)

Fig. 1. Typical example of 4 phases of the patient treatment: a) Patient before the treatment. b) At the end of the treatment. c) Two months after treatment. d) One year after treatment.

2.2 Technical results and trends

Our work is focused on the design, optimization and tests of the microwave applicators for medical applications, above all for hyperthermia cancer and BPH treatment. This means to design a microwave structure capable to:

- transfer EM energy into the biological tissue without power reflections back to the microwave generator,
- guarantee the best possible approximation of the area to be treated by the 3D distribution (coverage) of Specific Absorption Rate (SAR).

Our applicators (working at 434 MHz and at 2450 MHz) were used for the treatment of more than 500 patients with superficial or subcutaneous tumour. Now, following new trends in this field, we continue our research in the important directions of deep local and regional applicators. Most important technical fields of microwave thermotherapy development (covered also by our activities) can be specified as:

- Applicators: development and optimization of new applicators for more effective local, intracavitary and regional treatment,
- Treatment planning: mathematical and experimental modelling of the effective treatment
- Non-invasive temperature measurement: research of the possibilities of new techniques like Magnetic Resonance Imaging (MRI) and Ultrasound (US) for exact non-invasive measurements.
- Microwave medical diagnostics - e.g. Microwave Tomography (MT).

3. Applicators for microwave thermotherapy

Simulations of SAR distribution obtained by array of microwave applicators radiating at frequency 434 MHz will be described here. We will compare here the SAR distribution in a homogeneous agar phantom (which has similar dielectric characteristics to muscle tissue) and in an anatomical based biological model, which has been developed from a Computer Tomography (CT) scan.

3.1 Waveguide applicators

Wave guide applicators are based on microwave waveguide technology. Major advantage of waveguide applicator is that EM field in theirs aperture is roughly at 50% of its area very near to the case of EM plane wave, which is the wave with the best homogeneity and gives us the deepest penetration into the treated area.

Mostly rectangular and circular waveguides are being used to build microwave thermotherapy applicator. Examples of mentioned applicators are given in the Fig. 2. Typically they are operating at 434 MHz (depth of efficient treatment is between 4 and 6 cm), in case of deeper treatment lower frequency must be selected . Waveguide applicators displayed in Fig. 2a. are filled by dielectric material in order to decrease their cut off frequency. Air filled Evanescent mode applicator (Fig. 2b.) is excited under its cut-off frequency.

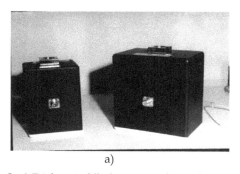
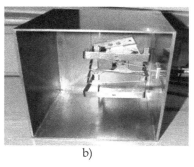

a)   b)

Fig. 2. a) Dielectric filled waveguide applicator, b) air filled Evanescent mode applicator.

On the next picture (Fig. 3.) there is a sketch of evanescent waveguide mode applicator working at 70 MHz, including its SAR distribution. There is a water bolus between aperture of the applicator and the agar phantom mimicking the biological tissue.

Interesting possibility how to achieve relatively sharp beam from external applicator is to use a focusing principle. The aperture of a standard rectangular waveguide applicator is then divided into 3 or 5 sectors with shifted excitation (i.e. different amplitude and phase). Another way how to focus microwave power is to use an array of external applicators, where amplitudes and phases of excitation of single applicators can be used for electronic steering of the focus area.

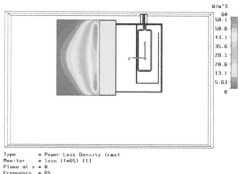

Fig. 3. Evanescent mode applicator and its calculated SAR pattern

3.2 Microwave stripline TEM applicators

Microwave stripline applicator with TEM (Transversal Electromagnetic Mode) is being described in the following. The TEM wave propagation depends on dielectric parameters, such as permittivity ε and permeability μ. The upper and bottom part of applicator consists of high conductivity material (copper). Transversal dimensions of the described applicator are 50 x 30 mm. Distance of exciting probe from short circuited section is 15 mm. Lateral sides of applicator are made from dielectric material, from acrylic glass, which is 2 mm thick. The second part of applicator consists of stripline horn. Dimensions of the horn aperture are 120 x 80 mm and length of applicator equals to two wavelengths. Wavelength depends on permittivity of environment (in our case $\varepsilon_{H20} = 78$). Whereas 70% of human body consists of water, applicator is filled with water. Advantage of this is better transfer of EM energy into human body and smaller dimensions of the applicator. This applicator was designed by the Finite Difference Time Domain (FDTD) simulator EM Field simulator (e.g. SEMCAD X).

3.3 Deep local heating applicators

Waveguide type applicators are very suitable for the deep local thermotherapy treatment based either on the principle of dielectric filled waveguide or on the principle of evanescent modes (i.e. waveguides excited below its cut-off frequency) - which is our specific solution and original contribution to the theory of microwave hyperthermia applicators. Technology of evanescent mode applicators enable us to design applicators with as small aperture as necessary also for relatively low frequencies e.g. from 10 to 100 MHz, needed for deep penetration into the biological tissue (i.e. up to 10 centimetres under the body surface). In theoretical and experimental evaluation, the grade of homogeneity of the temperature distribution in the target area has been tested, see the Fig. 4. Our mathematical approach is based on idea of waveguide TM_{01} (Transverse Magnetic) mode excited in the agar phantom under the given conditions (see the dashed lines). Measurement of SAR (full lines) has been done on agar phantom of the muscle tissue.

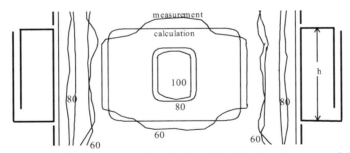

Fig. 4. Normalized SAR distribution (both calculated (full line) and measured (dashed line)) in the agar phantom.

3.4 New principles for the regional applicators

Goal of this work is the development of the new applicators with higher treatment effects. Methodological approach for the solution of the problem will be theoretical and experimental study of the new types of regional applicators. Our aim is to improve the present theoretical model to optimize the temperature distribution in the treated area.

We can design the regional applicators on the basis of the analytical description of the excited electromagnetic field for the case of simplified homogeneous model of the treated biological tissue. For a more realistic case of the non-homogeneous dielectric composition of the biological tissue the analytical calculation does not guarantee enough exact results. Therefore we would need to build the equipment for experimental tests of the applicators and we will study the possibilities of its numerical mathematical modelling.

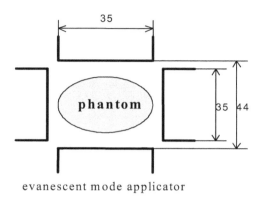

evanescent mode applicator

Fig. 5. Set up of proposed regional applicator (4 evanescent mode waveguides applicators)

Applicators must have perfect impedance matching for good protection of microwave generator against reflected power. For measurement of impedance matching a reflection parameter s_{11} is mostly used. This parameter shows, how much electromagnetic power is reflected back to generator. Electromagnetic field is inside discussed applicator excited at frequency of 434 MHz.

3.5 Anatomical model
To verify basic functionality of created applicator we can use a homogeneous agar phantom. This homogeneous phantom represents only one type of tissue in human body – in our case it represents muscle tissue. For further discussion we will use cylindrical agar phantom with diameter 8 cm, which can basically represent a human limb. In reality human body is very inhomogeneous, and therefore it is for hyperthermia treatment planning necessary to use anatomical precise 3D models with all types of biological tissues taken into account. 3D model thus can be created from segmentation of series of several scans from CT or MRI. Such scans are 2 dimensional transversal gray – scale cuts. After then is created 3D model imported to the program, which is used for hyperthermia treatment planning. This program must both cooperate well with a segmentation program and in the same moment to enable calculation of SAR distribution.

We can choose e.g. woman's calf (Fig. 6.) as an example to demonstrate EM simulations potential. Given anatomical model was created by segmentation program 3D – DOCTOR (vector-based 3D imaging, modelling and measurement software (Able Software Corp., 2011)). We should have available DICOM scans from CT (MRRF, 2010). DICOM scans hold the original quality of data. Model of woman's calf has resolution of 1 mm and mean voxel size is 1 x 1 x 1 mm.

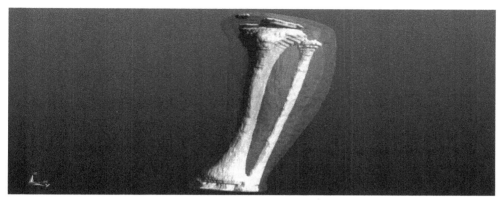

Fig. 6. 3D anatomical model of woman's calf

Each voxel was assigned to one of 3 different types of biological tissue, such as bone, muscle and fat with dielectric parameter shown in table (Table 1.).

Name	Conductivity [S/m]	Relative Permittivity [-]
Agar	0.80	54.00
Bone Cortical	0.09	13.07
Muscle	0.80	56.86
Fat	0.04	5.56

Table 2. Dielectric properties at frequency 434 MHz

3.6 Array of applicators

EM behaviour of arrays of 2, 3 and 4 stripline type applicators coupled to homogeneous cylindrical agar phantom and consequently on 3D anatomical model of woman's calf. Cylindrical agar phantom represents muscle tissue of human limb. In our case we simulated muscle tissue of woman's calf with diameter of 8 cm. The 3D anatomical model consists of 3 various types of tissue of woman's calf created from CT scans. All of here discussed arrays of applicators were simulated by FTDT program SEMCAD X.

3.6.1 Array of 2 microwave stripline applicators

Case of array of 2 applicators on cylindrical agar phantom coupled to 3D anatomical model of woman's calf is shown on following picture (Fig. 7.). From both normalized SAR distributions (Fig. 8.) it follows that this array of 2 applicators is suitable for treatment of tumor, which cover larger area near to surface of human limb.

3.6.2 Array of 3 microwave stripline applicators

The other possible configuration is array of 3 applicators coupled to homogeneous cylindrical agar phantom (Fig. 9a.). Consequently, we studied simulations of 3 applicators coupled to the 3D anatomical model (Fig. 9b.).

Another interesting case is shown on Fig. 10. –in this picture there are displayed interesting shapes of SAR distribution by change of phases of applicators and change of amplitude of one type of applicator located in the middle of all applicators.

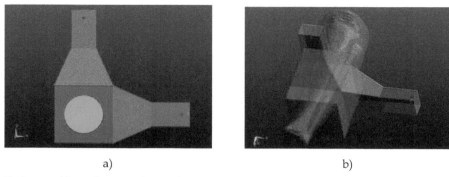

a)   b)

Fig. 7. Array of 2 applicators a) on cylindrical agar phantom, b) on anatomical model

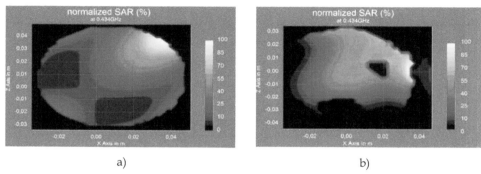

a)   b)

Fig. 8. Normalized SAR a) in agar phantom, b) in anatomical model

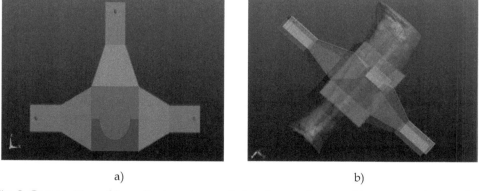

a)   b)

Fig. 9. Composition of 3 applicators a) on cylindrical agar phantom, b) on anatomical model

In homogeneous phantom were created 3 maxima, instead in anatomical model we can observe only one maximum of SAR distribution – that demonstrates very nice example of focussing possibilities. By setting of phases and/or amplitude of applicators we can accomplish required shape of SAR.

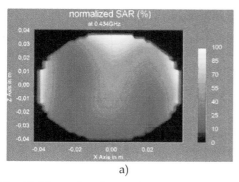 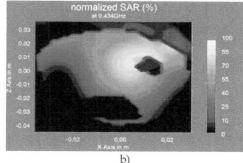

a)   b)

Fig. 10. Normalized SAR a) in agar phantom, b) in normalized SAR in anatomical model

3.6.3 Array of 4 microwave stripline applicators

By using 4 applicators we can see in following picture (Fig. 11.), that in both cases there is a very good focusing effect of SAR distribution near to the cylindrical axis.

By alternation of phases of several applicators we achieved better focusing in the middle of both homogeneous agar phantom and 3D anatomical model (Fig. 12.). Such array of 4 applicators could be used for treatment tumors located in the middle of human limb.

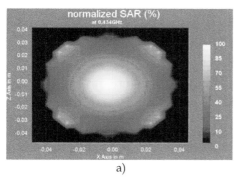 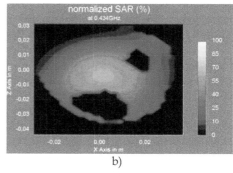

a)   b)

Fig. 12. Normalized SAR a) in agar phantom, b) in anatomical model

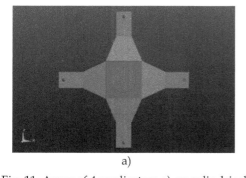 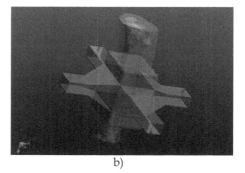

a)   b)

Fig. 11. Array of 4 applicators a) on cylindrical agar phantom, b) on anatomical model

4. Microwave applicators for „BPH" thermotherapy

In all above mentioned key activities we need to do numerical simulations of SAR and temperature 3D distribution. Temperature distribution inside area of biological tissue heated by microwave energy can be calculated from well known formula:

$$\rho_t c_t \frac{\partial T}{\partial t} = \gamma_t \Delta T - \chi(T - T_b) + q \qquad (1)$$

where t is the time.

$q = q(x,y,z,t)$	is energy delivered by EM field,
$T = T(x,y,z,t)$	is designates the temperature,
$Tb = Tb(x,y,z,t_o)$	is the temperature of blood,

Physical meaning and values of the here used constants for the case of high water contents tissue are:

$r_t = 0.965$ [g/cm3]	is density of biological tissue (BT).
$c_t = 3\ 586$ [mJ/g/C]	is specific heat of BT.
$k\ = 5.45$ [mW/cm3/C]	is blood flow and temperature capacity of BT.
$g_t = 5.84$ [mW/cm/C]	is spec. temp. conductivity of BT.

Possibilities of analytical solution of this equation are very limited to only a few cases - like e.g. "one dimensional" case of plane wave penetrating in homogeneous phantom. Therefore computers are to be used to solve this equation to obtain the temperature $T(x,y,z,t)$ time dependence and space distribution. For the treatment planning of microwave thermotherapy we use software product SEMCAD. Fig. 13 gives basic idea about SAR calculated for the case of the monopole intracavitary applicator.

4.1 Applicators for „BPH" treatment

We have investigated basic types of microwave intracavitary applicators suitable for BPH treatment, i.e. monopole, dipole and a helical coil structures. These applicators are designed to work either at 915 or at 434 MHz. We would like to discuss its effective heating depth, based on the comparison of the theoretical and experimental results. Basic mechanisms and parameters influencing (limiting) heating effective depth are described and explained in ref. (Vrba et al., 1996, 1999).

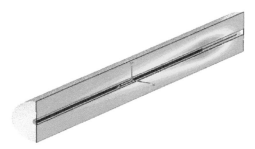

Fig. 13. Calculated SAR of BPH applicator

The basic type of intracavitary applicator is a monopole applicator. The construction of this applicator is very simple, but calculated and measured SAR distribution along the applicator is more complicated, than has been the first idea. SAR can be measured either in water phantom or by infrared camera.

4.2 Evaluation of BPH applicators

One of our tools for experimental evaluation of microwave applicators is the apparatus, which enable us to do 3D measurements of SAR distribution. It can be used for both local external and intracavitary applicators.

The basic part of this apparatus is big salt water phantom (water with 0.3% to 0.6% NaCl) and the measurement probe with the possibility of 3D scan around the applicators. As probes we use a Light Emitting Diodes (LED) with a fibber optic link connection to interface of the computer. The purpose of this link is to reduce influence of the metallic (i.e. conductive) components from the measured electromagnetic field. The schematics of the apparatus for 3D measurements of SAR distribution is shown in Fig. 14.

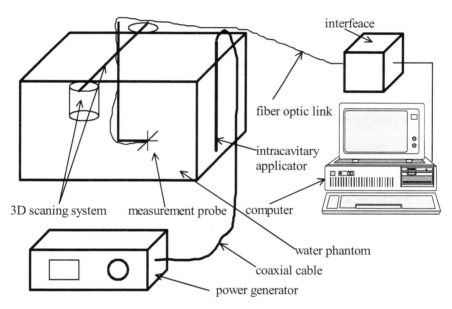

Fig. 14. Apparatus for 3D SAR measurements

During measurements of SAR along the applicator we have found, that typically there is not only a one main SAR maximum (first from the right side), but also a second and/or higher order maxima can be created, being produced by outside back wave propagating along the coaxial cable, see Fig. 15a. In Fig. 15b. SAR distribution improvement (i.e. reduction of second maximum) can be noticed for the case of dipole like applicator. To eliminate this second maximum and optimise the focusing of SAR in predetermined area of biological tissue needs to use the helical coil antenna structure.

After coil radius and length optimisation we have obtained very good results of SAR distribution, see Fig. 16a,b. Some problems can be with the antenna self-heating, but it can be reduced by cooler at the end of applicator tip.

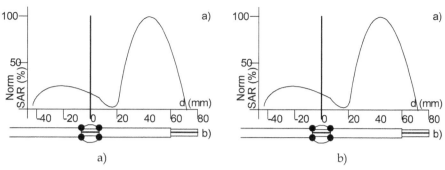

Fig. 15. a) Monopole applicator, b) Dipole applicator

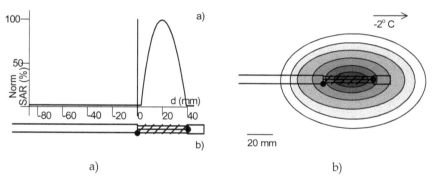

Fig. 16. a) Helical coil applicator, b) Temperature field around the helix

4.3 Effective treatment depth

We have studied the theoretical limits of intracavitary applicator heating depth. We have found the basic relation for determination of the limit of maximum heating depth for the case of "very long" intracavitary applicator. We suppose excitation of an ideal radial wave around radiating applicator.

Mentioned results can be simply interpreted by following figure, where on the horizontal axis is the working frequency of thermotherapy apparatus and on vertical axis there is effective depth of electromagnetic wave penetration. As a third parameter playing an important role there is a diameter of a discussed intracavitary applicator.

Very important is that in this case we are dealing with a radial wave, not the plane wave, and that's why the penetration depth is smaller than penetration depth of plane wave. Some works published in this field give too optimistic results. Measurements discussed without theoretical analysis can give results influenced by thermal conductivity of mostly used agar phantom of muscle tissue. As the real heating depth is typically a few millimetres (in the best case up to approx. 1 cm under the surface of the cavity), thermal conductivity of the phantom material can easily cause errors of several tenth of percents.

Ideal intracavitary applicator irradiates an ideal cylindrical wave into the biological tissue surrounding the cavity. According to our experience Fig. 17. gives very good approximation, i.e. the results with accuracy better than 5 % for higher frequencies (f >100 MHz) and/or bigger radii (R > 3mm). For lower frequencies (up to 100 MHz) combined with small radius of the cavity (R < 2 mm) the accuracy is cca 10 %. It is not possible to achieve a heating penetration depth (i.e. 50 % decrease) higher than R at any frequency and in any propagation medium. The small cavity radius plays a dominant role in the penetration depth.

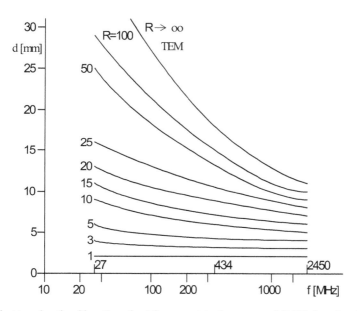

Fig. 17. Effective depth of heating d with respect to frequency f [MHz] and radius R [mm]

4.4 SAR measurements by infrared camera

Infrared camera is according to our experiences a very efficient tool for "SAR" measurements of microwave intracavitary applicators. In Fig. 18. there is the typical measured heating pattern of monopole (a), dipole (b), and helical coil antennas (c). This pattern can be obtained by heating suitable phantoms of biological tissue – mimicring the dielectric and thermal properties of the prostate tissue. Such phantoms can be made on the basis of agar or so called superstuff material. The pattern is colour-coded according to a linearly decreasing scale of white-yellow-red, where white is the maximum temperature. A diagrammatic catheter is inserted in each figure; the orientation of the bladder neck in a patient is indicated by a dashed line. Note the long back heating tails with a monopole antenna (Fig. 18a.) which is caused by microwave currents that flow backwards along the cable and cause the feeding cable to radiate. The radiation pattern from a dipole antenna (Fig. 18b.) is generally well confined without any excessive back heating. The dipole antenna is suitable for prostates with axial length > 40 mm. The helical coil antenna (Fig. 18c.) has the shortest and most focussed heating and would be the choice for small prostates, 25 – 40 mm in length.

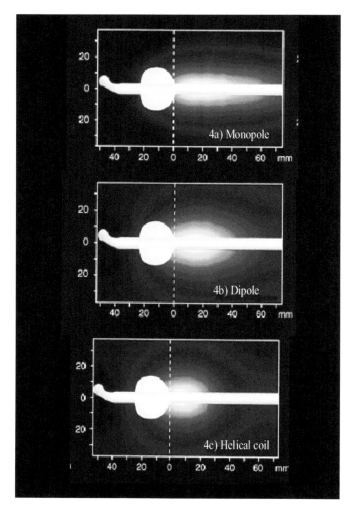

Fig. 18. The heating pattern for different antennas: a) the monopole, b) the dipole, c) the helical coil.

The pattern is colour-coded according to a linearly decreasing scale of white-yellow-red , where white is the maximum temperature. A diagrammatic catheter is inserted in each figure; the orientation of the bladder neck in a patient is indicated by a dashed line.

The pattern is colour-coded according to a linearly decreasing scale of white-yellow-red , where white is the maximum temperature. A diagrammatic catheter is inserted in each figure; the orientation of the bladder neck in a patient is indicated by a dashed line.

Moreover, by using infra-red camera we can follow a lot of other properties resp. behaviour of intracavitary applicators itself, like e.g. standing waves along feeding coaxial cable (i.e. the risk of existence of unwanted SAR and/or temperature maxima), possible overheating of some specific parts of tested applicator itself etc.

5. Technical equipment for research of biological effects of EM field

In present time four research institutions here in the Czech Republic run research projects focused on studies of interactions between EM field and biological systems. These institutions are technically supported by Dept. of EM Field of the Czech Technical University in Prague. In this contribution we would like to give more details about that projects and obtained technical results (i.e. description of developed exposition systems).

Three of discussed projects (1 in Germany and 2 here in Czech Republic) are basic research for simulation of the microwave hyperthermia treatment. Other two projects (both in Czech Republic are focused on simulation of the case of exposition by mobile phone.

In the modern view, cancer is intended as a complex illness, involving the cells that undergo to transformation, their environment, and the general responses at biochemical and biological levels induced in the host. Consequently, the anti-cancer treatment protocols need to be multi-modal to reach curative effects. Especially after the technical improvements achieved in the last 15 years by bio-medical engineering, microscopy devices, and molecular biology methods, the combinations of therapeutic procedures are growing in interest in basic and clinical research.

The combination of applied biological research together to the physical sciences can offer important perspectives in anticancer therapy (e.g. different methodologies and technical devices for application of energies to pathological tissues).

The modern bioengineering knowledge applied to traditional tools, as the microscopy, has largely renewed and expanded the fields of their applications (e.g.: in vivo imaging), pushing the interest for direct morpho-functional investigations of the biomedical problems.

5.1 Waveguide applicator

Very good results of EM field expositions in biological experiments can be obtained by simple but efficient waveguide applicators see example in Fig. 19. Waveguide offer a very big advantage – in approximately of fifty percents of its aperture the irradiated electromagnetic field is very near to a plane wave, which is basic assumption for good homogeneity of the heating and optimal treatment penetration.

Here described system is being used (shared) for research projects by two institutions (Institute of Radiation Oncology in Prague and Institute of Microbiology of the Czech Academy of Sciences).

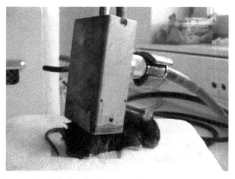

Fig. 19. Waveguide applicator for biological experiments

Aperture of this waveguide is 4.8 x 2.4 cm and it is excited at frequency 2.45 GHz. Effective heating is in the middle of the real aperture – its size is approximately 2.4 x 2.4 cm. Waveguide is filled by teflon to reduce its cut-off frequency. Power from generator is possible to control from 10 to 180 W, in these experiments we work between 10 and 20 W mostly.

5.2 Evaluation of waveguide applicator

To evaluate this applicator from technical point of view we made a series of experiments, see e.g. Fig. 20, where you can see example of measurement of temperature distribution by IR camera.

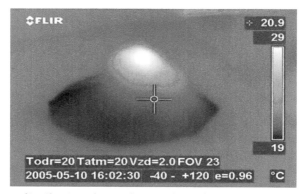

Fig. 20. Temperature distribution obtained on surface of a model of mouse

Here you can see temperature distribution obtained on surface of a model of mouse made from agar – with a simulated tumour on mouse back. Experiment has been done by heating phantom during 2 minutes delivering a power of 10 W. Maximum of temperature increase has been found approximately 10 °C. Similar results with different increase in temperature we have got also in other technical experiments on phantom or live mouse when power or heating time was changed.

Next Fig. 21. gives example of temperature increase on the surface of the phantom and 1 cm in that phantom. Temperature was measured by our 4-chanel thermometer. In this case with two thermo probes. Heating here is scheduled to 9 times repeated 30 s of heating and 30 s pause. Difference in temperature on the surface and under it is on the level of 1 °C. That means very good homogeneity of temperature distribution in the treated area during planned biological experiments.

5.3 Array applicator

The main goal of the planned biological experiment is a hyperthermia treatment of the experimentally induced pedicle tumours of the rat to verify the feasibility of ultrasound diagnostics and magnetic resonance imaging respectively to map the temperature distribution in the target area of the treatment. That means to heat effective volume of approximately cylindrical shape (diameter approx. 2 cm, height approx. 3 cm). Temperature to be reached is 41 °C or more (i.e. temperature increase of at least 4 °C from starting point 37 °C), time period of heating is 45 minutes.

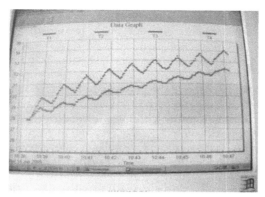

Fig. 21. Temperatures during experiments

Considering the necessary effective heating depth for the planned experiments, we have found 915 MHz to be suitable frequency. As an excellent compatibility of the applicator with non-invasive temperature measurement system (ultrasound or NMR) is a fundamental condition for our project, we should have to use non-magnetic metallic sheets of minimised dimensions to create the conductive elements of the applicator. Therefore the applicator itself (see Fig. 22.) is created by two inductive loops tuned to resonance by capacitive elements (Vrba, 1993). Dimensions of these resonant loops were designed by our software, developed for this purpose. Coupling between coaxial feeder and resonant loops (not shown in Fig. 22.) as well as a mutual coupling between resonating loops could be adjusted to optimum by microwave network analyser.

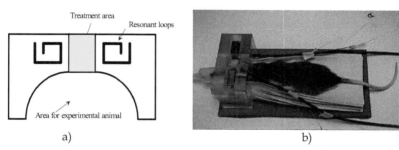

a)   b)

Fig. 22. a) Arrangement of discussed microwave hyperthermia applicator, b) Photograph of the discussed applicator

The position of the loops is fixed by perspex holder. There is a special cylindrical space for experimental animal in lower part of this perspex holder. As the heated tissue has a high dielectric losses, both loops are very well separated and so no significant resonance in heated area can occur. From this follows, that either the position of the loops with respect to heated area or the distance between the loops is not very critical.

First measurements to evaluate the basic properties of the discussed applicator were done on agar phantom of muscle tissue:

- evaluation of basic microwave properties (transfer of EM energy to the tissue, reflections),

- evaluation of compatibility with US and NMR,
- calculation and measurement of SAR and temperature distribution and its homogeneity.

Exact tuning of the resonant loops to frequency 915 MHz has been easy and we could optimise the coupling between the coaxial feeders and resonant loops as well, reflection coefficient less than 0.1. We have tested the power to be delivered to the applicator to obtain sufficient temperature increase (approximately 4 °C in less than 5 minutes is required). With power 10 W delivered to each loop for period of 2 minutes we succeeded to obtain the temperature increase of approximately 7 °C. To keep the increased temperature for a long time, 2 W in each loops were sufficient. Similar values were obtained during first experiments on rats also. Even with higher level of delivered microwave power we did not observe the change of resonant frequency (caused by increased temperature of the loops). This applicator has been developed for German Cancer Research Institute in Heidelberg. And it is being used there for a series of animal experiments to study effect of hyperthermia on tumours and possibility to combine hyperthermia with chemotherapy etc.

Compatibility of this applicator with a Magnetic resonance unit (MR) has been studied and it has been demonstrated. We have tested the influence of the applicators on US diagnostics and NMR imaging and the result of this evaluation shows very good compatibility. Only a negligible deterioration of the US images has been observed when the incident power was kept under 100 W.

Details about influence of microwave power on MR imaging are given in Fig. 23. We can see here a sequence of images of the discussed applicator made by MR unit for four different cases. First case (upper left) is image for the case without power excitation of the applicator. Second case (left down) a power of 10 W has been delivered to each loop. We can see quite clear configuration of the applicator set-up. Third case (upper right) gives situation when 20 W has been delivered to each loop. Slight noise but still quite a clear configuration of the applicator set-up can be observed. Fourths case (right down) gives situation when 40 W has been delivered to each loop. In this case noise disturbed the possibility to observe the configuration of the applicator.

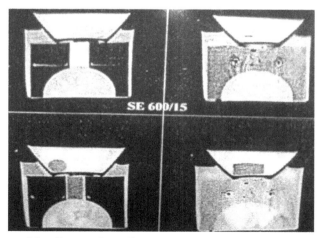

Fig. 23. MR images of the discussed applicator

In Fig. 25. we can see temperature vs. time measurement in the case of agar phantom inserted in the studied applicator. Next Fig. 26. shows experimental setup of applicator and simple exposure chambers installed at Medical Faculty of Charles University in Pilsen. 3D distribution of SAR distribution was verified numerically (Fig. 24).

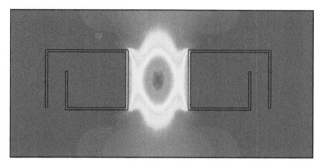

Fig. 24. Numerical SAR analysis.

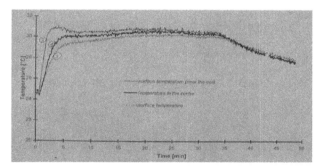

Fig. 25. Temperature measurements

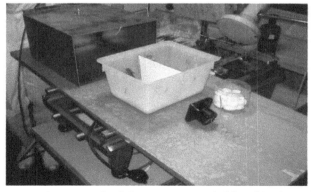

Fig. 26. Exposure system for research of electromagnetic field and biological system interactions

6. Measurement of the complex permittivity of the biological tissue as the possible imaging method

6.1 Introduction

This sub-chapter describes and evaluates a method for determining complex permittivity, and presents results of permittivity measurement of inhomogeneous agar phantom and living tissue. There are described different approaches for measurement of complex permittivity, in particular the non-invasive method of measuring complex permittivity at the end of the coaxial cable. Vector measurement of the reflection coefficient on the interface between probes and measured samples is performed with the aid of network analyzer in the frequency range from 300 kHz to 2 GHz. The results indicate that using the coaxial probe with dimensions of SMA (subminiature version A) connector is suitable in the frequency range approximately from 300 MHz to 10 GHz. In order to demonstrate the diagnostic potential of this method, measurements were first conducted on artificially created inhomogeneous agar phantom with added mixture of various dielectrics, followed by measurement of living biological tissue.

6.2 Complex permittivity

Relative permittivity, loss factor and conductivity are basic parameters for electromagnetic field modeling and simulations. Although these parameters could be found in the tables for many materials, their experimental determination is very often necessary (Hippel, 1954). Dielectric properties of biological tissues are determining factors for the dissipation of electromagnetic energy in the human body and therefore they are useful in hyperthermia cancer treatment. Measurement of the dielectric parameters of biological tissues is also a promising method in the medical diagnostics and imaging. Knowledge of the complex permittivity in an treated area, i.e. knowledge of the complex permittivity of healthy and tumor tissue, is very important for example in the diagnosing of tumor regions in the human body (Choi et al., 2004) or in the design of thermo-therapeutic applicators which transform electromagnetic energy into thermal energy in the tissue (Williams et al., 2008). Permittivity is known as

$$\varepsilon = \varepsilon_0 \varepsilon_c \qquad (2)$$

where ε_0 is free space permittivity and ε_c is complex relative permittivity. Complex relative permittivity can be written as

$$\varepsilon_c = \varepsilon_r - j\varepsilon_r \tan \delta \qquad (3)$$

where ε_r is real part of complex relative permittivity and $\tan \delta$ is loss factor.

6.3 Methods of complex permittivity measurement

The most commonly used method for measuring the complex permittivity is a method of measuring dielectric inserted into a dielectric waveguide. This method is very accurate, but unfortunately requires irreversible changes in the measured material. Another method used for measurement of complex permittivity is RLC measuring bridge. This method is very accurate but there are a few requirements on the quality of the interfaces of the measured material and the capacitor plates (Thompson, 1956). In most cases, this method is used as narrowband. The method of measurement in free space has its limitations in the demand for high-loss dielectrics measured. Electromagnetic wave through the material must be attenuated by at least 10 dB. Otherwise, standing waves will be created, which contribute significantly to the inaccuracy of this method. The method of measurement in cavity resonators gives us results with good accuracy. On the other hand, it is difficult to produce precise machining of the resonator and the measured material inserted inside (Ramachandraiah et al., 1975). Latest often used method for measuring complex permittivity measurement method is the open end of the waveguide, in our case, the coaxial cable. This method can be considered as very accurate. Moreover, we can achieve a good repetition of the results when we maintain the phase stability of the measuring coaxial cable (Tanaba & Joines, 1976). In this work, this application was selected for the main method for measuring complex permittivity of biological tissues because of its non-invasive nature.

6.3.1 Principle of reflection method

The reflection method represents measurement of reflection coefficient on the interface between two materials, on the open end of the coaxial line and the material under test. It is a well-known method for determining the dielectric parameters (Tanaba & Joines, 1976). This method is based on the fact that the reflection coefficient of an open-ended coaxial line depends on the dielectric parameters of material under test which is attached to it. For calculating the complex permittivity from the measured reflection coefficient, it is useful to use an equivalent circuit of an open-ended coaxial line. The probe translates changes in the permittivity of a material under test into changes of the input reflection coefficient of the probe. The surface of the sample of material under test must be in perfect contact with the probe. The thickness of a measured sample must be at least twice of equivalent penetration depth of the electromagnetic wave. This assures that the waves reflected from the material under test interface are attenuated (Stuchly et al., 1994).

6.4 Measurement probes

For measurement probes, we have adapted the standard N and SMA RF connectors from which the parts for connecting to a panel were removed. The measurement probes can be described by the equivalent circuit consisting of the coupling capacitance between the inner and outer conductor out of the coaxial structure and radiating conductance which represents propagation losses (Popovic el al., 2005). These capacitance and conductance are frequency and permittivity dependent.

6.4.1 N probe

Probe for measuring the complex permittivity of biological tissues has been adapted from a standard RF connector for coaxial cable N-type connector, see Fig. 27. The original proposed range of application was f_{BW} = 1 GHz, which together with the development of microwave technology is extended until today's f_{BW} = 12 GHz. N connector used in the construction of the probe is standard N 50Ω connector that can be used up to frequency f = 5 GHz. The measurements were kept with a high degree of the accuracy and repeatability. The measurement probe based on N connectors had significantly less bandwidth, and f_1 = 100 MHz and f_2 = 1 GHz.

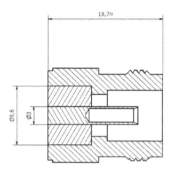
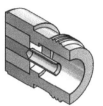

Fig. 27. Basic scheme of the N probe's dimensions

6.4.2 SMA probe

Probe for measuring the complex permittivity based on the SMA-connector was adapted from a standard 50 Ω SMA connector which was developed around 1960 when it was required to create a miniaturized version of the N connector with a higher frequency range of application. Today SMA connectors operate in the band up to f = 18 GHz. SMA connector used for the production of SMA probes, Fig. 28. shows low-cost, standard RF connectors with a usable bandwidth up to f = 12 GHz. This solution is appropriate for the purposes of our measurements because the highest frequency measured is equal to f = 2 GHz.

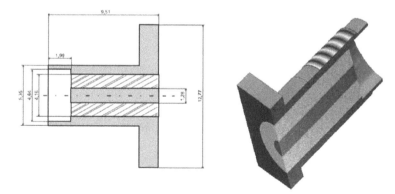

Fig. 28. Basic scheme of the SMA probe's dimensions

6.5 Measurement setup

A typical measurement setup using the reflection method on an open-ended coaxial line consists of the network analyzer, the coaxial probe and software. Our measurements were done with the aid of Agilent 6052 network analyzer in the frequency range from 300 MHz to 3 GHz. First the calibration of the vector network analyzer is performed. Then the calibration using a reference material is done. Finally, the reflection coefficient of material under test is measured. The complex permittivity of material under test is evaluated by the MATLAB.

6.5.1 Measurement on inhomogeneous agar phantom

The initial measurements on the inhomogeneous agar phantom were performed (Fig. 29.). As the simulations shows that the effective penetration depth in both cases, for N probe and SMA probe, is an interval of 4 mm to 2 mm depending on the frequency of measurement. Therefore, in this model of inhomogeneous agar phantom, strange dielectric immersion depths lies in the range from 4 mm to 1 mm. Thus, the purpose of this measurement was to detect strange dielectrics that are covered with an agar layer in terms of simulating the electrical parameters of human skin and soft tissue. Inhomogeneous agar phantom was covered with a regular square grid (30 points x 30 points), with the 900 points of measurement. Subsequently, measurements were taken at these points by the N probe and SMA-probe.

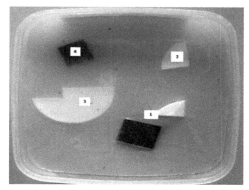

Fig. 29. Inhomogeneous agar phantom setup, the number shows the depth of strange dielectrics submersion

6.5.2 Measurement on biological tissue

The final verification of each experiment is necessary for practical usage. In our case, the experiment consisted of measuring the real biological tissue - the left upper limb of the first author (Fig. 30.). For this measurement, the SMA probe was used due to its ability to operate in higher bandwidth, and also because of its smaller size, and therefore a higher lateral resolution. The author's arm was marked with equidistant grid of measuring points, which then for-SMA probe measurements were carried out over a bandwidth of f_{MIN} = 300 MHz to f_{MAX} = 2 GHz. Measurements were carried out very quickly with a delay of 1s and 2s at each measuring point. The data was saved (with the help of an assistant) in CSV data format in the flash drive connected to the vector analyzer. Frequency sweep was set at 1600 points at a bandwidth of f_{MIN} = 300 MHz to f_{MAX} = 2 GHz and averaging was set to 16 in order to eliminate unwanted noise.

6.6 Results

The data presented here, obtained from measurements of the inhomogeneous phantom agar, are interpreted as a contour graph. Then there is the measurement on the left upper extremity of the author, which is displayed as contour graphs. All measurements were made in the band f_{MIN} = 300 MHz to f_{MAX} = 2 GHz, from whom were selected three representative frequencies f_1 = 500 MHz, f_2 = 1 GHz and f_3 = 2 GHz.

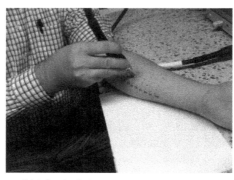

Fig. 30. Measurement on real biological tissue

6.6.1 Results of measurement on inhomogeneous agar phantom

For the measurement on inhomogeneous agar phantom was designed with a submerged object of Teflon ε_r = 2.1 and Bakelite ε_r = 4.1, immersed in a variable depth of 4 mm to 1 mm into the agar phantom. After solidify of the agar surface was applied spatially equidistant grid (30 x 30) with 900 data points.

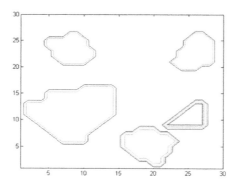

Fig. 31. Results of the measurement on inhomogeneous agar phantom (contour graph of real part of complex permittivity on frequency f = 500 MHz)

Measurements were performed by the SMA probe. Obtained values of the real part of complex permittivity have been rewritten into MATLAB and displayed as a contour graph image, see Fig. 31. The results of the measurement on the inhomogeneous agar phantom have shown the potential of imaging usability of this method for further investigations on real living tissue.

6.6.2 Results of measurement on biological tissue

Testing the imaging potential for complex permittivity measurement of biological tissue was finally performed on the left upper extremity of the author, see Fig. 30. SMA probe was used for this measurement. For a small separation of complex permittivity of biological tissue, these data are displayed only in the contour graph. It is very difficult to assess tissue formations without further visual assessment, using MRI and subsequent processing of data segmentation algorithms, but the Fig. 32a,b. shows that contours of real part of complex permittivity during the various measurements still occur in the same places. Among the limitations of the method, we can mention a small depth of penetration shown in Fig. 32c) at frequency f = 2000 MHz; as a result, we can register only the layer of skin. The actual depth of penetration can be improved by using of probes based on the waveguide thus having a greater radiating aperture that would better achieve the quasi-plane waves, but the loss of lateral resolution of the probe. Overcoming this eternal compromise can be achieved through a combination of two probes for a single measurement, one with an emphasis on greater penetration depth and the second for acceptable lateral resolution. When comparing the results of this measurement shown in Fig. 32., we can find among them a high degree of correlation pointing out that in real biological tissue this measuring method will able to detect coherent tissue structure having the same value of the real part of complex permittivity.

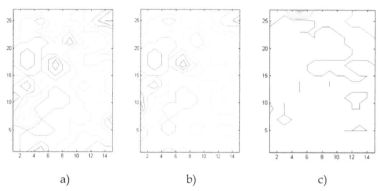

a)   b)   c)

Fig. 32. Results of the measurement on real biological tissue (contour graph of real part of complex permittivity on frequency a) f1 = 500 MHz, b) f2 = 1 GHz, c) f3 = 2 GHz

6.7 Evaluation

Measurements on inhomogeneous agar phantom showed the potential of this imaging method, because the strange dielectrical materials were detectable beneath the surface of agar. Based on this result, the measurement of the left upper extremity of the author was performed, and the contour map of the real part of complex permittivity shown the detectable difference between the tissues. The contour graphs of the real part of complex permittivity of biological tissue give us the hope for the future development that this method may be used as a imaging method. After proving more interaction on the pathological changes in tissues, such as growth of tumor tissue, we can consider this method for diagnostic purposes.

7. Conclusions

Research described

8. Acknowledgment

Research described in this chapter was supported by Grant Agency of the Czech Republic, projects: 102/08/H081:„Non-standard application of physical fields - analogy, modelling, verification and simulation" and P102/11/0649: „Research and measurements of signals generated by nanoparticles". Further by research program MSM6840770012: "Transdisciplinary Research in the Area of Biomedical Engineering II" of the CTU in Prague, sponsored by the Ministry of Education, Youth and Sports of the Czech Republic.

9. References

Able Software Corp. (2011). 3D-DOCTOR, 3D Imaging, Modeling, Rendering and Measurement Software, Available from: http://www.ablesw.com/3d-doctor

Bolmsjö, M.; Wagrell, L.; Hallin, A.; Eliasson, T.; Erlandsson, B.E. & Mattiasson, A. (1996). The heat is on - but how? A comparison of TUMT devices. *The Journal of Urology*, Vol.78, pp. 564-572

Choi, J.; Cho, Y. Lee, J. Yim, B.; Kang, K. & et al. (2004). Microwave detection of metastasized breast cancer cells in the lymph node, potential application for sentinel lymphadenectomy, In: Breast Cancer Research and Treatment, Vol.86, No.2, pp. 107-115, Springer, ISSN 0167-6806

De la Rosette, J.; D'Ancona, F. & Debruyne, F. (February 1997). Current status of thermotherapy of the prostate, *The Journal of Urology*, Vol.157, pp. 430-438

Franconi, C.; Vrba, J. & Montecchia, F. (1993). 27 MHz Hybrid Evanescent-Mode Applicators. *International Journal of Hyperthermia*, Vol.9, No.5, pp. 655 – 673

Hand, J. & James, J. R. (1986). *Physical Techniques in Clinical Hyperthermia*. Wiley, New York

Hippel, A. (1954). Dielectric Materials and Applications. Technology Press of MIT, Cambridge, 1954, pp. 71-75

Popovic, D.; McCartney, L.; Beasley, C.; Lazebnik, M.; Okoniewski, M.; Hagness, S.C. & Booske, J.H. (2005). Precision open-ended coaxial probes for in vivo and ex vivo dielectric spectroscopy of biological tissues at microwave frequencies. *IEEE Transactions on Microwave Theory and Techniques*, Vol.53, No.5, pp. 1713-1722, ISSN 0018-9480

Ramachandraiah, M. S. & Decreton, M. C. (December 1975). A Resonant Cavity Approach for the Nondestructive Determination of Complex Permittivity at Microwave Frequencies. *Instrumentation and Measurement, IEEE Transactions on Instrumentation and Measurement*, Vol.24, No.4, pp.287-291, ISSN 0018-9456

Tanaba, E. & Joines, W. T. (1976). A nondestructive method for measurement of the complex permittivity of dielectric materials at microwave frequency using an open-ended coaxial line resonator. *IEEE Trans. on Measurement and Instrumentation*, Vol.25, pp. 222-226, ISSN 0018-9480

Thompson, A. M. (November 1956). A bridge for the measurement of permittivity. *Proceedings of the IEE - Part B: Radio and Electronic Engineering*, Vol.103, No.12, pp. 704-707

Vrba, J.; Franconi, C. & Lapeš, M. (1996). Theoretical Limits for the Penetration Depth of the Intracavitary Applicat. *International Journal of Hyperthermia*, No.6., pp.737 – 742

Vrba, J.; Franconi, C.; Montecchia, F. & Vannucci, I. (May 1993). Evanescent-Mode Applicators for Hyperthermia. *IEEE Trans.on Biomedical Engineering*, Vol.40, No.5, pp. 397-407

Vrba, J.; Lapeš, M. & Oppl, L. (1999). Technical aspects of microwave thermotherapy. *Bioelectrochemistry and Bioenergetics*, Vol.48, pp. 305 – 309

Williams, T. C.; Sill, J.M. & Fear, E.C. (May 2008). Breast surface estimation for radar-based breast imaging systems. *IEEE Transactions on Biomedical Engineering*, Vol.55, No.6, pp. 1678-1686, ISSN 0018-9294

7

Photon Total Body Irradiation for Leukemia Transplantation Therapy: Rationale and Technique Options

Brent Herron, Alex Herron, Kathryn Howell,
Daniel Chin and Luann Roads
PSL Medical Center, Denver
USA

1. Introduction

Leukemia is a classification of disease in which the two major defects are unregulated proliferation and incomplete maturation of the hemopoietic progenitors (Scheinberg, Maslak, & Weiss, 2001). Leukemia originates in the marrow, although leukemia cells may infiltrate lymph nodes, liver, spleen, and other tissues. Scheinberg et al. (2001) describe the principal clinical manifestation is the decrease of red cells and platelets as a result of the suppression of normal hemopoiesis or turnover and repopulation of blood components. In the chronic leukemias, unregulated proliferation of leukemia cells and elevated white cell count dominate. Differentiation and maturation of the leukemia cells may be largely preserved. Scheinberg further characterizes acute leukemias with unregulated proliferation also, but the maturation of the leukemia progenitors is profoundly impaired.

Transplantation of blood products, in particular stem cells, has become a common treatment procedure for various types of leukemias since the early 1990's (Scheinberg, Maslak, & Weiss, 2001). Cells void of leukemia are transplanted into the leukemia patient. The purpose of the transplant is the repopulation of the non-cancerous cells. Urbano-Ispizua et al. (2002) describes the current practice of stem cell transplantation for hematological diseases, solid tumors and immune disorders. Definitions, abbreviations and classifications described in this review are summarized here.

Hemopoietic stem cell transplantation (HSCT) refers to any procedure where hemopoietic cells of any donor type and any source are given to a recipient with the intention of repopulation/replacing the hemopoietic system of the recipient in total or in part (Urbano-Ispizua et al., 2002). Human Leukocyte Antigen (HLA) matching is a six point scoring system that identifies antigens and antibodies for both donor and recipient. Allogenic and autologous implants are also characterized by Urbano-Ispizua, et al (2002). Allogenic implants are procedures in which the recipient receives stem cells from a related or unrelated donor whose HLA score is identical (HLA score=6) or nearly identical (HLA score=5) to the recipient. Autologous implants refer to procedures in which the recipient receives stem cells from a collection performed while the patient is in remission or leukemia-free.

Bone marrow and cerebral spinal fluid peripheral cells are standard sources of hemopoietic stem cells (Urbano-Ispizua et al, 2002). For autologous HSCT, peripheral blood has become the preferred choice in view of its more rapid hemopoietic reconstitution. For allogenic HSCT, both sources are used. Both methods have their specific advantages and disadvantages. There are marked differences in toxicity concerning the donors. For recipients, the final issue concerning long-term outcome remains open. Peripheral blood is associated with more rapid engraftment or repopulation in the recipient. Urbano-Ispizua (2002) warns of a major concern with allogenic transplantation with peripheral blood is the high incidence of chronic graft-versus-host disease. That is, the recipient's immune system rejects the donor cells. In general, cord blood transplantation is recommended when patients require allogenic transplantation and do not have an HLA identical or a one-antigen mismatched donor.

Both allogenic and autologous implants are performed subsequent to subjecting the leukemia patient to intensity conditioning regimens (Shank, 1998). Despite the classification of the patient as in remission or disease-free, there is still significant opportunity that undetected leukemia cells are still present and will repopulate along with the transplanted stem cells. Shank describes the conditioning regimen's intent is to reduce the likelihood of the leukemia cell re-growth. Conditioning regimens include intense chemotherapy or radiation therapy or a combination of both. The intensity of these treatments is severe. Shank cautions of the fine balance between transplant-related mortality and the risk of relapse or repopulation of the leukemia cells.

The role of radiation therapy in the preparation of patients for bone marrow transplantation is the primary focus of this chapter. The primary utilization of radiation in oncology management is the use of small (less than 100 sq.cm) beams or fields directed at localized solid tumors (Bentel, 1992). Since leukemia cells are present throughout the body, large fields encompassing the entire body are necessary. This type of radiation treatment is referred to as Total Body Irradiation (TBI) or sometimes as Magna Field Irradiation (Shank, 1998). In her review article, Shank cites sole use TBI did not eradicate all leukemia cells. The addition of chemotherapy such as cyclophosphamide (CY) provides a reduced recurrence rate. Shank notes that although a large number of regimens now combine chemotherapeutic agents with and without TBI for marrow ablation, combined therapy of CY and TBI remains the standard for comparison.

Irradiation holds several advantages over chemotherapy as a systemic agent (Shank, 1998). These advantages include a lack of crossreactivity with other agents, dose homogeneity independent of blood supply, no requirements for detoxification and excretion, and the ability to tailor dose distribution within the body by shielding areas of greater sensitivity or boosting the radiation dose in areas that may contain additional disease. This discussion will focus primarily on the clinical aspects of TBI. Technical aspects of providing these large fields will also be addressed..

2. Total body irradiation: Criteria and nuances

Bentel (1992) describes standard methodology of radiation oncology treatments. Standard radiation therapy treatments are provided utilizing a linear accelerator with x-ray energies approximately 100 times greater than conventional machines used for chest or dental x-rays. The accelerator is capable of rotating 360 degrees about a patient with the center of rotation placed within the tumor volume. Typically, 2-6 fields or beams are directed at the tumor volume from various angles. A criterion for field arrangement is accounting for dose uniformity within the tumor volume. That is, large variations in dose throughout the tumor are rarely acceptable. Bentel continues by specifying that additional beams will aid with dose uniformity. Beam angulation is determined by the desire to "spare" or reduce the radiation dose to non-malignant or non-cancerous tissue or organs. In most cases, the delivered radiation dose to the tumor is limited by normal tissue or organ tolerance in areas surrounding or close to the tumor volume (Bentel, 1997). Radiation doses are expressed in units of centigray (cGy) which is equivalent to the more common unit rad. Typical dose levels for standard non-TBI treatments are 4500-7000 cGy. Field dimensions are usually 100-200 sq.cm therefore; the fields are roughly 5 inches by 5 inches. Dose uniformity criteria is typically +/- 5%. The standard treatment distance from the housing of the accelerator is 100cm.

Van Dyk (2000) addresses the degree of accuracy required for total body irradiation treatments. As the specification of dose becomes less certain, disease control can be affected. In addition, undesirable radiation induced side effects can be pronounced. Van Dyk cites research that a 5% change in dose could result in a 20% change in the incidence of radiation pneumonitis. Under such circumstances, it is difficult to argue that +/- 5% accuracy is sufficient. Conversely, if the prescribed dose is well below the onset of radiation pneumonitis and if the dose is sufficient for adequate tumor control, then perhaps the guideline of +/- 5% accuracy can be relaxed and +/- 10% or even +/- 15% may be sufficiently accurate. The beam arrangement for total body irradiation is typically chosen with +/- 10% accuracy and uniformity criteria.

For large field radiotherapy, the delivery of a uniform dose of radiation over the entire target volume is not a trivial task. The irradiation method must be devised to produce radiation fields large enough to cover the entire body adequately. With this larger field size requirement, the patient is positioned further from the linear accelerator than the standard 100cm treatment distance. The increased distance takes advantage of the spread or divergence of the radiation field from the accelerator. The treatment distance can vary depending on the accelerator vault size, but is typically 350 to 500cm. The treatment distance for the TBI procedure represents a few additional problems (Lindsey & Deeg, 1998). These distances can be difficult to achieve in some linear accelerator vaults. Counter tops or other equipment will need to be removed. Since the patient will not be on the standard treatment couch at this extended distance, another adjustable patient support table must be acquired or fabricated.

Dose uniformity is a major concern for the TBI process and the technique option chosen (Bradley et al., 1998). Bentel (1992) describes the principle of radiation absorption. The absorption of radiation is exponentially proportional to the thickness of the different body sections of the patient. The variance between absorption and dose between thinner and thicker body sections is more pronounced as the x-ray energy is decreased. Therefore, higher x-ray energy aids the dose uniformity criteria. Fletcher describes a negative side to the use of higher x-ray energy. Unfortunately, higher x-ray energies provide decreased entrance dose with the first 2cm of the patient. That is, high energy x-rays will provide a more uniform dose in tissue only after the first 2cm. Therefore, the use of a x-ray energy greater than 4MV require the addition of an acrylic sheet placed in close proximity to the patient (Bradley et al., 1998). This acrylic sheet serves as a "beam spoiler" and produces scatter radiation that allows the entrance 2cm of tissue to receive a higher and more adequate dose.

Even with the use of high-energy x-rays and beam spoilers, the dose uniformity across the patient and from thicker to thinner body sections may not meet the +/- 10% criteria (Bredeson et al., 2002). Dose uniformity will improve if opposed beams are used. As shown and described in Figure 1, the beam can be directed from different sources (item d) or by changing the patient position from supine to prone. If a two-beam arrangement is utilized, half of the radiation dose is provided by one beam. The patient is rotated or the source of radiation is moved and the remaining dose is provided. Typically, two fields are adequate to provide acceptable dose homogeneity for TBI treatments (Bredeson et al., 2002).

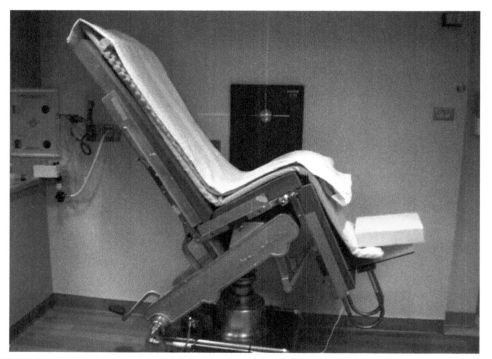

Fig. 1. Front view of TBI table used for opposed lateral treatments with couch sections angled at 45°.

Large variations in patient thickness, e.g. head thickness compared to shoulder thickness, pose problems with dose uniformity that multiple fields cannot resolve (Bredeson et al., 2002). Galvin and D'Angio and Walsh (2000) and Lin and Chu (2001) have described methods for compensating for the lack of patient thickness in certain areas such as the head or feet. The addition of rice bags or water-filled bags serves as adequate substitutes in these areas of decreased thickness. Rice or water exhibits the same attenuation characteristics as human tissue. Therefore, packing the patient or filling voids with these materials presents the patient as a uniform thickness. Therefore absorption variations are minimized.

The parameters used to characterize the x-ray beam at the standard 100cm distance will not necessarily apply to the extended distance (Van Dyk, 2000). Beam profiles and output calibration of the linear accelerator at the treatment position will need to be measured.

Verification of the attenuation of the beam should be made with anthropomorphic or tissue equivalent phantoms. Scatter radiation from other components within the room, such as walls and equipment, will apply to this extended distance large field treatment and should be accounted.

One of the major complications of large field radiotherapy is radiation pneumonitis (Corns et al., 2000). For total lung radiation, this syndrome is lethal in 80% of the patients who develop it. Because of this effect, Corns et al. (2000) warns that it is imperative that the dose to the lung be precisely controlled to ensure the probability of its occurrence is minimal. Even in standard radiation treatments, a calculation of the lung dose requires density corrections to the standard attenuation data (Bentel, 1992). The lower density lungs will transmit more radiation than regular more dense tissue. Several methods have been developed to correct for the lower density lung tissue and provide an accurate accounting of dose in this region (Bentel, 1992). Unfortunately, these calculations vary in ease of use as well as in the resulting correction factor. Van Dyk (2000) has calculated the correction factor from four of the most popular methodologies and observed a +/-12% variation. Despite this variation in accounting accuracy, methods of lung dose reduction is often required (Van Dyk, 2000).

When a prescribed tumor dose is well above lung tolerance, the dose to lung will have to be reduced to minimize the probability of lung complication. Several methods can be used to reduce the dose. The techniques vary in complexity of design and application. All techniques incorporate one common concept: the use of an attenuator (Van Dyk, 2000). The attenuator absorbs radiation prior to delivering dose to the lungs. The decreased dose delivered to the lungs coupled with the increased transmission of dose within the lungs because of their lower density provides a dose comparable to rest of the body. Van Dyk describes several methods for the design of these attenuators. These methods vary from shielding the lungs with arm positioning to full or partial-transmission shielding blocks based on Computerized Tomography scans.

3. Representative Total Body Irradiation program

A representative TBI program is described here as an aid to the development of similar programs. Room modifications, technique selection, energy choice, and equipment necessary to achieve adequate dose uniformity in a comfortable setting are included in this discussion.

3.1 Accelerator room

TBI treatments should be performed with a high energy accelerator capable of providing photons of 15MV or greater. Lower x-ray energies can be utilized, but as the energy is decreased, dose homogeneity becomes more difficult to achieve with opposed fields. The distance to the closest wall with the gantry angled at 90 or 270 degrees will dictate the maximum field size to encompass the patient. Offset of the isocenter in the treatment vault design may allow for a greater treatment distance. Unfortunately, the desire to add TBI to the radiation therapy services may occur after a vault has been constructed. Most vaults are configured with a 20 foot width. Without an isocenter offset, this room width provides a source-wall distance of approximately 4m. Our institution's vault design provided a source-wall distance of slightly less than 4m. A 40x40 cm^2 field at 1m projects to 1.58m^2 without collimator rotation and 2.2m^2 with a 45° collimator rotation. Only a minor room modification may be necessary to provide audio and visual communication with a patient positioned at this location.

3.2 Opposed lateral field TBI table

A portable surgical couch was obtained from a medical equipment reclamation firm. This modified couch is utilized for providing TBI treatments with opposed lateral fields. It is the technique of choice where treatment goals include dose uniformity without specific organ blocking. Figure 1 is a front view schematic of the couch arrangement. The effective length of the patient was reduced as sections of the couch are angled 45°. Four inch urethane foam cushions are used to separate the patient from any metal located on the couch. An additional egg crate cushion is provided for patient comfort. The couch height is adjusted vertically to coincide with the isocenter height of 1.3m.

After patient positioning, four beam spoiler plates constructed of ¼" lexan polycarbonate are inserted into aluminum slots added to the couch. The width of the treatment table including the lexan polycarbonate plates is 52cm. Factoring in couch clearance to the wall, the source-tray distance for these lateral treatments is 374 cm. Our wall choice required a gantry angle selection of 270° (IEC). A collimator position of 20° and 340° is used for right lateral and left lateral fields, respectively.

Prior to treatment, a head and neck missing tissue compensator is positioned. An acrylic compensator is secured to a tray and supported with the accelerator hand support which is affixed to the accelerator couch rail (Fig. 2). The compensator angle position can be pivoted on the tray to match each patient. The compensator tray is rotated for the opposing lateral treatment and the couch longitudinal position is adjusted accordingly. The compensator bottom is curved to match the alignment between the patient neck and shoulders.

Tissue-equivalent rice bolus is used for additional missing tissue compensation for the body below the patient neck level. Figure 3 demonstrates the bolus placement. Since the patient's torso represents the widest section of the patient, bolus is typically only provided below the waist level between and around the legs and feet. The rice bag placement essentially makes the patient separation constant below the neck level and matching the maximum torso separation. Since the dose prescription point is typically at mid-depth at the umbilicus level. Tubes of rice and smaller individual plastic bags of rice with disposable outer covering are used for this aspect of patient preparation.

This treatment assumes that the treatment goal is to provide the same dose to the lungs as provided at the mid-umbilicus level. Prior to treatment, a lateral separation is determined at the nipple level. Previous chest x-ray review for over 50 patients revealed a relationship between this separation and the lateral width of the lungs. Of the lateral tissue separation, 77-83% of the tissue was comprised by the lower density lungs. Rather than measuring the lung width with a chest x-ray on each patient, we calculate the lung thickness as 80% of the full tissue thickness and assume a lung physical density of $0.35g/cm^3$. An effective thickness at this level is determined.

The arms are positioned at the patient's side thus adding higher density thickness to the chest area (Fig. 3.). The arm separation is determined and added to the effective thickness. This total is compared to umbilicus separation. If additional thickness is needed at the arm level to meet the thickness uniformity criterion of +/-1cm, additional "bolus with skin" (CIVCO, Orange City, IA) is added around the arm in 0.5cm increments until this criterion is met. A simple spreadsheet is used to perform these calculations as well as print setup instructions.

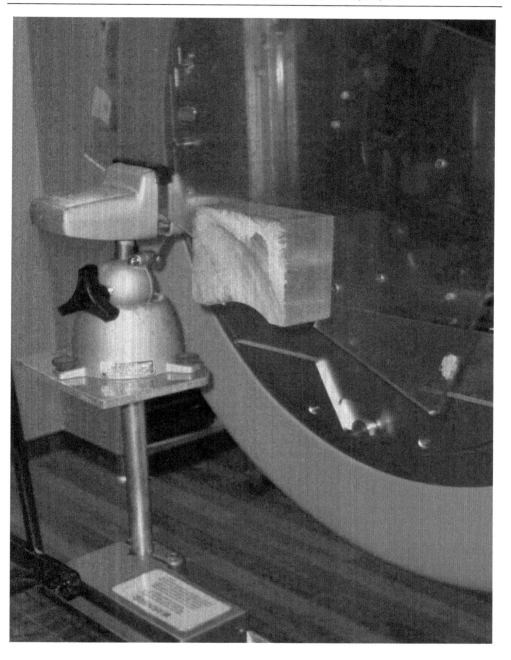

Fig. 2. Acrylic head and neck compensator mounted on post connected to accelerator couch rail arm support.

Monitor unit settings are calculated for the mid-depth at the umbilicus level. In-vivo entrance and exit dosimeters are placed at the head, neck, nipple, umbilicus, knee and ankle levels. After delivery of one half of the fractional dose, the patient remains positioned and the table is rotated 180°. The collimator is rotated to correspond to the new lateral orientation. The head and neck compensator is repositioned. The remainder of the treatment is provided. The dose rate from the accelerator is reduced between 100-200MU/min at isocenter. This machine dose rate reduction, the measured distance correction output factor, and attenuation will provide a dose delivery near 7cGy/minute. Dose rate has been determined to have a significant effect on lung toxicity. Most treatment protocols require dose delivery less than 10cGy/minute. Treatment times are approximately 15 minutes per field. This method of TBI delivery offers a uniform dose, easy and reproducible field arrangement, and a comfortable patient setup.

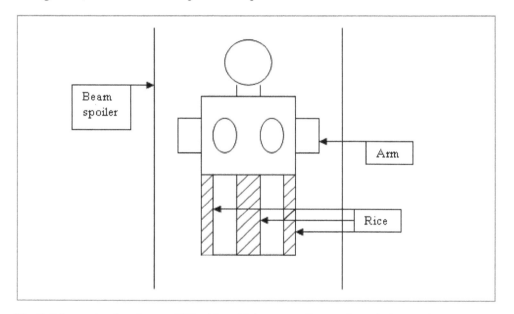

Fig. 3. Schematic of patient on TBI table with beam spoilers and rice bolus in place.

3.3 AP/PA TBI treatment stand
The opposed lateral field TBI table method does not allow for partial transmission blocking of the lung or liver as required by various protocols. Towards this goal, an alternative stand was developed to accommodate AP/PA field arrangement, cerrobend blocking, and verification of block placement in a reproducible and comfortable environment for the patient. The initial design of this stand utilized specifications described previously.[6,7] Over the years, significant modifications to these designs have been made largely to accommodate weak patients who had difficulty standing for lengthy periods. The majority of patients presenting for TBI have received a chemotherapy regimen as a complementary preparation before the transplant.

The current version of the AP/PA TBI stand is pictured in Figure 4. Detailed drawings describing the construction of this stand are available from the authors to aid in duplicating this construction. The stand begins with a 29"(w)x29"(l)x27"(h) wooden platform. This height allows field coverage at the treatment distance with the accelerator gantry positioned at 272° and a collimator rotation of 45°. A patient rehabilitation walker was affixed to the platform after wheel removal. The cushioned arm supports can be positioned at varying levels to accommodate different patient heights.

A fabric harness is attached around the patient's waist and thighs. This harness is then attached with plastic buckles to the frame of the walker support. The harness system provides the patient significant stability and tolerance for the required lengthy standing time for this procedure. Patients have experienced episodes of significant weakness or even fainting and the harness system allowed potential injury to be avoided before care could be offered to the patient.

Additional patient support and comfort is provided by an adjustable bicycle seat attached to a slide affixed to the platform. The current seat arrangement represents the evolution from a seat supported from the platform rear to a single post from the platform middle. Other stools were investigated and rejected due to adjustment restrictions or beam attenuation.

The blocking support is attached to a portable beam spoiler (Fig. 5). The plastic spoiler is fabricated with 3/8" lexan polycarbonate and supported on a mobile assembly that is positioned directly in front of the patient after configuring the patient on the harness and stool. Angle iron is placed on the sides of the beam spoiler away from the beam to provide additional rigidity when the blocks are added. Again, detailed drawings are available from the authors upon request.

The cerrobend partial transmission blocks are affixed to a separate ¼" lexan tray. The blocking tray is supported on a tray slot placed on each side of the bam spoiler. The thickness of the transmission blocks is calculated utilizing attenuation properties measured previously. The block thickness also varies with the patient separation and the desired transmitted dose, 8 or 10Gy. Typical thickness varies between 2-4cm of cerrobend and is determined using a simple spreadsheet calculation.

The positioning of the block is verified with imaging. In our case, we utilize the Kodak ACR 2000 CR system. However, a film cassette requiring chemical processing could also be used. Fig. 4 also shows a cassette holder attached to the rear of the platform. This spring-loaded cassette holder allows easy height adjustment and was obtained from a medical equipment reclamation service for less than $50. If lateral adjustment in block placement is necessary after imaging, the blocking tray can be adjusted horizontally using a top-loaded bearing system. This adjustment provides +/- 7cm adjustment. Refer to the appendix for details. Two worm screws are added to the sides of the block assembly and vertical adjustment is accomplished by cranking up or down along this mechanism. After an acceptable image is obtained, the block shadow is traced onto the patient's surface for subsequent fractions.

As with the opposed lateral TBI treatment, the accelerator output rate is adjusted such that the midline dose rate is less than 10cGy/minute. Entrance and exit in-vivo dosimeters are placed to verify dose uniformity. Since the hands and forearms are not placed at the patient's side, but on the cushioned arm supports, there was a concern about dose uniformity in this region. Measurements confirm uniformity within +/- 5% as the hands and forearms are closer to the beam during the anterior field treatment and further from the beam during the posterior field delivery.

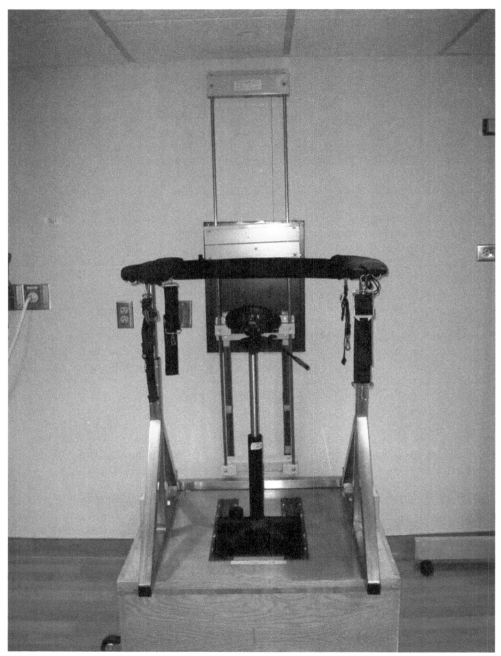

Fig. 4. Front view of TBI stand used for AP/PA fields.

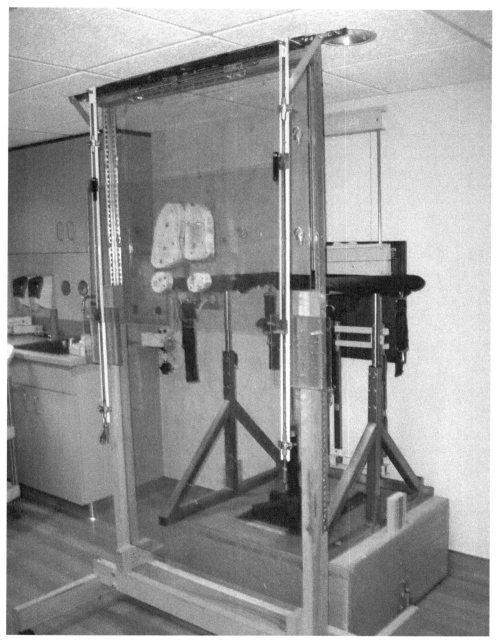

Fig. 5. Front view of mobile spoiler and blocking mechanism used in conjunction with TBI stand.

3.4 Combination of treatment methods

Despite efforts to provide a comfortable treatment in the TBI stand, the opposed lateral TBI table still is viewed as the most comfortable for patients and easy to set up. Patients receiving TBI that requires dose reduction to the lungs and/or liver are treated using a combination of these two techniques. All current protocols requiring dose reduction to these organs require treatments to be administered over four days or 8 fractions. We routinely treat 4 fractions with the AP/PA TBI stand technique and 4 fractions with the opposed lateral TBI table option.

4. Radiobiological considerations for Total Body Irradiation

The techniques and methodology described in the previous section account for the physical criteria and limitations for the TBI procedure. The actual dose prescription and dose delivery schedule also play an important role in the success of the procedure (Shank, 1999). Normal lymphocytes are among the most radiosensitive cells and become profoundly depleted with TBI (Shank, 1999). In addition to finding that TBI was more immunosuppressive than CY, Shank describes early animal studies that found the degree of immunosuppression was a function of the total radiation dose. Dividing the treatment into multiple fractions over several days required an increase in total dose to achieve consistent results. Shank states the need for an increased dose over a fractionated schedule implies repair processes occurring between fractions.

Radiobiologists categorize the repair process from fractionated radiation treatments as repair, reoxygenation, redistribution and repopulation (Evans, 2000). In the context of TBI as applied to bone marrow transplantation, Evans states repair and repopulation are probably the most significant of these processes and can be best explained with a cell survival curve as shown in Figure 6. The slope of a survival curve can describe the radiation sensitivity of a particular cell type. The slope of the curve, termed D_o and the shoulder region, termed D_q, quantify significant parameters of a cells response to radiation. Cells from different tissues have different D_o's and D_q's as illustrated in Figure 6.

It has been generally accepted that a small shoulder (D_q) is typical of bone marrow stem cells and leukemia cells (Evans, 2002). Therefore, these cells have a limited ability to repair damage. In contrast, cells of lung tissue and intestinal epithelial cells have survival curves with must broader shoulders (D_q), implying a greater repair capacity. The second important repair process is repopulation. Evans defines repopulation as the proliferation of cells between dose fractions. Rapidly dividing tissues, like the intestine, can increase their normal proliferation rate after a radiation treatment. Slowly dividing tissues such as the lung and vascular tissues tend not to proliferate at a higher rate after radiation. Therefore, during a fractionated radiation therapy regimen, Evans speculates that both repair and repopulation may occur between fractions. Repair of the leukemia cells is minimal. The separation of the leukemia cell survival curve from the lung cell survival curve increases the therapeutic ratio and supports fractionation. Shank (1998) attempted to calculate the optimal TBI schedule including fraction dose, number of fractions, and total dose. In addition, Shank reviews some clinical trials with regards to percentage relapse with different TBI schedules. Shank summarizes her findings that the greatest leukemia cell kill with minimum morbidity will occur with a highly fractionated radiotherapy regimen. A total dose of 1400-1500 cGy delivered over 10-13 fractions may be optimal.

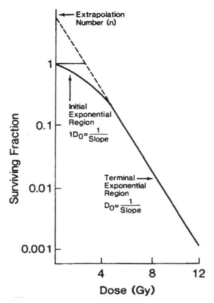

Fig. 6. A typical survival curve for mammalian cells exhibiting an initial shoulder followed by an exponential region. An initial shoulder characterizes the curve with some slope to it ($1D_o$), the exponential slope (D_o), n (extrapolation number) and D_q.

5. Effectiveness of TBI for various leukemias

Leukemia is a broad classification for several types of this disease. This variety of leukemias differs based on pathological examination of cell definition. Bredeson et al. (2002) provide a summary and results of clinical trials including TBI. Patients with acute myeloid leukemia (AML) have shown to be fairly responsive to stem cell transplants with TBI preparation. Results of randomized studies comparing TBI containing regimens with total chemotherapy preparatory regimens indicate a 75% actuarial survival with TBI compared to 51% without. Relapse rates are lower with the TBI regimens as well. 14% relapsed within 2 years with TBI while 34% relapsed under chemotherapy regimens.

Bredeson et al. (2002) reports acute lymphoblastic leukemia (ALL) results show significant improvement with TBI regimens. 52% disease-free survival rates are reported when TBI is utilized as compared to 37% with chemotherapy alone. The percentage relapse is nearly identical from both types of regimens. Studies of treatments for chronic myeloid leukemia patients show fairly high yet identical disease-free survival rates. Nearly 80% survival rates were reported for both protocols. Relapse rates were indistinguishably different.

6. Discussion and summary

Leukemia is a disease classification for an imbalance within the hemopoietic system. Acute leukemias are characterized with unregulated cell growth while chronic leukemias exhibit incomplete maturation of cells and some increase proliferation. Bone marrow or stem cell transplantation is a viable treatment option for the leukemia patient. Stem cells collected from an HLA matching donor or cells collected from the patient while in remission are provided to the leukemia recipient. The clinical desire of the transplant is repopulation and re-growth of the stem cells triggering a balanced regulated hemopoietic system.

Preparative regimens for marrow transplantation are required to rid the leukemia patient of any microscopic disease. Rigorous protocols of chemotherapy or radiation therapy combined with chemotherapy are provided prior to transplantation to reduce relapse. Radiotherapy includes fractionated treatments delivered to the total body (TBI). TBI treatments pose several concern issues in methodology and fractionation. High-energy fields with opposing beam arrangements lead to improved dose uniformity. Acrylic plates can serve as beam spoilers to increase the dose to an adequate dose for shallow depths. The lung tissue is sensitive to radiation and limits the dose delivered to the rest of the body. Accurate lung dose calculations are necessary to determine if attenuators are necessary to reduce the total lung dose. Fractionation of the TBI dose requires an increase in the total dose delivered as repair and repopulation occurs between fractions. Repair processes are minimal for the leukemia cell and therefore the therapeutic ratio is enhanced. Analysis of the disease-free survival rates and evaluation of the percentage of patients relapsing or recurring measure the effect of these preparatory regimens. TBI shows a marked improvement in both factors for AML and ALL. Studies reviewing the effects of treatments for CML show excellent results for both chemotherapy only protocols and TBI-chemotherapy combined protocols.

Over the last 35 years, TBI delivery protocols have evolved due to toxicity concerns. Radiation-induced toxicity is influenced by the dose rate and total dose. The total dose was predominantly restricted by pulmonary toxicity from interstitial pneumonitis. Single fraction TBI was replaced with fractionated and hyperfractionated techniques. Radiobiological principles of preferential normal tissue repair with fractionation forecast improved anti-leukemic effects without increasing toxicity. Dose rate was considered a strong factor in the causation of interstitial pneumonitis and most protocols restrict the delivery dose rate to less than 10 cGy/min. TBI protocols vary with the primary malignancy and complementary chemotherapy conditioning regimen. Current TBI protocols include: a single fraction of 200 Gy; two BID fractions of 2 Gy/fraction; eight BID fractions of 1.5 Gy/fraction with or without lung and liver dose reduction to 8-10 Gy; and eight BID fractions of 1.65 Gy/fraction with or without partial transmission blocking of the lung and liver.

Factors influencing large field treatment technique choice include dose homogeneity, accurate and reproducible delivery, ease of set up, treatment room limitations, and the treatment protocol used. For example, if a reduced organ dose is required with blocking, an AP/PA treatment technique is required. Different techniques have been described recently including those utilizing tomotherapy or translational couch options. Two methods of comfortable total body irradiation using conventional linear accelerators without machine modifications are presented here. A technique for lateral treatments and a process for AP/PA treatments with blocking are described. Techniques described here enhance other reported design specifications. The technique options represent an evolution in our process and should aid facilities looking to begin a TBI program or facilities desiring modifications to adjust to different treatment protocols.

Dose uniformity is the primary criterion when creating a treatment technique. The use of beam spoilers, strategically placed bolus, missing tissue compensators, and opposed fields with high energy x-rays will accomplish the uniformity goal. While dose uniformity is the major priority in developing a suitable treatment technique, patient comfort and support are equally important. Patients presenting for TBI are often weak and recovering from other chemotherapy treatments as part of the preparatory program for transplant. Two treatment options, opposed laterals and AP/PA fields and associated apparatus have been presented. The limitation of dose delivered to the lung/liver is specified in several protocols and is accomplished with partial transmission blocks placed in conjunction with AP/PA fields. Both techniques were designed to insure accurate dose delivery, comfortable patient support, and easy patient setup. Calculation spreadsheets referenced in this manuscript are available by contacting the authors.

7. Appendix

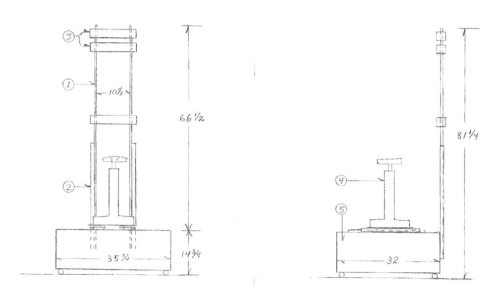

Legend: 1. 5/8" stainless steel rod, 2. Angle iron for stabilization and support, 3. Adjustable cassette holder, 4. Double track system support for bicycle seat placement, 5. Platform with ¾"plywood on oak framework

Fig. A-1 Front and side view of AP/PA stand .

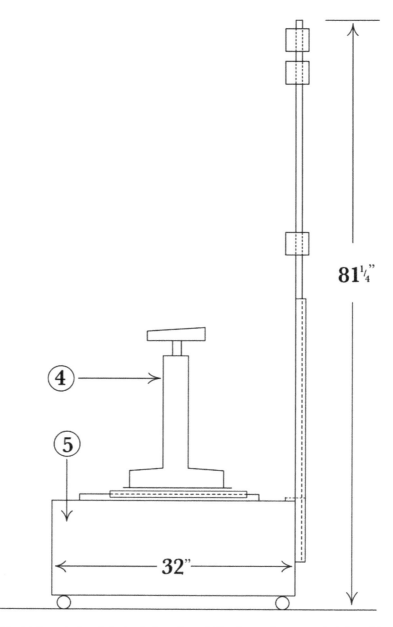

Legend: 1. 5/8" stainless steel rod, 2. Angle iron for stabilization and support, 3. Adjustable cassette holder, 4. Double track system support for bicycle seat placement, 5. Platform with ¾"plywood on oak framework

Fig. A-2 AP/PA Stand Side View

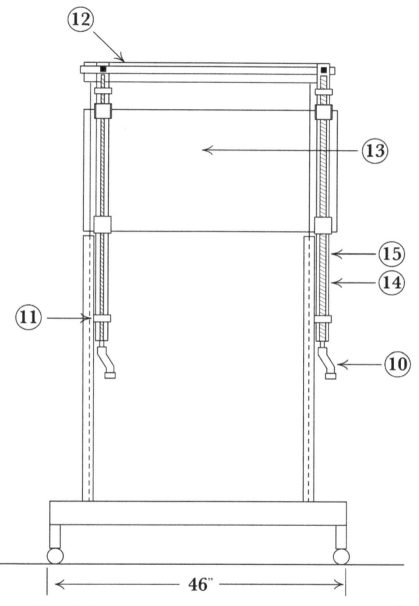

Legend: 6. 1-1/2"x3-1/2" Oak frame support, 7. Lexan beam spoiler, 8. Support for block tray with galvanized metal support, 9. Galvanized metal lock, 10. Crank, 11. Bearing location & cap (2 bearings/crank), 12. Ball bearing track for horizontal block adjustment, 13. ¼" block tray, 14. 7/16" thread rod, 15. ¼" channel for rod adjustment system

Fig. A-3 AP/PA Beam Spoiler and Blocking Support Front View

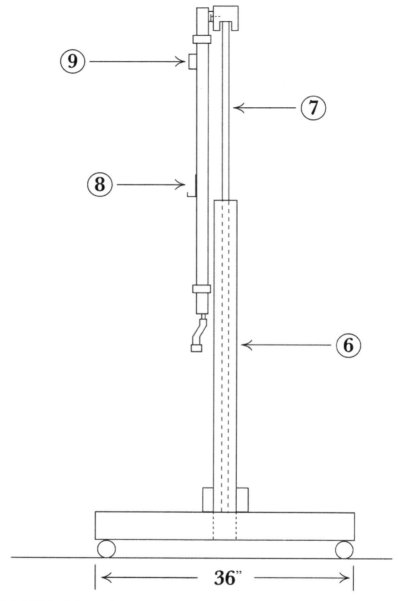

Legend: 6. 1-1/2"x3-1/2" Oak frame support, 7. Lexan beam spoiler, 8. Support for block tray with galvanized metal support, 9. Galvanized metal lock, 10. Crank, 11. Bearing location & cap (2 bearings/crank), 12. Ball bearing track for horizontal block adjustment, 13. ¼" block tray, 14. 7/16" thread rod, 15. ¼" channel for rod adjustment system

Fig. A-4 AP/PA Beam Spoiler and Blocking Support Side View

8. Acknowledgement

The authors express their gratitude to Craig Nicholson for his thoughtful efforts and insight in the construction of the AP/PA stand and the beam spoiler/block support system.

9. References

Bentel, G. (1992). *Radiation Therapy Planning* (4th ed.). New York, NY: Macmillan.

Bradley, J., Reft, C., Goldman, S., Rubin, C., Nachman, J., Larson, R., et al. (1998). High-energy total body irradiation as preparation for bone marrow transplantation in leukemia patients: treatment technique and related complications. *International Journal of Radiation Oncology, Biology and Physics, 40*, 391-396.

Bredeson, C., Perry G., Martens C., McDiarmid S., Bence-Bruckler, I. Atkins, H., et al. (2002). Outpatient total body irradiation as a component of a comprehensive outpatient transplant program. *Bone Marrow Transplantation, 29*, 667-671.

Corns, R., Evans, M., Olivares M., Syke, L., & Pogorsak, E. (2000). Designing attenuators for total body irradiation using virtual simulation. *Medical Dosimetry, 25*, 27-31.

Evans, R. (2000). Radiobiological considerations in magna-field irradiation. *International Journal of Radiation, Oncology, Biology and Physics, 43*, 1907-1911.

Galvin, J., D'Angio, G., & Walsh, G. (1999). Use of tissue compensators to improve dose uniformity for total body irradiation. *International Journal of Radiation Oncology, Biology and Physics, 42*, 767-771.

Lin, J., & Chu, T. (2001). Dose compensation of the total body irradiation therapy. *Applied Radiation Isotopes, 55*, 623-630.

Lindsley, K. & Deeg, H.J. (1998). Total body irradiation for marrow or stem-cell transplantation. *Cancer Investigation, 16*, 424-425.

Serota, F., Burkey, E., August, C., & D'Angio, G. (1998). Total body irradiation as preparation for bone marrow transplantation in treatment of acute leukemia and aplastic anemia. *International Journal of Radiation Oncology, Biology and Physics, 12*, 1941-1949.

Shank, B. (1999). Techniques of magna-field irradiation. *International Journal of Radiation Oncology, Biology and Physics, 42*, 1925-1931.

Shank, B. (1998). Total body irradiation for marrow or stem-cell transplantation. *Cancer Investigation, 16*, 397-404.

Scheinberg, D., Maslak, P., & Weiss, M. (2001). Acute leukemias. In V.T. DeVita & S. Hellman & S. Rosenberg (Eds.), *Cancer-Principles and Practice of Oncology*, (6th ed.), (pp. 2404-2432). Philadelphia, PA: J.B. Lippincott.

Urbano-Ispizua, A., Schmitz, N., de Witte, T., Frassoni, F., Rosti, G., Schrezenmeier, H., et al. (2002). Allogenic and autologous transplantation for hematologic diseases, solid tumors, and immune disorders: definitions and current practice. *Bone Marrow Transplantation, 29*, 639-646.

Van Dyk, J. (2000). Magna-field irradiation: physical considerations. *International Journal of Radiation Oncology, Biology and Physics, 43*, 1913-1918.

8

Non-Invasive Devices for Early Detection of Breast Tissue Oncological Abnormalities Using Microwave Radio Thermometry

Tahir H. Shah, Elias Siores and Chronis Daskalakis
Institute of Materials Research and Innovation (IMRI),
University of Bolton
United Kingdom

1. Introduction

Breast cancer is the most common cancer in women worldwide, comprising 16% of all female cancers and is the leading cause of cancer-related deaths in women ages 40-55. Each year in the U.S.A. over 180,000 women are diagnosed with breast cancer and 46,000 women die of this disease. One in twelve women in the United Kingdom develops breast cancer and the annual death toll stands at around 14,000. Over 33,000 new cases are being monitored year on year basis in the UK. In all, 10%-11% of all women can expect to be affected by breast cancer at some time during their lives. The causes of most breast cancers are not yet fully understood. Sixty years ago, MacDonald proposed that the biological behaviour of a neoplasm is established during its preclinical growth phase (MacDonald, 1951). This view is supported by some data on the behaviour of metastatic lesions such as poor cytological differentiation, lymphatic permeation, blood vessel invasion and the invasion of the surrounding soft tissue by the tumour (Nealon et al, 1979). Screening and early diagnosis are currently the most effective ways to reduce mortality from this disease. Early diagnosis and treatment are the keys to surviving breast cancer. Breast cancer survival rates vary greatly worldwide, ranging from over 80% in North America, Sweden and Japan to around 60% in middle-income countries and below 40% in low-income countries. It is believed that the low survival rates in less developed countries are mainly due to the lack of early detection programmes, resulting in a high proportion of women presenting with late-stage disease, as well as by the lack of adequate diagnosis and treatment facilities. Studies from the American National Cancer Institute show that 96 percent of women whose breast cancer is detected early live five or more years after treatment. Early diagnosis remains an important detection strategy, particularly in low- and middle-income countries where the disease is diagnosed in late stages and resources are very limited. There is some evidence that this strategy can produce "down staging" of the disease to stages that are more amenable to less aggressive treatment. Therefore, thousands of lives and considerable healthcare costs could be saved each year with treatment if early symptoms of breast cancer are detected. Taking full advantage of early diagnosis and treatment means that screening technology should have the characteristics that have high detection success rate, speed of procedure, comfort to the subject and very low health risk.

The principal aim of early breast cancer detection is to identify the disease at a more curable stage and thus improve the prognosis and other vital clinical outcomes. Currently breast cancer detection is a three part procedure. The first part is identification of the abnormality in the breast tissue either by physical examination or by an imaging technique. Secondly, the abnormality is diagnosed as a benign or a malignant condition by using additional diagnostic methods or by biopsy and microscopic examination of the tissue morphology. The third part is concerned with biochemical characterisation of the malignant tissue in order to stage the cancer according to the size of the tumour and extent of invasion and metastasis. Of particular importance is the ability to clearly distinguish between malignant and benign tumours and early detection. This then determines the prognosis and appropriate course of treatment. A review of the published literature shows that all current breast cancer detection techniques have limited capability and surgery is often required to establish the true nature of the tumour.

Currently, the frontline strategies for breast cancer detection still depend essentially on clinical and self-examination and mammograms. The limitations of mammography, with its reported sensitivity rate often below 70% are recognized (Sickles, 1984) and the proposed value of self-breast examination is being queried (Thomas et al, 1997). Mammography is accepted as the most reliable and cost-effective imaging technique, however, its contribution continues to be challenged with persistent false-negative results - ranging up to 30% (Moskowitz, 1983 & Elmore et al, 1884). However, most of the research and development activity related to cancer detection and diagnosis is focussed on the analysis of the existing condition and is costly, time-consuming and requires trained personnel to use the equipment. Furthermore, the incidence of the earliest form of breast cancer, Ductal Carcinoma in Situ (DCIS), has increased significantly over the last few years in the United States and this seems to be directly related to successful screening programmes. This clearly shows that there is a need and scope for developing early breast cancer detection techniques that are simple, quick and can be used by women by themselves.

In this chapter a review of some of the most promising techniques that are being developed for breast cancer detection is presented. A comparison of the various breast cancer detection techniques that are in the developmental stages with the established procedures has been carried out and a state-of-the-art in all the areas is briefly described and the concept of a wearable breast cancer detection device - the 'smart bra'- is also discussed. Particular emphasis has been placed on the non-invasive thermometry based methodologies for early detection of the oncological condition. When infrared thermography was first introduced in medicine, the instrumentation was not sensitive enough to detect the subtle changes in temperature that are involved in diseases such as breast cancer. However, more recently the sensitivity of infrared instrumentation has greatly improved and the IR thermography imaging is being developed and used to monitor the health of the breast and detection of cancerous tumours. Recent literature shows that the technique has the ability to detect tumours that are 3cm in size and are located deeper than 7 cm from the skin surface and tumours smaller than 0.5 cm can be detected if they are close to the surface of the skin. Non-invasive techniques based on profiling of the breast tissue using microwave radiometry are also being developed and investigated as early warning systems for breast cancer. These techniques involve the measurement of the passive electromagnetic thermal radiation emitted from human body using suitable combination of microwave antenna internal temperature sensor and infrared surface temperature sensor, with an appropriate configuration to determine the temperature profile of the concerned area of the body.

Microwave radiometry principles can be employed to obtain sensor information from subcutaneous tissues up to a few centimetres in depth. The device based on these principles can provide an early breast cancer detection/warning technique that is simple, quick and may also be used for diagnosis of other types of cancers such as prostate cancer in men.

The evidence indicates that screening mammography, when correctly performed at recommended intervals and combined with appropriate interventions, can reduce, but not eliminate, breast cancer mortality. This conclusion is based on evidence of efficacy in clinical trials and evidence of effectiveness in the general population. The "ideal" breast cancer screening tool has not yet been developed. All of the tests available for the screening and diagnosis of breast cancer have different strengths and limitations. The ideal test would combine the following characteristics:

- The test should present a low risk of harm from screening
- The test should have high degrees of specificity and sensitivity (low rates of false-positive and false-negative results).
- The test results should have uniform high quality and repeatability.
- Interpretation of test results should be straightforward (objective).
- The test should be simple to perform.
- The test should be non-invasive.
- The test should be able to detect breast cancer at a stage that is curable with available treatments.
- The test should have the ability to distinguish life-threatening lesions from those that are not likely to progress.
- The test should be cost-effective (usually considered <$50,000 per quality-adjusted life year saved).
- The test should be widely available.
- The test should be acceptable to women.

Each modality has different strengths and limitations therefore it seems to be feasible to adopt a multi modality approach in order to achieve the optimum methodology for the detection and diagnosis of the breast tissue oncological abnormalities.

1.1 Anatomy and physiology of female breast

It is important to consider the physiology of the breast, as the changes seen in the breast during a woman's life will have an effect on the properties of the tissues. The female breast is a complex and sensitive organ, which is composed of a mass of glandular, fatty, and fibrous tissues positioned over the pectoral muscles of the chest wall and attached to the chest wall by fibrous strands called Cooper's ligaments (Figure 1). A layer of fatty tissue surrounds the breast glands and extends throughout the breast. The fatty tissue gives the breast a soft consistency. The glandular tissues of the breast house the lobules and the ducts. The female breast has a network of arteries and capillaries that carry oxygen- and nutrient-rich blood to the breasts. The axillary artery extends from the armpit and supplies blood to the outer half of the breast. The internal mammary artery, which extends down from the neck, supplies blood to the inner part of the breast. The breast also contains lymph vessels. The lymphatic system is part of the immune system and is composed of blood vessels, lymph ducts and lymph nodes. Clusters of lymph nodes are located under the arm, above the collarbone, behind the breastbone and in various other parts of the body.

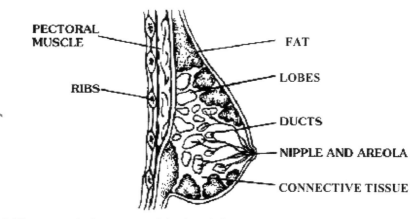

Fig. 1. The anatomical structure of the female breast

The shape and appearance of female breast undergo a number of changes as a woman ages. In young women, the breast skin stretches and expands as the breasts grow, creating a rounded appearance. Young women tend to have denser breasts, due to the presence of more glandular tissue, than older women. The denser breasts lead to poorer contrast between healthy and diseased tissue in x-ray mammography. However the occurrence of breast cancer in younger women is low, with 80 % of breast cancers occurring in women over the age of 50. The growth of breast tissue is mainly influenced by the relative concentrations of progesterone and oestrogen in the body. During each menstrual cycle, breast tissue tends to swell due to variation in the oestrogen and progesterone levels. The milk glands and ducts enlarge resulting in retention of water by the breast. During menstruation, breasts may temporarily appear swollen and this can give rise to breast pain, tenderness, or they may feel lumpy. At menopause, a woman's body stops producing oestrogen and progesterone, which causes a variety of symptoms in many women including hot flushes, night sweats, mood changes and vaginal dryness. During this period breasts also undergo many changes, such as mentioned earlier for the menstrual cycle, and sometimes appearance of cysts may be observed. The glandular tissue tends to shrink after menopause and is replaced with fatty tissue. The breasts also tend to increase in size and droop because the fibrous tissue loses its strength. The breasts become less dense after menopause, which makes the detection of breast cancer often easier in older women. A woman's risk of breast cancer increases with age thus all women are recommended for breast cancer screening at regular interval beyond the age of 40.

1.2 Main types of breast cancer

Treatment of cancer depends on the type and stage of the cancer along with other issues such as the individual circumstances of the patient. Mostly breast cancer develops in the glandular tissue and is classified as adenocarcinoma, which is a cancer of the epithelium that originates in the glandular tissue. The common types of breast cancers are:

Carcinoma in situ: This term is used for early stage cancer, when it is confined to the place where it started. In breast cancer, it means that the cancer is confined to the ducts or the lobules, depending on where it started. It has not gone into the fatty tissues in the breast nor spread to other organs in the body.

Ductal carcinoma in situ (DCIS): This is the most common type of non-invasive breast cancer. DCIS means that the cancer is confined to the ducts. It has not spread through the walls of the ducts into the fatty tissue of the breast. Over 70% of breast cancers are ductal carcinomas, which are associated with the milk ducts. Nearly all women with cancer at this stage can be cured.

Infiltrating (invasive) ductal carcinoma (IDC): This type of cancer starts in a duct and breaks through the wall of the duct, and invades the fatty tissue of the breast (Figure 2), then spreading to other parts of the body. IDC is the most common type of breast cancer. It accounts for about 80% of invasive breast cancers.

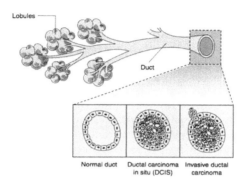

Fig. 2. Growth of ductal carcinoma

Lobular carcinoma in situ (LCIS): This condition begins in the milk-making glands but does not go through the wall of the lobules. Although not a true cancer, having LCIS increases a woman's risk of getting cancer later. For this reason, it is important that women with LCIS follow the screening guidelines for breast cancer. 10% - 15% are lobular carcinomas associated with the lobes, and the rest are relatively rare forms of cancer such as of the connective tissue.

Infiltrating (invasive) lobular carcinoma (ILC): This type of cancer starts in the lobules and can spread to other parts of the body (Figure 3). About 10% of invasive breast cancers are of this type.

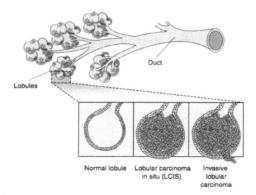

Fig. 3. Growth of lobular carcinoma

Benign conditions: There are many lesions and conditions that are non-cancerous but still affect the health of the breast and could be mistaken for cancer. These include fibroadenomas, cysts, mastalgia, breast calcifications, duct ectasia and periductal mastitis, fat necrosis, hyperplasia, intraductal papilloma, phyllodes tumour and sclerosing adenosis.

2. Current breast cancer detection modalities and their limitations

Breast is susceptible to a range of pathologic conditions. The most serious of these is breast cancer, which is widely recognised as the most common cancer in women. Other breast conditions include mastalgia, which is referred to a variety of conditions that cause breast pain, and benign lesions such as fibroadenomas and cysts. These conditions are not fatal but they are a source of undesirable symptoms and considerable anxiety for the patients. Improved methods for early detection and diagnosis of breast disease are essential to decrease mortality rates due to cancer. In addition a greater understanding of the physiology of the breast is needed to aid in the diagnosis of disease and in improving treatments.

The breast cancer detection is a three part procedure. The first part is the identification of the abnormality in the breast tissue either by physical examination or by an imaging technique. Secondly the abnormality is diagnosed as a benign or malignant condition by using additional diagnostic methods or by biopsy and microscopic examination of the tissue morphology. The third part is concerned with biochemical characterisation of the malignant tissue in order to stage the cancer according to the size of the tumour and extent of invasion and metastasis. This then determines the prognosis and appropriate course of treatment. The most commonly used imaging modalities are described in the following sections.

The main strategy of breast cancer detection is based on clinical examination and mammography. Mammography is considered to be the 'gold standard' test for breast cancer detection and diagnosis and is accepted as the most cost-effective imaging modality. The performance of a screening test is evaluated by three related measurements: sensitivity, specificity, and a positive predictive value. The sensitivity of a screening test is the proportion of people with the disease who test positive. Specificity is the proportion of people without the disease who test negative. The positive predictive value is the proportion of individuals with a positive screening test result who actually have the disease. In the development of optimum detection modality, there is often a trade-off between sensitivity and specificity, with an increase in one leading to a decrease in the other. The contribution of mammography continues to be challenged with persistent false-negative rates ranging up to 30%. The clinical examination has been challenged with reported sensitivity rates often below 65%. There is also variability in radiologists' interpretation of mammograms with decreasing sensitivity in younger patients and those on oestrogen replacement therapy. In addition, recent data suggests that denser and less informative mammography images are precisely those associated with an increased cancer risk (Boyd et al, 1995). It has also been suggested that mammography procedure cannot be performed by an inexperienced technician or radiologist. With the current emphasis on earlier detection, there is now renewed interest in the development of complimentary imaging techniques that can also exploit the metabolic, immunological, and vascular changes associated with early tumour growth. While promising, techniques such as Doppler ultrasound and MRI are associated with a number of disadvantages, which include the following:

- Duration of the test,

- Limited accessibility,
- Need of intravenous access,
- Patient discomfort,
- Restricted imaging area,
- Difficult interpretation
- Limited availability of the technology

These modalities are in fact more suited as the second-line options to pursue the already abnormal screening evaluations. This stepwise approach currently results in the non-recognition, and thus delayed utilization of any second-line technology in approximately 10% of established breast cancers (Moskowitz, 1995). This view is supported by another study of infrared screening of breast cancer [Keyserlignk & Ahlgren, 1998). A list of the established breast cancer detection modalities approved by FDA is given in Table 1.

Modality	Description
Full-field digital mammography	Detector responds to X-ray exposure, sends electronic signal to computer to be digitized and processed. Separates detector and image display.
Computer-assisted detection	Computer programs to aid in identification of suspicious mammograms and classification as benign or malignant.
Ultrasound : Compound imaging and Three-dimensional ultrasound imaging	Uses high-frequency sound waves to generate an image.
Magnetic resonance imaging (MRI)	Makes use of the property of nuclear magnetic resonance (NMR) to image nuclei of atoms inside the body. Image generated by signals from excitation of nuclear particles in a magnetic field. Breast tumours show increased uptake of contrast agent.
Scintimammography	Image created with radioactive tracers, which concentrate more in cancer tissues than in normal tissues.
Positron emission tomography (PET)	Uses tracers such as labelled glucose to identify regions in the body with altered metabolic activity.
Infrared Thermography	Measures heat emitted by the body. Tumours can raise skin surface temperature, which is detected by infrared cameras. Dynamic area telethermometry detects changes in blood flow.
Electrical impedance imaging	Measures voltage at skin surface while passing small current through breast. Changes in cancerous tissue decrease impedance of tissue.

Table 1. FDA approved modalities for breast cancer detection

2.1 X-ray mammography

X-ray mammography is the most common method of imaging the breast at present. The technique involves the breast being compressed between two plates with an x-ray film placed underneath and low energy x-rays are then passed through the breast and the images are recorded. The best contrast between soft tissues is achieved at low energies and hence these are used in x-ray mammography. The x-rays are produced by an electron beam irradiating either a tungsten or molybdenum target depending on the size of the breast to be imaged. At low energies, the transmission is low causing a high dose to the patient. Thus a compromise between contrast and dose is necessary. This problem is reduced by compression of the breast. The breast is compressed to between 2 and 8 cm enabling a high contrast whilst keeping the dose within an acceptable level. Contrast is dependent on the thickness of the breast and the difference in linear attenuation coefficient (μ) between the tissue types. The value of μ is dependent on the atomic number of the material. Thus tissues with higher atomic numbers will produce a higher attenuation than others (e.g. microcalcifications).

The established sensitivity of mammography is higher than 91% (Brem et al 2003), which is greater than any other imaging modality for breast cancer detection. This is the main reason for the use of mammography in screening programmes. The reported specificity of the technique is quite variable and is considered to be in the region of 72% (Bone et al 1997). This means that nearly a quarter of the benign lesions are diagnosed as suspicious, which leads to unnecessary invasive procedures, biopsies, in order to establish the true nature of the lesion. Furthermore, the sensitivity of mammography for younger women is lower than that for older women. Younger women have denser breasts and less adipose tissue. Adipose tissue provides a greater contrast to calcifications than denser fibrous tissue and so mammography is more successful in older women.

Nearly one quarter of all invasive breast cancers are not detected by x-ray mammography in women aged between 40-49 years. However, the statistics for women above the age of 50 years are significantly better (1 in 10). Treatment of women with undetected invasive cancers, because of false-negative results, may be delayed. Many mammographic abnormalities may not be cancer, but will prompt additional testing and anxiety. Approximately 10 percent of all screening mammograms are read as abnormal. This will result in additional diagnostic tests such as diagnostic mammography, ultrasound, needle aspiration, core biopsy, or surgical biopsy. Given the lower incidence of breast cancer in 40- to 49-year-old women compared with that in older women, false-positive examinations are more common in younger women and the proportion of true-positive examinations increases with increasing age. There is concern that women having abnormal mammograms, both true-positive and false-positive, experience psychosocial stresses, including anxiety, fear, and inconvenience. There is the concern that experiencing a false-positive mammogram may affect subsequent willingness of the patient to undergo future screening mammography at ages when it is of greatest benefit.

The main advantages of x-ray mammography are that the technique has good resolution and microcalcifications can easily be observed. Furthermore, the relatively fast imaging time allows many women to be scanned in one screening session. The major drawbacks of the modality are the use of ionising radiation, which is potentially harmful for the patient and the operator, and interpreting mammograms can be difficult due to differences in the appearance of the normal breast for each woman. The sensitivity is high (91.4% (Brem et al, 2003) but is not 100% and also the specificity is relatively low for some types of tumours.

Particularly, the sensitivity is lower for women with dense breast tissue (e.g. younger women) and breast implants can affect the accuracy of mammography, as silicone implants are not transparent to X-rays. The disadvantages of compressing the breast are that it is, at best, uncomfortable and for many women with sensitive breasts it can be very painful. This limits the maximum time feasible for the imaging process. Also the spatial accuracy of the image can be distorted so that it is difficult to exactly locate an identified lesion.

The risk of radiation-induced breast cancer has long been a concern and has driven the efforts to reduce the radiation dose per examination. Radiation has been shown to cause breast cancer in women, and the risk is proportional to the dose. Especially the younger women are at a greater risk for breast cancer due to the exposure to radiation. Radiation related breast cancers occur at least 10 years after exposure. However, breast cancer as a result of the radiation dose associated with mammography has not been established. Radiation from yearly mammograms during ages 40-49 has been estimated as possibly causing one additional breast cancer death per 10,000 women.

2.2 Magnetic resonance imaging (MRI)

The principal imaging modality used for the detection of breast tissue abnormalities is x-ray mammography, which has a high sensitivity, but suffers from a relatively poor specificity for some tumours and breast types, leading to unnecessary biopsies. Thus there is a need for an imaging technique that can non-invasively distinguish between malignant and benign lesions. At the present, magnetic resonance imaging (MRI) and ultrasound (US) can provide additional diagnostic information for this purpose.

The theory of MRI is based on the fact that the nuclei of some atoms have a property known as spin. Such nuclei act like tiny current loops and consequently generate a magnetic field (or magnetic moment), along the spin axis. Under normal circumstances these moments have no fixed orientation so there is no overall magnetic field. When an external magnetic field is applied, the moments will align in certain directions. In the case of hydrogen nuclei, which are the most abundant nuclei in the human body, two discrete energy levels are created. An MRI detection system consists of a magnet, magnetic gradient coils, a radio frequency transmitter and receiver, and a computer that controls the acquisition of signals and computes the MR images obtained. When an atomic nucleus is exposed to a static magnetic field, it resonates when a varying electromagnetic field is applied at an appropriate frequency and an image is computed from the resonance signals.

The signal in MRI arises from the rotating magnetisation, but it decays due to two different relaxation processes. The first process is the spin-lattice relaxation. The second relaxation process is the spin-spin relaxation. During spin-spin relaxation, the detected signal decays over a period of time. However, the spins are also subject to inhomogeneities in the magnetic field causing the signal to decay faster than the natural time period. Part of the signal can be obtained due to the spin-echo effect. This involves the application of a further RF pulse which causes the spins to be flipped by 180°. This means that the phase-position of each spin has been inverted and so nuclei that were precessing faster are now behind spins that were precessing at a slower rate. At the echo time TE, the spins will catch each other up and a peak in the signal will be detected. An MRI exam of the breast typically takes between 30 and 60 minutes. Diffusion and perfusion MRI are relatively new procedures. Diffusion MRI measures the mobility of water protons whereas perfusion MRI measures the rate at which blood is delivered to tissue. Both of these factors vary in malignant tissues as compared with benign tissue and therefore can be used as indicators for cancer.

The injection of a contrast agent can enhance the ability of MRI to detect specific features or in the case of dynamic contrast-enhancement MRI the functionality of the tissue can be investigated. The contrast agents used are paramagnetic agents with gadolinium (Gd-DTPA) being the most common. The increased vascularity of tumours produces a preferential uptake of contrast agent and the technique can be used to improve their contrast from surrounding normal tissue. In dynamic contrast-enhancement MRI, scans are repeatedly acquired following the contrast injection and the dynamic nature of contrast uptake can be examined, which may improve the differentiation of benign and malignant disease.

The main advantages of MRI are that the modality is suitable for women with denser breasts and the technique is non-ionising. It is possible to take images in any orientation and determine multi-focal cancers. The technique can also show breast implants and ruptures. The disadvantages of MRI are that a contrast agent is required to provide adequate specificity and that it is immobile, expensive, and unsuitable for some women. The modality cannot image calcifications and can induce feelings of claustrophobia, and require long scan times in comparison to x-ray mammography.

2.3 Ultrasound

Ultrasound is defined as a frequency of sound above the threshold of human hearing (i.e. > 20 kHz). The frequency range used in medical ultrasound imaging is 1 – 15 MHz. This allows wavelengths less than 1 mm to be measured and thus produces good spatial resolution. Ultrasound waves interact with tissue in a variety of ways but it is the reflection and transmission at interfaces between tissues of different acoustic impedance that is utilised in medical imaging. If there is a large acoustic mismatch between two tissues then a large fraction of the ultrasound intensity will be reflected. If there is a small difference in the acoustic impedance then most of the intensity will be transmitted. The time between pulse generation and the detection of an echo provides the depth of the reflecting interface, and thus images can be generated. Measuring the magnitude and time difference between different reflected signals can be used to determine the type, depth and size of different tissues.

Ultrasound pulses are generated and detected by a hand-held transducer, based on an array of small piezoelectric crystals. The very low acoustic impedance of air means that any boundary between air and tissue results in a near 100% reflection, so to ensure that the ultrasound waves are coupled into the body an impedance matching gel is used between the breast and the transducer. As there is a large difference between the acoustic impedance of a liquid filled cyst and normal breast tissue, around 23% of the ultrasound wave is reflected at such a boundary, making this technique particularly useful for the diagnosis of such a lesion. The small differences in acoustic impedance between adipose tissue and glandular tissue mean that this technique is of particular use for younger women with denser breasts, where x-ray mammography is often unsuitable. Doppler ultrasound utilises Doppler shifts from Rayleigh backscattered ultrasound waves to determine the velocity at which red blood cells are moving. Doppler ultrasound can be used to monitor blood flow and as a result can be used as an indicator of vascularisation of a malignant tumour in the breast.

Ultrasound is relatively inexpensive and a versatile technique. It can provide excellent contrast resolution, which means suspicious areas are easy to differentiate from normal tissue. X-ray mammograms are frequently followed up with ultrasound imaging to determine whether a lesion that appeared on a mammogram is a cyst or a solid mass. Since a fluid-filled cyst has a different sound signature than a solid mass, radiologists can reliably use ultrasound to identify cysts, which are commonly found in breasts. The technique can be used for younger women and women with breast implants and is entirely safe, and can be used repeatedly. The main disadvantages of the modality are the lack of fine detail, difficulty in detection of microcalcifications, poor ability to see deep lesions and inability to differentiate between certain types of solid breast masses.

2.4 Scintimammography

Scintimammography or nuclear medicine imaging is sometimes used alongside x-ray mammography in the diagnosis of breast disease since this technique is able to determine if a located lesion is malignant. The technique involves injection of a radioactive tracer into the patient. The tracer emits radiation, which is detected using a gamma camera. Appropriate image reconstruction algorithms enable the distribution of the tracer within the body to be mapped. Since the tracer accumulates differently in malignant and benign tissues it can be used to distinguish between the two conditions. Several radioactive compounds have been investigated, although only one, technetium-99m sestamibi (MIBI), is approved by FDA for use in breast imaging. A nuclear medicine investigation of the breast usually takes between 45 and 60 minutes. In a typical examination, the radioactive tracer (Tc-99m sestamibi) is injected into the patient's arm. The patient lies face down on a special table with her breast suspended through a hole. The images of the breast are taken from several angles using a gamma camera.

The advantages of scintimammography are that it can be used on patients with dense breasts and it can image large palpable lesions that do not appear with other imaging modalities. The modality involves the use of ionising substance that is injected into a patient (invasive) and is time consuming. Whilst it is 90% accurate for abnormalities over 1cm it is only 40- 60% accurate for smaller size abnormalities. The technique can be used to test tissue remaining from a mastectomy and can also be used to check for metastases in the auxiliary lymph nodes.

3. Techniques under development for breast cancer detection

There are several modalities that are at early stages of development but have a considerable potential as breast cancer detection devices. Majority of the imaging technologies for the breast are based on physical, mechanical, electrical, chemical and biological characteristics of the breast tissue. These detection techniques are based on their response to various tissue properties as listed in Table 2.

In an article about controversy over breast cancer screening, Reidy argued that death from malignancy rather than detection of malignancy should be a point of reference in evaluating any screening modality, since fast growing tumours, although detected while small, may have already metastasised. As a result, the number of malignancy related deaths have not altered regardless of their detection stage (Reidy, 1988). This has led to the view that the development of any new breast cancer detection modality must recognise the existence of three biologically distinct breast cancer patient subgroups. Firstly, there is a group of patients, which have slow-growing population of malignant cells that show ability to metastasise until very late. The second group comprises of patients with rapidly growing tumours that can lead to the development of micrometastases long before the tumour is detectable using the current modalities. Finally, there is the group of patients that have moderately fast growing tumours that may or may not be metastatic at the time of detection. The current breast cancer detection modalities are more valuable for the last group of patients. Some of the more likely modalities that can be developed as breast cancer diagnostic tools, which appear to be based on the recognition of the above points, are described in Table 3 and briefly discussed in the following sections.

Mode of Imaging	Tissue Property
Physical	Photon attenuation
	Temperature
Electrical	Conductivity
	Dielectric coefficient
	Impedance
Mechanical	Architecture
	Elasticity
Biological	Protein (expression/function)
	Perfusion

Table 2. Properties of breast tissue exploited by different modes of imaging

Modality	Description
Magnetic resonance spectroscopy	Use of magnetic resonance spectra and "functional" molecular markers to measure biochemical components of cells and tissues.
Optical imaging	Use of fibre-optic probes to obtain spectral measurements of elastically scattered light from tissue. Generates spectral signatures that reflect architectural changes at cellular and sub-cellular levels.
Optical tomography	Use of light to image the breast
Electrical potential measurements	Measurement of electrical potential at the skin surface. Proliferation of epithelial tissue disrupts normal polarization
Electronic palpation	Quantitative palpation of breast using pressure sensors.
Thermo acoustic computed tomography	Breast is irradiated with radio waves, causing different thermal expansion of tissue and generating sound waves, from which a three-dimensional image is constructed.
Microwave imaging	Transmits low-power microwaves into tissue and collects backscattered energy to create three-dimensional image. Higher water content in malignant tissues causes more scatter
Hall effect imaging	Induces vibrations by passing electric pulse through tissue while exposed to a magnetic field.
Magneto mammography	Tags cancerous tissue with magnetic agents that are imaged with SQUID magnetometers.

Table 3. Modalities under development for breast cancer detection

3.1 Optical imaging

Near infrared imaging is a simple method to determine the optical properties of tissues. It involves placing a light source onto the surface of the tissue and detecting the diffusely reflected light via a fibre/ detector placed some distance from the source. Measurements made in this manner can be used to determine the concentration of different chromophores such as oxy (HbO2) and de-oxy (Hb) haemoglobin within tissue. Optical imaging provides a potential alternative modality to the current breast cancer detection techniques. Diffuse optical tomography (DOT) and spectroscopy (DOS) are non-invasive techniques used to measure the optical properties of tissues. In the near-infrared (NIR) spectral window of 600 - 1000 nm, photon propagation in tissues is dominated by scattering rather than absorption. Photons experience multiple scattering events as they propagate deeply into tissue (up to 10 cm). The technique is based on the study of functional processes and provides several unique measurable parameters with potential to enhance breast tumour sensitivity and specificity. Optical tomography provides a distinction between different tissues based on their optical properties obtained from measurements of transmitted light. The presence of various substances in biological tissues contributes to the absorption of light. Tissue optical absorption coefficients provide access to blood dynamics, total haemoglobin concentration, blood oxygen saturation, water concentration and lipid content. These tissue properties are often substantially different in rapidly growing tumours; for example, high concentrations of haemoglobin with low oxygen saturation are suggestive of rapidly growing tumours due to their high metabolic demand. (Vaupel et al, 1991, 1998 & Weidner, et al 1992). The main substances of interest in optical imaging of breast tissue are water, lipids, haemoglobin and melanin. Of particular interest is the facility to exploit the differences between the absorption spectra of oxy-haemoglobin and deoxy-haemoglobin at near infrared wavelengths to produce images of blood volume and oxygen saturation (Cheng et al, 2003 & Jiang et al, 2003).

Optical tomography involves transillumination of the breast using near infrared (NIR) light. Characteristic absorption by oxy- and deoxy- haemoglobin at NIR wavelengths can be exploited to yield oxygen saturation and blood volume information. This information can provide a distinction between the high vascularisation often associated with malignant lesions and benign or normal breast tissue. Cutler demonstrated the first use of light for breast imaging in 1929 (Cutler, 1929), but it was not until the mid 1980s that interest in the subject became widespread due to the emergence of new source and detector technologies (Hebden et al, 1997). The research activity in this field was further enhanced by the developments in computing technology, which allowed the use of algorithms to reconstruct images representing the optical properties contained within a three-dimensional volume. The constant improvement in processing speeds and detectors has made optical tomography a potential safe alternative imaging technique that, in combination with conventional imaging techniques, can provide greater specificity for breast cancer diagnosis. In a recent study, a 32 channel time-correlated single photon counting system has been utilised to perform the test (Yates, 2005). Specific data extracted from a histogram of the times of flight of photons across the breast is used to reconstruct images of the optical properties. The reconstruction is performed using a non-linear, finite element based algorithm. One system is based on two rings of different diameters to which source and detector bundles are attached. Images displaying heterogeneous features that are unique to specific healthy tissues and reproducible are presented. Pre-diagnosed benign lesions can be identified but they are not always the most dominant feature. A single tumour is identified as a dominant increase in absorption. The second system based on a hemisphere filled with a coupling fluid can also be used. Preliminary findings suggest second method provides superior information to the ring system due to its three dimensional capability and its ability to provide consistent coupling.

3.2 Electrical impedance based modalities

Trans-scan (T-scan) and electrical impedance tomography (EIT) modalities are based on the principle that tissues have different conductivities depending on their cell structure and pathology. Cancerous tissue causes alterations in the intracellular and extracellular fluid compartments, cell membrane surface area, ionic permeability, and membrane associated water layers. These histological biochemical changes within the cancerous tissue give rise to measurable changes in tissue electrical impedance. When a small alternating current is placed across the breast, the increase in electrical conductance and capacitance of the cancer tissue distorts the electric field within the breast and the resulting impedance map can be used to highlight a malignant area.

3.2.1 Trans-scan (T-scan)

T-scan is an imaging technique that utilises the inherent differences in electrical impedance between neoplastic and normal tissue and maps noninvasively the distribution of the breast tissue electrical impedance and capacitance. It is a simple device that utilises measurements of electric impedance to distinguish between benign and malignant lesions. The methodology measures low-level bioelectric currents to produce real-time images of the electric impedance properties of the breast. It is considered that a T-scan used in addition to x-ray mammography can increase the specificity of breast cancer diagnosis. During a T-scan 1.0 to 2.5 mA of AC electrical current are generated by the system and conducted through the body via a metallic wand held by the patient. The scanning probe is then moved over the breast, and the current at the surface is measured. This information is then used to construct an image, which is immediately displayed on a computer screen. A gel is used between the skin and the scanning probe to improve the conductivity.

The technique employs relatively small and inexpensive devices and can detect small cancers down to 1 mm. The limitations of the method are that depth information is not available and microcalcifications cannot be detected. Furthermore T-scan cannot be used on patients with pacemakers and is less sensitive to larger tumours. The sensitivity and specificity of the T-scan have not yet been fully investigated, although values of 78% and 53 % respectively have been reported (Tetlow & Hubbard, 2000). T-scan has also been evaluated for symptomatic patients and women with screen-detected abnormalities. Patients undergoing both mammographic and T-scan examinations, which subsequently underwent excision or core biopsy, were retrospectively analysed. The results suggested that the T-scan is a useful addition to the assessment of patients, increasing diagnostic accuracy in terms of both sensitivity and specificity (Barter & Hicks, 2000).

3.2.2 Electrical impedance tomography (EIT)

EIT uses the same principles as a T-scan but utilises a number of measurements obtained by applying different current distributions to reconstruct an image of the electric impedance of the whole breast. The quantities measured by EIT are related to the electric impedance at low frequencies via the Laplace equation. The solution of the Laplace equation is very sensitive to noise in the measurements and so normalisation techniques are used. Most in-vivo images use linear approximating techniques which attempt to find a solution for a small change in resistivity from a known starting value. Until recently, this change in resistivity was measured over time, and so EIT images displayed physiological function. More recently anatomical images have been produced using the same reconstruction technique, but by imaging changes with frequency (Osterman, et al, 2000).

The advantages of using electric impedance devices are that they are much smaller and cheaper than other imaging modalities and use non-ionising radiation. Also in principle it is possible for EIT to produce thousands of images per second. Its main limitations are low resolution and large variation of images between subjects. The EIT technique still requires further research and development before it is approved for the detection of breast cancer.

3.3 Modalities based on histological examination and biomarkers
3.3.1 Fine needle biopsy

If a breast lesion appears to be suspicious or is undefined following examination using the imaging methods described then the patient will undergo a biopsy. There are two degrees of biopsy: fine needle aspiration cytology and core biopsy. In the first biopsy technique a fine needle and syringe are used to obtain a small sample of cells from the suspicious area. If this sample is insufficient or the diagnosis remains inconclusive a core biopsy may be needed which requires a larger needle to remove a larger sample of cells. In both cases the procedure is painful and involves the extraction of potentially diseased tissue through healthy tissue. This is one of the main reasons for a considerable research activity for the development of non-invasive imaging techniques with greater specificity that can reduce the need for biopsy.

3.3.2 Ductal lavage

Ductal lavage is a relatively newer technique used to detect pre-cancerous and cancerous breast cell changes in women who are at high risk for developing breast cancer. It is estimated that over 95% of breast cancers begin in the cells lining the breast ducts. Ductal lavage involves analysing cells that have effectively been washed out from the breast ducts using a breast pump or aspirator. The cells are studied under a microscope to determine whether they have malignant characteristics before they develop into breast cancer. This technique is still in its early stages of development and is a similar idea to the Pap smear used to test for cervical cancer.

3.3.3 Tumour markers

These are substances produced by cancer cells and sometimes normal cells. They can be found in large amounts in the blood or urine of some patients with cancer. Less often, they can also be found in large amounts in the blood or urine of people who do not have cancer. There are many different kinds of tumour markers. Some are produced only by a single type of cancer. Others can be produced by several types of cancer. Most tumour markers used today are proteins or parts of proteins. They are detected by combining the patient's blood or urine with antibodies made to react with that specific protein. The results of any tumour marker test are considered with other laboratory test results and a thorough medical history and physical examination. The American Society of Clinical Oncology first published evidence-based clinical practice guidelines for the use of tumour markers in breast cancer in

1996, which are updated at regular intervals. Thirteen categories of breast tumour markers have been considered that showed evidence of clinical utility and were recommended for use in practice. These include: CA 15-3, CA 27.29, carcinoembryonic antigen, oestrogen receptor, progesterone receptor, human epidermal growth factor receptor 2, urokinase plasminogen activator, plasminogen activator inhibitor 1, and certain multiparameter gene expression assays. Not all applications for these markers were supported, however. The following categories demonstrated insufficient evidence to support routine use in clinical practice: DNA/ploidy by flow cytometry, p53, cathepsin D, cyclin E, proteomics, certain multiparameter assays, detection of bone marrow micrometastases, and circulating tumour cells (Harris et.al, 2007). However, as yet, there are no tumour markers that are useful for diagnosis of early stage breast cancer.

3.4 Thermal imaging techniques (TITs) for breast cancer detection

Thermography is based on the principle that metabolism and blood vessel proliferation in both pre-cancerous tissue and the area surrounding a developing breast cancer is almost always higher than in normal breast tissue. Developing tumours increase circulation to their cells by enlarging existing blood vessels and creating new ones in a process called neovascularisation or angiogenesis. This uncontrolled proliferation is considered to be of critical importance in the development of neoplastic condition. The tumour mass is unable to grow to a detectable size (2 mm^3) without the establishment of a new blood supply, since passive diffusion of nutrients and waste products is not sufficient for the growing tumour's metabolic requirements. Angiogenesis is induced as a result of the release of a variety of angiogenic peptides that may be produced by the neoplastic cells. These newly developed blood vessels are quite porous and provide easy access to the circulating immediately adjacent tumour cells. For this reason the propensity to metastasise has been related to the number of micro vessels found in a growing mass of tumour. (Nathanson et al, 2000; Wade & Kozolowski, 2007). This process frequently results in an increase in regional temperature of the breast and forms the basis of the thermal modalities for the detection of breast cancer.

The first recorded use of thermo-biological diagnostics can be found in the writings of Hippocrates around 480 B.C. Mud slurry was spread over the patient and allowed to dry. The body areas that dried first were thought to indicate underlying organ pathology. Since then continued research and clinical observations proved that certain temperatures related to the human body were indeed indicative of normal and abnormal physiological processes. There are two thermal based modalities that could have a very significant impact on the detection and diagnosis of breast cancer. These are named as infrared thermography and microwave radiometry. Both techniques detect the changes in the physiology of the tissue rather than evaluating the changes in the tissue anatomical and dielectric features. Figure 4 illustrates that the physiological changes (preclinical phase) in the tissue begin nearly eight years earlier before they become apparent in the form of mass of malignant tumour (Lundgren, 1981).

Although thermography is an appealing method of screening for breast cancer, research over the past 20 years has failed to produce a system that is reliable for such a purpose and therefore thermography is not a widely used modality. However, it is expected that advances such as computerised thermal imaging will provide significant improvement in the cancer detection rate but this remains to be seen. Furthermore, attenuation of infrared radiation in tissue is high. For this reason thermography will only ever be able to provide information on the surface temperature variations and so no depth information is available. This is a severe limitation of infrared thermography in detecting breast cancer.

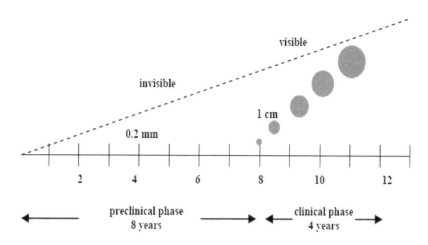

Fig. 4. Kinetics of tumour growth ((Lundgren, 1981)

3.4.1 Infrared thermography

Infrared thermal imaging has been used for several decades to monitor the temperature distribution over human skin. Abnormalities such as malignancies, inflammation, and infection cause localized increases in temperature that appear as hot spots or asymmetrical patterns in an infrared thermogram. Thermography, alternatively termed thermometry has been pursued for many years as a technique for breast cancer detection. Studies of thermography have focused on a range of potential uses, including diagnosis, prognosis, and risk indication and as an adjunct to existing technologies; however, the results have been inconsistent and scientific consensus has been difficult to achieve. The research activity in infrared thermography as cancer detection technique was diminished in the 1970s, but the recent technological advances have renewed the interest in the modality. Digital infrared cameras have much-improved spatial and thermal resolutions, and libraries of image processing routines are available to analyze images captured both statically and dynamically.

As an addition to the breast health screening process, infrared imaging has a significant role to play. Due to the technique's unique ability to image the metabolic aspects of the breast, very early warning signals have been observed in long-term studies. A breast tumour can raise the temperature of the skin surface by as much as 3 ^{0}C compared with the temperature of the skin surface of a woman with normal tissue probably due to the elevated rates of tumour metabolism and elevated levels of vascularity and perfusion. It is for this reason that an abnormal infrared image may be the single most important marker of high risk for the existence of or future development of breast cancer. Furthermore, the proven sensitivity, specificity, and prognostic value of the modality, makes infrared imaging one of the frontline methods for breast cancer screening. The diagnosis of cancer is based on the difference in temperature relative to that for the contralateral breast, which serves as a built-in control. The procedure is non-invasive and does not require compression of the breast or radiation exposure.

3.4.2 Microwave radio thermometry (MRT)

The National Cancer Institute (NCI) in the United States of America has funded numerous research projects to improve conventional and develop new technologies to detect, diagnose, and characterize breast cancer. According to the U.S. Institute of Medicine, an ideal breast screening tool is a low risk device that is sensitive to tumours, detects breast cancer at a curable stage, non-invasive, simple to use, cost effective and widely available. The device should also involve minimal discomfort to the user and provides easy to interpret, objective and consistent results. Of particular importance is the ability to clearly distinguish between malignant and benign tumours and early detection. A brief review of the published literature shows that all techniques have limited capability in these respects and surgery is required to establish the nature of the tumour. The research in this area is time consuming since the ultimate test of a technique beyond the proof of concept stage must be clinical trials.

Microwave radio thermometry (MRT) is a modality that uses non ionising electromagnetic radiation for cancer detection in humans. The technique has attracted a great deal of research in the last three decades. An electromagnetic imaging method can be active or passive. In an active system, one or more antennas radiate onto the body, where the electromagnetic field is scattered by tissue dielectric inhomogeneities and then received by the same or other antennas. In multi-frequency active imaging, data is collected at various frequencies and for various locations of the antennas outside the body [Liu et al, 2002; Meaney et al, 2000]. Field data are known terms in the inverse scattering problem, whose solution attempts a retrieval of the contrast of an eventual dielectric anomaly with respect to the background permittivity of healthy tissues. On the other hand time-domain systems exploit higher frequencies and wide-band antennas showing some similarity to ground penetrating radar [Fear & Stuchly, 2000; Li et al, 2004].

Thermal imaging methods include both infrared and microwave radiometry modalities. Both methods detect physiological tissue response, rather than evaluating anatomic dielectric features. Heat is released from the body on the whole electromagnetic spectrum with a maximum at infrared frequencies. There are several physiological features that are related to malignant tissue, which may contribute to the infrared signal. These include increased blood flow in the area surrounding a malignancy, angiogenesis, and the release of vasoactive mediators. The infrared imaging system uses a camera that is highly sensitive to infrared radiation in the appropriate spectrum. Microwave radiometry is based on the measurement of the electromagnetic field spontaneously emitted by a body in the microwave frequency range [Bardati & Solimini, 1983; Edrich, 1979; Leroy et al, 1998; Meyer et al, 1979]. Charged particles in motion are primary sources of incoherent thermal radiation propagating inside the body, where it is partially absorbed and partially radiated externally. Antennas located in the vicinity of the body collect and changes the radiation to an electrical current that fluctuates in the receiver's input unit. Assuming that the body is in a thermodynamic equilibrium, the spectral content of the radiometric signal can be related to the local temperature distribution in the body, allowing its retrieval to be attempted from radiometric data collected at different frequencies and for various antenna positions. A thermal anomaly may be a significant indicator of a malignancy.

The fundamental basis for developing a microwave imaging technique for detecting breast cancer is the significant contrast in the dielectric properties, at microwave frequencies, of normal and malignant breast tissue, as evidenced by experimentally measured data [Li et al, 2005; Bardati et al 2002]. The estimated malignant-to-normal breast tissue contrast is between 2:1 and 10:1, depending on the density and water content of the different tissues. Therefore, microwave modality does not offer the potential for the high spatial resolution provided by X-rays, but it does permit exceptionally high contrast with respect to physical or physiological factors of clinical interest, such as water content, vascularisation or angiogenesis, blood-flow rate, and temperature. Microwave imaging techniques result in a three-dimensional (3-D) volumetric mapping of the relevant tissue properties, and thus offer in situ 3-D positioning of the tissue abnormalities. Furthermore, microwave attenuation in normal breast tissue is low enough to make signal propagation through even large breast volumes quite feasible (~ 4 cm). For these reasons, microwave breast imaging has the potential to overcome some of the limitations of conventional breast cancer screening modalities.

Microwave systems in use or under development may be categorised into three types: passive, active or hybrid. However, the passive technique has been investigated for many years, with clinical trials undertaken with the availability of commercial units that are currently used mainly in conjunction with mammography. The passive method detects regions of increased temperature due to the tumour from the very small "natural" microwave signal from the breast (black body radiation as given by Planck's law). The signals detected are very low and require sensitive electronic systems. Temperature differentials between adjacent areas on the breast are taken as an indication of an abnormality, using a similar area on the other breast as a reference – the approach is somewhat empirical. The increased tumour temperature is thought to arise from "vascularisation" (angiogenesis). There is a great deal of ongoing research, which is related to the development of thermal models of the breast to relate the measured temperature differentials with temperature rises located in the tissue. There is also a considerable focus for the last few years in the USA on the development of detecting antennas. There is evidence that the passive MRT technique can detect malignant tissue abnormality at an early stage, but as yet this cannot be taken as an established fact.

Current understandings of the underlying pathological mechanisms for increased temperature in breast cancer are that breast cancer cells produce nitric oxide, which interferes with the normal neuronal (nervous system) control of breast tissue blood vessel flow by causing regional vasodilation in the early stages of cancerous cell growth, and enhancing angiogenesis in the later stages. The subsequent increased blood flow in the area causes a temperature increase relative to the normal breast temperature, and even deep breast lesions may also contribute to the detectable increase in the heat evolved. These changes relate to physiological breast processes. It is believed that in healthy individuals, temperature is generally symmetrical across the midline of the body. Subjective interpretation of many diagnostic imaging modalities, including microwave thermometry and infrared thermography, rely on the normal contralateral images are relatively symmetrical, and the likelihood that small asymmetries may indicate a tissue abnormalities. Therefore, in breast cancer, thermography/thermometry detects disease by identifying areas of asymmetric temperature distribution on the breast surface.

Microwave radiometry is used for diagnosis of diseases by measuring small changes of internal tissue temperature. The detection and diagnosis is conducted by measuring the intensity of natural electromagnetic radiation of patient's internal tissues at microwave frequencies. The intensity of radiation is proportional to the temperature of the tissues. Cancerous tumours have a significantly different index of refraction and the internal tissue temperature often changes due to inflammation changes in the blood supply or with increased metabolism of cells during oncological transformation of tissues. Microwave radiometry measures the emission of natural radiation from the body in the microwave, or centrimetric, region of the electromagnetic spectrum. All materials above absolute zero emit natural, thermally generated electromagnetic radiation. At body temperature of 37°C the maximum intensity of radiation occurs in the infrared part of the spectrum at wavelengths close to 10 μmeters (Fraseri et al, 1987).

Microwave thermometry may be envisioned as the microwave analogue of infrared thermography (Barrett, et al, 1980). Whereas infrared thermography uses wavelengths of 10 mm (typical), microwave thermometry makes use of much longer wavelengths, typically 1 - 20 cm; this leads to important and fundamental differences between the two techniques as described in the literature(Barrett & Myers, 1975a, 1975b; Barrett et al, 1977, 1980). Microwave radiation is capable of penetrating human tissue and therefore the emission provides information related to subcutaneous conditions within the body. The intensity of microwave emission is linearly proportional to the temperature of the emitter. Therefore, microwave thermometry provides information related to internal body temperatures. The depth of penetration, and hence the depth from which microwave radiation may escape from the body, depends on the wavelength, the dielectric properties of the tissue and the water content of the tissue. Furthermore, the frequency used for microwave breast imaging needs to be low enough to provide adequate depth of penetration, but high enough to allow the use of small antenna array elements. The final resolution of the image depends on both the number of antenna array elements and the frequency. In general, resolution increases with frequency and the number of antenna array elements. In order to obtain useful images, there must be significant contrast between normal and malignant tissue and the greatest contrast in breast tissue occurs in the frequency range 600 MHz-1 GHz.

The distinctive feature of microwave radiometry is an extremely low signal strength entering input of the antenna from the biological tissues. This signal strength is approximately 10^{-13} Watt. While conducting the measurement it is necessary to distinguish temperatures differing on a tenth part of degree, which corresponds to signal strength to be 10^{-16} Watt. Therefore the special circuits are required for receipt, amplification and treatment of signals. So far, the application of microwave radiometry has been directed at the early detection and diagnosis of breast cancer. Present breast cancer detection techniques, other than radiometry, require that the tumour must have significant mass and contrast with respect to the surrounding tissue (i.e., palpation physical examination, mammography and ultrasound). This results in approximately 85 percent of all determinations of breast disease undergoing extensive surgical procedures. Early detection could lead to a more conservative treatment and a positive attitude toward detection. The diagnosis of breast cancer at a smaller size or earlier stage will allow a woman more choice in selecting among various treatment options.

The passive MRT method is a non-invasive, non-ionizing procedure that determines the thermal activity of the tissue rather than mass and therefore when used in conjunction with one or more other detection modalities, could provide early indication of breast with good accuracy. The determination of thermal activity is a measurement of tumour activity, or growth rate, providing data beyond the physical parameters (i.e., size and depth determined by mammography). Suspicious results found by screening using microwave radiometry could then be referred for further investigation by mammography and other appropriate techniques. Medical microwave radiometry has a number of positive characteristics as follows:

- Early diagnosis of diseases;
- Possibility of non-invasive detection of disease in internal organs before the appearance of structural changes that can be detected by X rays or ultrasound;
- Completely harmless for the patients of all age and with any diseases as well as for medical staff;
- Possibility to conduct the investigation repeatedly (control of treatment):
- Depth of anomaly detection is from 3 to 10 cm;
- Accuracy of measuring the internal averaged temperature ± 0,2 ⁰C
- Simplicity of the device handling, the procedure may be conducted by the secondary medical staff.
- Time measuring of one point: 5 – 15 sec.

3.5 The concept of the smart bra as an early warning system for breast cancer

The concept of wearable early warning system for breast cancer is under investigation at the Institute of Materials Research and Innovation (IMRI), University of Bolton. The researchers are working on the development of a wearable system that integrates the passive microwave antennae with textile structures. The basic concept of this approach is to present the microwave antennas to the breast in the form of a 'Smart Bra'. Work on developing antenna systems and microelectronics is being carried out. Miniaturisation of the radiometer, antennae and electronics and there integration with appropriate textile structures are the main thrusts of the research and development programmes in progress. It remains to be established how much of the electronics would be mounted on the bra and how critical accurate positioning of the sensors would be. The incorporation of the electronics is the critical part of the research and development programme. Work is also in progress on the development of wearable breast cancer device at De Montfort University, Leicester, UK. This is a low frequency active electrical impedance tomography (EIT) based system, which utilises the differences in electrical properties between healthy and malignant breast tissues and the researchers have introduced the concept of a "Smart Bra" which allows the impedance tomography to be carried out conveniently and rapidly. However, the microwave radio thermometry modality being adopted by the Bolton team is non-contact and passive whereas the EIT is an active modality albeit at low power levels. In the following sections the concept of MRT based wearable early warning system for breast cancer is described.

The microwave radiometer is a device which measures the intensity of electromagnetic radiation from human body in microwave wave length. The noise power at the input of the microwave receiver is proportional to the internal temperature of human body. An array of receivers can resolve the local temperature inside the breast in 3-D and hence provide a signature of local temperature differences inside the breast. The geometrical resolution is determined by the element number and the bandwidth and frequency of operation. Tumour detection relies on temperature difference resolution, which is a function of the noise figure of the receiver, its stability and the bandwidth as well as the test integration time (Skou, 2006).

Traditional microwave radiometers for breast cancer detection known from literature and available on the market are rather large and heavy in weight. Today, only one relatively compact model of microwave radiometer (RTM-01-RES) is available in the market. The radiometer receives energy-emissions from the human body using an infrared sensor and a microwave sensor. The weight of internal temperature sensor is rather high and consequently it is not possible to incorporate such a device in a self-powered wearable system. It is therefore necessary to design miniature balance zero Microwave Radiometer and the Microwave Multi-Channel Electron Switch (MMCES). Miniaturization is essential for both technical reasons, achieving direct coupling to antenna and good stability, as well as for integration into textiles for maximum comfort. In traditional microwave systems antennae are fabricated on rigid substrates, as wires or as hollow structures. Antennae on textiles have been demonstrated earlier but only with limited design variations, mainly as microstrip patch or slot antennae (Klemm et al, 2004, 2005; Locher, 2006; Klemm & Troester, 2005, 2006; Behdad, 2004; & Alomainy et al, 2005). There is a need to explore different structures especially in view of multi-frequency or wideband operation.

The relevant accuracy of measuring the noise power at the input of the receiver is $\sim 10^{-3}$. The dielectric constant of a person may change dramatically from 5.5 for fat breast to 50 for muscle. Therefore, the reflection coefficient between antenna and human body tissue may change significantly and as a result about 10% of energy may be reflected from the antenna. However, the accuracy of noise power measurement should remain unchanged. In order to solve this problem it is necessary to use zero balance radiometer with compensation of reflections between antenna and human body tissue. This principle is used in most modern microwave radiometers (Leroy et al, 1998, Hand et al, 2001 & Lee et al, 2002). An overview of microwave radiometry is given in a recent publication (Hand et al, 2001). The balance multi-frequency microwave radiometer has also been described (Leroy et al, 1998). These researchers used 5 frequencies in calculating the temperature profile in the brain. It is very important to use multi-frequency radiometer in order to visualize the temperature inside body. But the increase in the number of frequencies increases the sizes and the weight of the radiometer and decreases the noise imperviousness of the device. The radiation from human body is very small therefore the noise immunity is one of the critical parameters of the microwave radiometer.

It is expected that the multi frequency radiometer will have better accuracy for breast cancer detection in comparison with a single channel radiometer, but it is not evident that the sensitivity will increase greatly. Thousands of measurements during 10 years with the microwave radiometer (RTM-01-RES) have shown that there are about 10 % of breast cancer patients who have no skin temperature increase or brightness temperature increase (Burdina et al, 2005). Thus the probability that these patients will have temperature increase at another frequency is not very high. Due to the weight and sizes limitations for a wearable system, there is no reason to use more than two frequencies. Furthermore, skin temperature information is very important for breast cancer detection.

The fluctuation error of radiometer is dependent on time of integration, the bandwidth and losses of the microwave part of the receiver. Usually for the receiver's bandwidth of 500-600 MHz the measurement time is 5 seconds and fluctuation error is 0.1°C. The increase of bandwidth may decrease the fluctuation error. Another possibility to decrease the fluctuation error is to increase the integration time. Monolithic microwave integrated circuit (MMIC) provides the opportunity to increase the bandwidth of microwave device greatly. Furthermore, for wearable, self-examination devices the time of measurement is not a very important factor, therefore, the fluctuation error may be minimized by choosing the proper value of integration time.

It may be possible to combine a single channel microwave radiometer and a MMCES. In this case, the results of brightness temperature measurement will highly depend on the environment temperature, due to the losses in the MMCES. To overcome this problem, it is necessary to use balance zero radiometer and balance the losses of MMCES and losses of reference noise source. In this situation the losses of MMCES do not decrease the performance of radiometer. Furthermore, it is possible to minimise the losses in MMCES by the utilization of integrated radiometer front-ends. The integration requires the design and fabrication of microwave monolithic integrated circuits with ultra low-noise performance. This can be achieved using state-of-the-art MMIC fabrication processes. Such components are very compact (few square millimetres) and therefore minimize losses and temperature variations. The employed fabrication processes can achieve amplifiers with noise figure below NF<0.5 dB with high gain resulting in excellent radiometer performance (Dabrowski et al, 2004). However, these devices are either large and operate at cryogenic temperatures or are relatively narrowband. There is a need to especially focus on the development of wideband for multi-frequency receiver in order to improve the overall system performance. Yet, another possibility is the introduction of multi-receiver system alleviating the need for an MMCES. This however requires identical channel operation, which can only be fabricated using identical components. In the development of MMIC for the radiometer front-end such a technique becomes feasible.

Introduction of microelectronic microwave components close to the antenna requires appropriate textile integration technologies. This aspect has been dealt within various publications both with woven and nonwoven materials (Catrysse et al, 2004; Coosemans et al, 2005; Hermans et al, 2005; Van Langenhove et al, 2003a, 2003b; Scilingo et al, 2005 & Paradiso et al, 2005). However, only little data is available on the microwave properties of different woven and nonwoven materials (Locher, 2006). Interconnection to the microwave monolithic integrated circuit is an important area of research and development. One possible approach is the implementation of ribbon type interconnects, which can efficiently be used for power supply and low frequency output signals. The active components need to be developed with MMIC operating over a wide range. Low-noise amplifiers determine the overall noise performance of the receivers. Very wideband performance has been demonstrated in GaAs and CMOS technologies, respectively (Nosal, 2001; Jung et al, 2006; Xu et al, 2005 & Wang et al, 2005). However, in most cases a noise figure NF>1.0 dB over a frequency range of DC – 10 GHz has been achieved. There is a need to design amplifiers complying with the frequency range of DC – 10 GHz, but exhibiting a noise figure NF < 1.0 dB with an associated gain of G > 30 dB. These parameters are well beyond the state-of-the-art today. There is a need to develop MMIC components that can be used for the assembly of the microwave radiometer system. Figure 5 shows one possible functional scheme of Multi-Channel Microwave Radiometer.

Multi-Channel Microwave Radiometer's development consists of the following stages.

- Designing of Multi-Channel switch.
- Designing of Radiometer's microwave parts
- Designing of radiometer's digital part and analog low-frequency part of feedback circuit.
- Software design for visualization of the measurements and for the radiometer's microcontrollers.

Microwave radiometer consists of an electronic switch, circulator, isolator, low-noise amplifier, filter, amplitude detector and miniature reference noise source with the temperature sensor. All of these components parts must be designed in miniature sizes using MMIC and plastic materials.

There are two critical parameters which define Radiometer's quality:

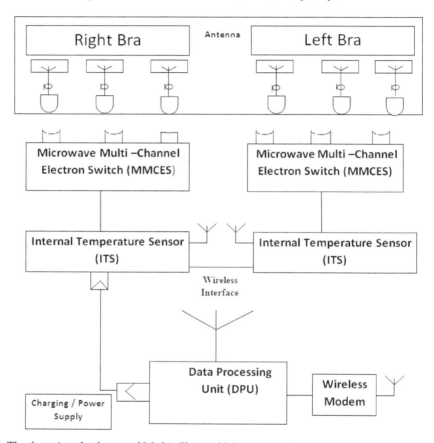

Fig. 5. The functional scheme of Multi-Channel Microwave Radiometer

1.   Brightness temperature error when the reflection's coefficient of antenna changes.
2.   Brightness temperature error when the environment's temperature changes.

The over arching aim of the research in progress on the development of wearable breast cancer detection system is to deliver a miniaturized microwave technology, Multi-frequency Microwave Radiometry (MFMWR), which is a totally non-invasive and passive method for cancer detection. It is proposed to use microwave radiometry (MWR) to detect the "hot spots" (the cancerous regions) in the breast tissue. This technology was initially used in the field of astrophysics, measuring the minute amounts of microwave energy emitted by stars and planets. The same principle can be used for medical diagnostics (Chaudhary, 1984), as anything that can absorb radiation also emits radiation. In MWR, the power in the

microwave region of the natural thermal radiation from body tissues is measured to obtain
the brightness temperature of the tissue under observation. The brightness temperature at
an antenna centre frequency f_i is,

$$T_{B,i} = \frac{P_i}{k\,df_i} = \frac{(1-R_i)\,P_{tissue,i}}{k\,df_i} = (1-R_i)\,T_{B,tissue,i} \tag{1}$$

Where $P_{tissue,i}$ is the thermal radiation power emitted by the tissue, P_i is the power received
by the antenna in a bandwidth df_i around f_i, R_i is the power reflection coefficient at the skin-
antenna interface at f_i and k is Boltzmann's constant.

According to the Rayleigh-Jeans law, at microwave frequency f_i, the thermal radiation
intensity is proportional to the absolute temperature, so that

$$T_{B,i} = \int_{\Omega} W_i\,T(r)\,dv \tag{2}$$

where $T(r)$ is the absolute temperature in a tissue volume of dv located at r, $W_i(r)$ is the
receiving antenna's weighting function and the integration is over the antenna's field of
view Ω.

It can be seen that (equation 1) that the brightness temperature $T_{B,i}$ is dependent upon the
temperature in the tissue $T_{B,tissue,i}$ and the reflection coefficient R. For balance zero
radiometer with the compensation of the reflection on the border antenna and tissue the
reflection from the tissue is compensated by thermal radiation of the radiometer and the
brightness temperature is independent of reflection coefficient R. Therefore, for non-
invasive detection of temperature abnormalities it is possible measure the power radiation P
from the tissue.

Thus the measured brightness temperature at frequency f_i,

$$T_{B,i} = \frac{\displaystyle\int_{\Omega} W_i\,T(r)\,dv}{1-R_i} \tag{3}$$

The receiving antenna's weighting function depends upon its operating frequency and
microwave attenuating properties of the tissues, as well as antenna characteristics. Microwave
reflections occur at interfaces between different tissue regions and between these regions and
the measuring equipment. Since the attenuation of microwaves in tissue and the antenna
characteristics are frequency dependent, the temperature-depth profile within the tissue
beneath the antenna can be found using a multi-frequency radiometer and a stable solution to
the inverse problem of retrieving the temperature-depth dependence from a set of measured
brightness temperatures. The human body's tissues have different permittivities therefore the
reflection coefficient of the antenna for diverse people or in different tissues can reach 10%.
This fact can decrease noise power at the input on the radiometer. But brightness temperature
cannot change in spite of the fact that the brightness temperature is proportional to noise
power at the input on the radiometer. This problem can be overcome by balance zero
radiometer with sliding scheme of the reflections compensation.

Evidently the temperature of microwave part of the radiometer may change greatly. This
leads to noise power change at the input of the radiometer. If the front-end loss of

radiometer is about 1 dB, one degree change in the environment temperature will lead to brightness temperature change in 0.4 degree. This is why the radiometer input circuits temperature is usually stabilized. But this is not feasible for the wearable self-powered detection system because of the power demand. For balanced radiometer it is possible to optimize parameters of input circuit including Multi-Channel Switch and the reference noise source circuit to minimize error due to environment temperature changes. However, if the losses of microwave part of radiometer do not change in time, the error due to environment temperature change can be compensated. For this purpose it is necessary to measure the front-end temperature. This principle was successfully used in industrial single-channel radiometer (RTM-01-RES) and can be applied to the multi-channel radiometer. For this purpose it is important to measure antenna array temperature and to transmit this information to the radiometer. Software is a need for visualisation of the results of the measurements and the database storage in the control centre. It is vital that radiometer should monitor the function of its various components appropriately, estimate the measurement error and transmit this information to the central database by wireless connection. This allows the estimation of the radiometer's accuracy automatically. Fabrication of the breast cancer microwave screening system also requires the development of the hardware for the system.

Microwave thermometry is the detection of microwave radiation from the human body and may be considered as the microwave equivalent of infrared thermography. Infrared thermography typically uses wavelengths of 10 μmetre, whereas in microwave thermometry much longer wavelengths are employed (1 -20 cm). The other major differences between the two modalities can be summarised as following:

- Microwave radiation is capable of penetrating human tissue and therefore the emissions can provide useful thermal signals related to the subcutaneous conditions within the body. On the other hand, infrared radiation is not able to penetrate such depths and therefore is able to detect conditions close to the surface i.e. skin.
- The intensity of microwave emission is linearly proportional to the temperature of the emitter. Therefore a measurement of the emission may be easily related to the temperature of the emitter. Infrared intensity measurements may also be related to the body temperature but this relationship is somewhat nonlinear.
- Microwave emission gives coarser spatial resolution (~ 1cm) than infrared because of its longer wavelength than infrared (~1mm). This supposes that microwave thermography provides information about internal body temperatures. The depth of penetration, and hence the depth from which microwave radiation may escape from the body, depends on the wavelength, the dielectric properties of the tissue, and, most importantly, on the water content of the tissue.

Development of a wearable, self-powered early warning system for breast cancer will also require the production of textile structures that are flexible, comfortable, breathable, light and suitable for integration with the materials developed to perform various functions to operate the cancer detecting devices produced. Conducting fibres and filaments are needed to produce fabrics using a range of mechanical conversion methods, particularly knitting, crochet or braiding to produce the developmental materials. The structures then need to be characterised and optimised. Conducting fabrics can also be prepared using chemical methods, including coating, printing and lamination. Wet chemical methods and dry methods can be employed for this purpose. The integrated textile structures must be tested for their efficiency, durability, launderability, mechanical and comfort properties. Finally, the integrated textiles need to be converted into wearable structures to act as cancer detection devices.

4. Conclusions

At present x-ray mammography is the most commonly used breast imaging technique and is the only modality used for routine screening. X-ray mammography has become the "gold standard" for breast imaging. The technique has a high sensitivity and is able to detect very small tumours and calcifications. The main limitations of x-ray mammography are that it has a poor specificity for some tumour types and that it is unsuitable for use on women with dense breasts. In addition, x-ray mammography uses ionising radiation and usually causes considerable discomfort to the patient. Thus there is potential for an alternative technique to replace x-ray mammography or to be used as an additional resource to improve the overall specificity of the diagnosis. As discussed MRI, ultrasound and Nuclear medicine are currently used to provide additional diagnostic information, but all have their limitations and are not alternatives to mammography. Other techniques are currently being investigated such as EIT and infrared thermography but as yet these have severe limitations in resolution and specificity. Thus there still remains a niche for an additional imaging modality to aid in the early detection and diagnosis of breast tissue oncological abnormalities.

Microwave radiometry (MRT) appears to be an attractive alternative modality for breast imaging. MRT can be used effectively in breast cancer investigation. The method has many advantages over the currently used breast cancer detection techniques:

- Oncological changes in tissues could be detected earlier using MRT as compared to the classical methods based on ultrasounds and ionising radiation
- Breast cancer detection is made at a curable stage
- The technique is non-invasive and non-hazardous both to the patient and the device operator.
- MRT is easy to use, cheap and fast
- Involves no risk for patients of any age
- Involves a minimum discomfort for patient, easily accepted by women - is easy to interpret and objective.

The MRT can be used repeatedly to improve cancer detection rates and monitor the progress of cancer treatment. Using microwave radiometry in conjunction with other traditional modalities can significantly improve the diagnosis, especially for the patients with fast growing tumours. Studies show that breast thermometry has the ability to warn a woman that a cancer may be forming many years before any other test can detect the condition. The major gaps in knowledge can be addressed by more robust research on the technologically advanced microwave thermometry devices and large-scale, prospective randomised trials for population screening and diagnostic testing of breast cancer. The MRT system components can be miniaturised and integrated with textiles to produce wearable early warning systems for breast cancer.

5. References

Alomainy, A.; Hao, Y.; Parini, C. & Hall, P. (2005). Comparison Between Two Different Antennas for UWB Onbody Propagation Measurements', *IEEE Antennas and Wireless Propagation Letters*, Vol. 4, pp. 31-34

Bardati, D.; Marrocco, G. & Tognolatti, P. (2002). New-born-infant Brain Temperature Measurement by Microwave Radiometry, *Antennas and Propagation Society International Symposium, 2002. IEEE*,Vol.1, pp. 811,

Barrett, A et al, (1980)Microwave Thermography in the Detection of Breast Cancer', *AJR*, Vol.134, pp. 365-368.

Barrett, A. & Myers, P. (1975). Microwave Thermography', *Bibl Radiol,* Vol.6, pp. 45-56

Barrett, A. & Myers, P. (1975). Subcutaneous Temperatures: A Method of Noninvasive Sensing, *Science, Vol.*1 90, pp.669-671

Barrett, A.; Myers, P. & N L Sadowsky, N. (1977). Detection of Breast Cancer by Microwave Radiometry, *Radio Science, Vol.*1 2, pp.167-171

Barrett, A.; Myers, P. & N L Sadowsky, N. (1980), Microwave Thermography of Normal and Cancerous Breast Tissue. *Conference on thermal characteristics of tumors: applications in detection and treatment*, New York, March, 979. Ann NY Acad Sci.

Barter, S & IP Hicks (2000). Electrical Impedance Imaging of the Breast (TranScan TS 2000): Initial UK Experience. *Breast Cancer Res, Symposium Mammographicum 2000.* Vol. 2, (Suppl 2):A11

Behdad, N. (2004). A Wideband Multiresonant Single-Element Slot Antenna. *Antennas and Wireless Propagation Letters,* Vol. 3, pp.5-8

Boyd, N.; Byng, J. & Jong, R. (1995). Quantitative Classification of Mammographic Densities and Breast Cancer Risk. *J. Natl Cancer Inst.*, Vol.87, pp. 670

Burdina, L. et al. (2005).Tikhomirova «Microwave Radiometry in Algorithm Complex Diagnosis of Breast Diseases', *Modern Oncology*, 2005, V6, №1, p.8-9 (in Russian)

Brem, R.; Kieper, D.; Rapelyea, J. & Majewski, S. (2003). Evaluation of a High-Resolution, Breast-Specific, Small-Field-of-View Gamma Camera for the Detection of Breast Cancer. *Nuclear Instruments and Methods in Physics Research A* Vol.497, (2003), pp. 39–45

Catrysse, M. et al (2004). Towards the Integration of Textile Sensors in a Wireless Monitoring Suit. *Sensors and Actuators.* Vol. A114, pp. 302-311, 2004

Chaudhary, S.; R. K. Mishra.; Swarup, A. & Thomas, J. (1984). Dielectric Properties of Normal and Malignant Human Breast Tissues at Radiowave and Microwave Frequencies. *Indian J. Biochem. Biophys.* Vol.21, pp. 76–79

Cheng, X.; Mao, J.; Bush, R.; Kopans, D.; Moore, R. & Chorlton, M. (2003). Breast Cancer Detection by Mapping Hemoglobin Concentration and Oxygen Saturation. *Applied Optics,* Vol.42, pp. 6412-6421

Coosemans, J.; Hermans, B. & Puers, R. (2005). Integrating Wireless ECG Monitoring in Textiles', *International Conference on Solid-State Sensors and Actuators, Transducers 05*, pp. 228-232, June 5-9, 2005

Cutler, M. (1929). Transillumination as an Aid in the Diagnosis of Breast Lesions. *Surg Gynecol Obstet,* Vol. 48, pp. 721-729

Dabrowski, J. et al, 'Design and Performance of Low Noise Cascode IC for Wireless Applications', *15th International Conference on Microwaves, Radar and Wireless Communications*, Vol. 3, pp. 882-885, May 2004

Elmore, J.; Wells, F. & Carol, M. (1994). Variability in Radiologists Interpretation of Mammograms. *NEJM.* Vol. 331, No.22, pp. 1493

Fraseri, S et al. (1987). Microwave Thermography – An Index of Inflammatory Joint Disease. *British Journal of Rheumatology.* Vol. 261, pp. 37-39

Hand, J. Van Leeuwen,G.; Mizushina, G.; Van de Kamer, J.; Maruyama, K.; Sugiura, T.; Azzopardi, D. & Edwards, A. (2001). Monitoring of Deep Brain Temperature in Infants Using Multi-Frequency Microwave Radiometry and Thermal Modelling. *Phys. Med. Biol.* Vol.46, pp. 1885–1903

Harris, L.; Fritsche, H.; Mennel, R.; Norton, L.; Ravdin, P.; Taube, S.; Somerfield, M.; Hayes,
    D.; Bast, R (2007). Update of Recommendations for the Use of Tumor Markers in
    Breast Cancer. *J. Clinical Oncology*, Vol. 25, No. 33, pp. 5287-5312

Hebden, J.; Arridge, S. & Delpy, D. (1997). Optical Imaging in Medicine: I. Experimental
    Techniques. *Phys.Med.Biol.*, Vol. 42, pp. 825-840

Hermans, B.; Coosemans, J. & Puers, R. (2005). Integration of Sensors and Electronics in
    Textile for use in Infant Medicine. *European Microlectronics and Packaging Conference
    and Exhibition*, pp. 588-592, June 12-15, 2005

Jiang, S.; Pogue, B.; McBride, T. & Paulsen, K. (2003). Quantitative Analysis of Near-infrared
    Tomography: Sensitivity to the Tissue-simulating Precalibration Phantom. *Journal
    of Biomedical Optics*, Vol.8, pp. 308-315

Jung, J. et al, 'Ultra-Wideband Low Noise Amplifier Using a Cascode Feedback Topology',
    IEEE Silicon Monolithic Integrated Circuits in RF Systems, 2006. pp. 202-205

Keyserlignk, J. & Ahlgren, P (1998). Infrared Imaging of the Breast: Initial Reappraisal Using
    High Resolution Digital Technology in 100 Successive Cases of Stage 1 and 2 Breast
    Cancer. *Breast J*. Vol.4, pp.245-251

Klemm, M.; Locher,I. & Troster, G. (2004). A novel circularly polarized textile antenna for
    wearable applications. *The 34rd European Microwave Conference (EuMC)*, pp.11-14, 2004.

Klemm,M.; Kovcs,I.; Pedersen, G. & Troster, G. (2005). *Novel* small-size directional antenna
    for UWB WBAN/WPAN applications', *IEEE Trans. on Antennas and Propagation*.
    Vol. 53, No. 12 pp. 3884- 3896

Klemm, M & Troester, G. (2006). EM Energy Absorption in the Human Body Tissues due to
    UWB Antennas', *Progress In Electromagnetics Research*. Vol. 62, pp.261-280

Klemm, M. & Troster, G. (2005). Integration of Electrically Small UWB Antennas for Body-
    Worn Sensor Applications. *IEE Wideband and Multi-band Antennas and Arrays*, 2005,
    pp.141-146.

Lee, J.; Kim, K.; Lee, S.; Eom, S. & Troitsky, R. (2002). A Novel Design of Thermal Anomaly
    for Mammary Gland Tumor Phantom for Microwave Radiometer', *IEEE Trans.
    Biomed. Engineering*. Vol. 49, pp.694-699

Leroy, Y. Bocquet, B. & Mamouni, A. (1998). Non-invasive Microwave Radiometry
    Thermometry. *Physiol. Meas*, Vol.19, pp.127-148

Li, X.; Bond, E.; Van Veen, B. & Hagness, S. (2005). An Overview of Ultra Wide Band
    Microwave Imaging via Space-Time Beam Forming for Early-Stage Breast Cancer
    Detection. *IEEE Antennas and Propagation Magazine*. Vol. 47, No. 1, pp. 19-34

Locher, I. (2006). Technologies for System-on-Textile Integration. *PhD Thesis*, ETH Zürich,
    Zürich, Switzerland, 2006

Lundgren, B. (1981). Observations on Growth Rate of Breast Carcinomas and its Possible
    Implications for Lead Time. *Cancer*. Vol. 47, pp. 2769

MacDonald, I. (1951) Biological Predeterminism in Human Cancer. *Surg Gaenecol Obstet*. Vol.
    92, pp. 443-452

Moskowitz, M. (1983). Screening for Breast Cancer. How Effective are our Tests? *CA Cancer J
    Clin*. Vol. 33, pp. 26-39

Moskowitz, M.(1995). Breast imaging, In:*Cancer of the Breast*, W.L Donegan & J.S. Spratt,
    (Eds.), , 206–239, Saunders, New York

Nathanson, S.; Zarbo,R.; Wachna, D.; Spence, C.; Andrzejewski, T. & Abrams, J. (2000).
    Microvessels That Predict Axillary Lymph Node Metastases in Patients with Breast
    Cancer. *Arch Surg*. Vol. 135, pp.586-594

Nealon T., Kongho A., Grossi C.(1979). Pathological Identification of Poor Prognosis of Stage I (T.N.M.) Cancer of the Breast. Ann. Surg, 1979:190, 129-32

Nosal, Z. (2001). Simple Model for Dynamic Range Estimate of GaAs Amplifiers', *IEEE-MTTS, Proc. Intern. Microwave Symp.* 2001

Osterman, K.; Kerner, T.; Williams, D.; Hartov, A.; Poplack, S. & Paulsen, K . (2000). Multifrequency Electrical Impedance Imaging: Preliminary In Vivo Experience in the Breast, *J. Phys Meas,* Vol.21, pp. 67-77

Paradiso, R.; Loriga, G. & Taccini, N.(2005). A Wearable Health Care System Based on Knitted Integrated Sensors', *IEEE Tran. Information Technology in Biomedicine.* Vol. 9, No. 3, pp. 337-344.

Reidy, J.(1988). Controversy Over Breast Cancer Detection. Br. Med. J. Vol. 297, pp. 932-3

Scilingo, E.; Gemignani, A.; Paradiso, R.; Taccini, N.; Ghelarducci, B. & De Rossi, D. (2005). Performance Evaluation of Sensing Fabrics for Monitoring Physiological and Biomechanical Variables. *IEEE Tran. Information Technology in Biomedicine,* Vol. 9, No. 3, pp. 345-352

Sickles, E. (1984). Mammographic Features of Early Breast Cancer. *Am J Roentgenol.* Vol.143, pp.461-464

Skou, N & Le Vine, D. (2006). *Microwave Radiometer Systems, Design and Analysis.* Artech House, ISBN 978-1-58053-974-6

Tetlow, R & Hubbard, A. (2000). Preliminary Results of a Pilot Study into the Diagnostic Value of T-scan in Detecting Breast Malignancies. *Breast Cancer Research Breast Cancer Res.,* Vol.2:A13

Thomas, D.; Gao, D.; Self,S.; Allison, C.; Tao, Y.; Mahloch, J.; Ray, R.; Qin, Q.; Presley, R. & Porter, P.   (1997). Randomized Trial of Breast Self-Examination in Shanghai. Methodology and Preliminary Results, *J Natl Cancer Inst.* Vol. 5, pp. 355-65.

Van Langenhove, L. et al, 'Textile electrodes for monitoring cardio-respiratory signals', *European Conference on Protective Clothing,* Montreux, Switzerland, CDROM poster no. 27, May 21-24, 2003.

Van Langenhove, L.; Hertleer, C.; Catrysse, M.; Puers, R.; Van Egmond, H. & Matthys, D. (2003). The use of textile electrodes in a hospital environment', *AUTEX - World Textile Conference.* pp. 286-290, ISBN 83-89003-32-5, Gdansk, Poland, June 25-27, 2003

Vaupel, P.; Schlenger, K.; Knoop, C. & Hockel. M. (1991). Oxygenation of Human Tumors: Evaluation of Tissue Oxygen Distribution in Breast Cancers by Computerized O_2 Tension Measurements. *Cancer Res.* Vol.51, No.12, pp.3316–22

Vaupel, P.; Thews, O.; Kelleher, D. &. Hoeckel. M.(1998). Current Status of Knowledge and Critical Issues in Tumor Oxygenation, *Adv. Exp. Med. Biol.* Vol.454, pp.591–602

Wade T. & Kozlowski, P. (2007). Longitudinal Studies of Angiogenesis in Hormone-Dependent Shionogi Tumors. *Neoplasia.* Vol.9, No.7, pp 563–568

Wang, Y.; Duster, J. & Kornegay, K. (2005). Design of an Ultra-wideband Low Noise Amplifier in 0.13m CMOS. *IEEE International Symposium on Circuits and Systems,* May 2005.

Weidner, N.; Folkman, J.; Pozza, F.; Bevilacqua, P.; Allred, E.; Moore, D.; Meli, S. & Gasparini, G. (1992). Tumor Angiogenesis: A New Significant and Independent Prognostic Indicator in Early-Stage Breast Carcinoma. *J. Natl. Cancer Inst.,* Vol. 84, No.24, pp. 1875–87

Xu, J. Woestenburg, B.; Geralt bij de Vaate, J. & Serdijn, W. (2005). GaAs 0.5 dB NF dual-loop negative-feedback broadband low-noise amplifier IC. *IEE Electronics Letters.* Vol. 41, No. 14, pp. 780 - 782

9

Immunophenotyping of the Blast Cells in Correlations with the Molecular Genetics Analyses for Diagnostic and Clinical Stratification of Patients with Acute Myeloid Leukemia: Single Center Experience

Irina Panovska-Stavridis
University Clinic of Hematology, Skopje
Republic of Macedonia

1. Introduction

1.1 Acute leukemias

Acute leukemias are a heterogeneous group of malignancies that result from the malignant transformation of immature hematopoietic cells followed by clonal proliferation and accumulation of the transformed cells. They are characterized by aberrant differentiation and maturation of the malignant cells, with a maturation arrest and accumulation of more than 20% of leukemic blast in the bone marrow (Lichtman et al., 2010).

The natural history of acute leukemia and the response to therapy varies according to the type of blast involved in the leukemic process. Although in many instances the lineage assignment of the different types of blast cells may be recognized by simple morphological and cytochemical stains, it is necessary to employ immunological analyses with monoclonal antibodies and cytogenetic or molecular biological techniques to identify their particular differentiation features (Haferlach et al., 2007).

Acute leukemias are primarily characterized according to their differentiation along the myeloid and lymphoid lineage and they are divided into two main groups: acute myeloid leukemia (AML) and acute lymphoblastic leukemia (ALL). In 10% to 20% of patients, the leukemic cells have characteristics of both myeloid and lymphoid cells (Lichtman et al.,2010).

The classification of the acute leukemias underwent many changes in recent years. The French-American-British (FAB) classification of AML and ALL was based on cytomorphological and cytohemistry details only. Since then, the diagnostic of acute leukemias had undergone a complete change and the routine diagnostic work-up incorporated immunophenotyping by multiparameter flow cytometry, classical cytogenetics, molecular cytogenetics (comprising diverse fluorescence in situ hybridization techniques and comparative genomic hybridization) and molecular genetics (mostly polymerase chain reaction (PCR)-based techniques and sequencing) (Bennet et al., 1997; First MIC Cooperative Study Group, 1985; Haferlach et al., 2007).

According to the proceedings in diagnostic methods and the improved understanding of the diversity of acute leukemia subtypes, the latest World Health Organization (WHO) classification of acute leukemias incorporates and interrelates morphology, cytogenetics, molecular genetics and immunologic markers and pays major attention on the importance of genetic events in the classification, prognosis and therapy of the AMLs. Its prognostic relevance is most clearly demonstrated in the AMLs characterized by recurrent chromosome translocation: t(15,17), t(8,21) and inv(16)/t(16,16) which generally have a favorable prognosis when treated with appropriate therapeutic agents. All other genetic events identified among AMLs had strong prognostic meaning but did not influence on the therapeutic decision (Swerdlow et al., 2008).

In the WHO classification of precursor B-cell and T-cell neoplasms, immunophenotying of the malignant cells plays a decisive role in the diagnosis, prognosis and clinical stratification of patients (Swerdlow et al., 2008).

Correct diagnosis of the diverse subtypes of AML and ALL play a central role for individual clinical risk stratification and therapeutic decisions.

1.2 Acute myeloid leukemia

Acute myeloid leukemia (AML) is one of the most common types of leukemia in adults. It is characterized by limited myeloid differentiation of the malignant cells. The malignant cells characteristically undergo maturation arrest at the level of the early myloblast or promyelocyte, although varying proportions of mature hematopoietic cells are leukemia derived. The cells that display myeloid markers include morphology, Auer rods (aberrant primary granules), cytochemistry (Sudan black, myeloperoxidase, or nonspecific esterase), and cell surface antigens (Lichtman et al., 2010).

AML encompasses a family of hematologic malignancies that can be categorized according to their cytogenetic and associated genetic abnormalities, which have major prognostic importance. During recent years, considerable progress has been made in deciphering the molecular genetics and epigenetic basis of AML and in defining new diagnostic and prognostic markers. A growing number of recurring genetic changes have been recognized in the new WHO classification of AML. Furthermore, novel therapies are now being developed that target some of the genetic lesions and the treatment increasingly is being individualized by prognostic groups, with a goal of developing treatment tailored to the molecular basis of the patient's malignancy (Swerdlow et al., 2008).

1.2.1 WHO classification of AML

The current WHO classification of AML reflects the fact that an increasing number of new clinico-pathologenetic entities of AML are categorized based upon their underlying cytogenetic or molecular genetic abnormalities (Swerdlow et al., 2008). A number of recurrent genetic abnormalities are adequately defined and are recognized as entities of AML. The subgroup "AML with recurrent genetic abnormalities" is comprised of entities that are defined with seven recurrent balanced translocations and inversions, and their variants. Two entities from this group: "AML with t(8;21)(q22;q22); AML1/ETO" and "AML with inv(16)(p13.1q22) or t(16;16)(p13.1;q22); CBFβ/MYH11" are considered as AML regardless of bone marrow blast counts. In "APL with t(15;17)(q22;q12); PML/RARα," RARα translocations with other partner genes are recognized separately. The former category "AML with 11q23 (MLL) abnormalities" is redefined in "AML with t(9;11)(p22;q23); MLLT3/MLL", and now is a unique entity. Three new cytogenetically defined entities also are incorporated: "AML with t(6;9)(p23;q34);DEK-NUP214", "AML with inv(3)(q21q26.2) or t(3;3)(q21;q26.2); RPN1-EVI1"; and "AML (megakaryoblastic) with t(1;22)(p13;q13); RBM15-MKL1," a rare leukemia most commonly occurring in infants (Vardiman et al., 2008).

Moreover, two new provisional entities defined by the presence of gene mutations between the group of cytogenetically normal AML (CN-AML) were added, "AML with mutated NPM1 (nucleophosmin)," and "AML with mutated CEBPA [CCAAT/enhancer binding protein(C/EBP), alpha]." There is growing evidence that these two gene mutations represent primary genetic lesions (so-called class II mutations), that impair hematopoietic differentiation, and when present alone in AML have favorable prognostic meaning. Mutations in the FMS-related tyrosine kinase 3 (FLT3) gene are found in many AML subtypes and are considered as class I mutations conferring a proliferation and/or survival advantage. AML with FLT3 mutations are not considered as a distinct entity, although determining the presence of those mutations is recommended by WHO because they have prognostic significance. The former subgroup termed "AML with multilineage dysplasia" is now designated "AML with myelodysplasia-related changes." Dysplasia in 50% or more of cells, in 2 or more hematopoietic cell lineages, was the diagnostic criterion for the former subset (Schhlenk et al, 2008; Vardiman et al.,2008)

However, the clinical significance of this morphologic feature has been questioned. AMLs are now categorized as "AML with myelodysplasia-related changes" if (1) they have a previous history of myelodysplastic syndrome (MDS) or myelodysplastic/myeloproliferative neoplasm (MDS/MPN) and evolve to AML with a marrow or blood blast count of 20% or more; (2) they have a myelodysplasia-related cytogenetic abnormality; or (3) if 50% or more of cells in 2 or more myeloid lineages are dysplastic (Swerdlow et al., 2008).

"Therapy-related myeloid neoplasms" has remained a distinct entity; however, since most patients have received treatment using both alkylating agents and drugs that target topoisomerase II for prior malignancy, a division according to the type of previous therapy is not often feasible. Therefore, therapy-related myeloid neoplasms are no longer subcategorized. Myeloid proliferations related to Down syndrome are now listed as distinct entities (Döhner et al., 2010).

A previous FAB classification is recognized in WHO classification as the entity AML, not otherwise specified. In this subgroup one can find the morphologic separation of AML according to the immaturity of leukemic cells as well as according to the hematopoietic lineage involved. This subtype of AML is reserved for the patients without the known cytogenetic or molecular genetic abnormalities. In some of them, there are markers associated with prognostic significance (Swerdlow et al., 2008; Vardiman et al, 2008).

The rare forms of AML and acute leukemia of ambiguous lineage recognized in WHO classification are also associated with poor prognosis (Döhner et al., 2010; Vardiman et al., 2008).

1.3 Diagnostic procedures

The diagnosis of the diverse subtypes of AML is a major challenge for modern hematology. Modern therapeutic concepts of AML are based on individual risk stratification in diagnosis and during follow-up. In the 1970s cytomorphology and cytochemistry represented the only available diagnostic tools. Nowadays, the routine diagnostic setting is completely changed and it consists of classic cytogenetics, molecular cytogenetics, molecular genetics and immunophenotyping by multi-parameter flow cytometry (Döhner et al., 2010).

1.3.1 Cytomorphology

First steps in the diagnostic work-up of a patient with suspected AML is a morphological evaluation of a classical bone marrow aspirate and a peripheral blood smear by using a May-Grunwald-Giemsa or a Wright-Giemsa stain. It is recommended that at least 200 leukocytes on blood smears and 500 nucleated cells on marrow smears to be counted. For a diagnosis of AML, a marrow or blood blast count of 20% or more is required, except for AML with t(15;17), t(8;21), inv(16) or t(16;16), and some cases of erythroleukemia. Myeloblasts, monoblasts, and megakaryoblasts are included in the blast count. Erythroblasts are not counted as blasts except in the rare instance of pure erythroid leukemia (Bennet et al,1997; Döhner et al., 2010; Panovska-Stavridis et al., 2008).

1.3.2 Cytochemistry

Lineage involvement could be identified with cytochemistry by using myeloperoxidase (MPO) or Sudan black B (SBB) and nonspecific esterase (NSE) stains. Detection of MPO (if present in > 3% of blasts) indicates myeloid differentiation, but its absence does not exclude a myeloid lineage because early myeloblasts and monoblasts may lack MPO. SBB staining parallels MPO but is less specific. NSE stains show diffuse cytoplasmic activity in monoblasts (usually 80% are positive) and monocytes (usually 20% positive). In acute erythroid leukemia, a periodic acid-Schiff (PAS) stain may show large globules of PAS positivity (Bennet et al,1997; Döhner et al., 2010, Panovska-Stavridis et al., 2008).

1.3.3 Immunophenotyping

Application of immunophenotyping together with the cytomorpohology and cytohemistry has a crucial role in the initial diagnosis of all cases with a suspected or proven diagnosis of acute leukemias. Immunophenotyping allows the discrimination of different cell population on the basis of their size, granularity, and antigen expression patterns. Flow cytometry is a powerful technology for characterization and analysis of cells. It simultaneously measures and analyzes multiple physical characteristics of single particles, usually cells, as they move in a fluid stream through a beam of light through an optical and/or electronic detection apparatus. Flow cytometry uses the principles of light scattering, light excitation, and emission of fluorochrome molecules to generate specific multi-parameter data from particles and cells in the size range of 0.5nm to 40nm diameter (Panovska-Stavridis et al., 2008).

The applied methodology detects cell surface antigens in a suspension of viable cells and cytoplasmic and nuclear antigens in previously fixed and stabilized cell suspension with the application of monoclonal antibodies conjugated with different fluorochromes. It permits simultaneous detection (multiparameter analyzes) of more than two membrane and nuclear or cytoplasmic antigens by means of double or multiple immunostaining (Bain et al., 2002; Bene et al., 1995; Döhner et al., 2010; Panovska-Stavridis et al., 2008).

1.3.4 Cytogenetics

Chromosome abnormalities are detected in approximately 55% of adult AML. Conventional cytogenetic analyses are part of the standard diagnostic approach of a patient suspected with AML. This allows the identification of genetics entities that deserve targeted treatments

like acute promyelocytic leukemia (APL). Also, it allows the distinction of the disease with
widely different prognosis. For example AML t(8;21)(q22;q22) with favorable risk versus
AML abn 3q26 with adverse risk (Döhner et al., 2010; Grimwade D.,2001).

1.3.5 Molecular genetics

Numerous genetic abnormalities that escape cytogenetic detection like gene mutations and
gene expression abnormalities are more recently discovered among CN-AML. Molecular
diagnosis by reverse transcriptase- polymerase chain reaction (RT-PCR) for the frequent gene
fusions, such as AML1/ETO, CBFβ/MYH11, MLLT3/MLL, DEK/NUP214, can also be useful
in certain circumstances. RT-PCR, for which standardized protocols are already published, is
also an excellent option to detect recurrent cytogenetic rearrangements, if chromosome
morphology is of poor quality, or if there is typical marrow morphology but the suspected
cytogenetic abnormality is not present. (Gabert et al., 2003; Beillard et al, 2003).

1.4 Prognostic factors

Prognostic factors of an AML case may be subdivided into those related to patient
characteristics and general health condition and those related to characteristics particular to
the AML clone. The former subset usually predicts treatment-related mortality (TRM) and
becomes more important as patient age increases while the latter predicts resistance to, at
least, conventional therapy.

1.4.1 Patient-related factors

Age, comorbidities, performance status and genetic variation in the drug metabolism are the
main prognostic factors related to patients with AML. Increasing age is an important
independent adverse prognostic factor (Appelbaum et al., 2006). Nonetheless, calendar age
alone should not be a reason for not offering potentially curative therapy to an older patient
because age is not the most important prognostic factor for either TRM or resistance to
therapy. Currently all patients under the age of 60 are candidates to receive standard
intensive chemotherapy and according to prognostic factors stem cell transplantation or
intensive chemotherapy as postremission therapy. It has to be stressed that age as a factor is
not only dependent on so-called „calendar age". Recently many older patients with a good
clinical status have been successfully treated with intensive chemotherapy. Attention should
be given to a careful evaluation and documentation of comorbidities. Comorbidity scoring is
a current field of investigation and should contribute to a better definition of the patient
considered "unfit" for intensive chemotherapy (Piccirillo et al., 2004; Sorror et al., 2005).

1.4.2 AML-related factors

According to the AML working party of European Leukemia Net, several important and
independent prognostic factors have been recognized: white blood cell counts, existence of
prior MDS or AML with MDS features, previous cytotoxic therapy for another malignancy,
and cytogenetic and molecular abnormalities in leukemic cells (Döhner et al., 2010).

1.4.2.1 Cytogenetics

Chromosome abnormalities are detected in approximately 55% of adult AML. Although, there
is a diversity of cytogenetic entities of AML, the karyotype of the leukemic cells is the strongest
prognostic factor for response to induction therapy and for survival for AML patients

(Swerdlow et al., 2008). Younger adult patients are commonly categorized into 3 risk groups, favorable, intermediate, or adverse. The favorable group is represented by the reciprocal translocations t(15;17)/PML/RARα, t(8;21)/AML1/ETO, and inv(16)/CBFβ/MYH11, which are associated with a favorable prognosis In contrast, AML associated with t(9;11)(p22;q23) shows an inferior prognosis. These subgroups represent the first hierarchy of the WHO classification of AML, emphasizing that these subtypes represent distinct biologic entities. The second subgroup of AML patients shows a normal karyotype and an intermediate prognosis. However, from molecular aspects, this subgroup is very heterogeneous. Lately, there are emerging data suggesting that two genetics entities from this group, the AML with mutation of NPM1 gene without FLT3 mutations and AML with mutation in CEBPA gene should be moved from the intermediate prognosis group to the favorable group of AML. Those two entities are also added to the new WHO classification (Schlenk et al., 2008). The third (prognostically unfavorable) subgroup includes mostly unbalanced karyotypes characterized by a gain or loss of larger chromosomal regions. Within these, an especially complex aberrant karyotype, which occurs in 10% to 12% of patients and that is defined by ≥3 chromosomal anomalies shows a very unfavorable prognosis. Cytogenetics is further helpful to delineate patients with therapy related AML (t-AML), who are classified as third hierarchy in the WHO classification, and developed either after treatment with alkylating agents often associated with cytogenetic aberrations involving 5q-, −7, or p53 and complex aberrant karyotype or are showing MLL/11q23 or other balanced cytogenetic aberrations which are in frequent association to previous treatment with topoisomerase II inhibitors One striking observation is the increasing incidence of adverse versus favorable cytogenetic abnormalities with increasing age. This, at least in part, contributes to the poorer outcome of AML in older adults. (Byrd et al., 2002; Schlenk et al., 2008, Swerdlow et al., 2008)

1.4.2.2 Molecular genetics

Nowadays, considerable progress has been made in elucidating the molecular pathogenesis of acute leukemias that resulted in identification of new molecular diagnostic and prognostic markers. Gene mutations and deregulated gene expression have been identified that allow us to interpret the genetic diversity within defined cytogenetic groups, in particular the large and heterogeneous group of patients with CN-AML. Risk stratification by molecular markers in patients from the former group of AML plays an increasing role at diagnosis. The most relevant markers, which can be detected alone or in coincidence with other mutation are NPM1 mutations that is detected in approximately 40% of cases, MLL-PTD in 6%, NRAs in 8-10%, CEBPA in 10% and FLT3-TKD mutations in 6% of CN-AML. Thus, a rather of limited number of markers further subclassifies more than 85% of CN-AML. Data from the literature suggest that those markers have different prognosis regarding the outcome of the disease and they all indicate that in the near future molecular screening may allow " targeted allogeneic stem cell transplantation (alloSCT)" in AML patients with normal karyotype (Schlenk et al., 2008; Koreth et al, 2009).

There is a growing list of the new genetic abnormalities with clinical value that are being investigated. These genetic events perturb diverse cellular pathways and functions, and they often confer a profound impact upon the clinical phenotype of the disease and treatment response.

It is anticipated that advances in molecular technology will reveal additional markers that will result in more precise classification of this heterogeneous complex of disorders (Löwenberg B., 2008b; Haferlach T., 2008)

1.5 Treatment

The parallel progress of the development of the diagnostic techniques improvement of the classification and therapeutical approach lead acute leukemia which were for the first time described before 150 years, and in the 1970s were still fatal disease nowadays to have overall 5 years survival rates of up to 40%. (Appelbaum et al, 2001).

Despite heterogeneity of the disease, with the exception of acute promyelocytic leukemia, this disease has been treated with a "one size fits all" approach. Although, the vast majority of AML patients can be individually characterized on the basis of the distinct chromosomal aberrations and molecular markers, treatment of AML is still based on quite unspecific cytotoxic therapy. For almost 40 years, the use of continuous infusion of cytarabine combined with another agent, usually an anthracycline, the "3+7" regimen, has been the mainstay of therapy (Yates et al, 1973). Response rates for induction with standard chemotherapy ranged from 70% to 80% for adults aged less than 60years which are enrolled in clinical trials and average in 50% for patients older than 60 years (Lichtman et al.,2010) .

Alternative consolidation therapies by applying additional chemotherapy, autologous stem cell transplantation (autoSCT) or alloSCT based on the initial cytogenetic and molecular studies are available (Cornelissen J.J.et al.(2007); Fernandez H.F.,2010; Koreth et al, 2009)

As more sophisticated molecular techniques have become available, it is clear that it is still possible to detect residual disease when all morphological and functional criteria for remission are met. Techniques such as "real–time"-quantitative polymerase chain reaction (RQ-PCR) are capable of detection at a level of 1 in 10^4 or 1 in 10^5 residual cells, but such markers are available for only a minority of cases in which the molecular lesion has been characterized(Freeman et al., 2008).

AlloSCT is the most effective antileukemic modality that is characterized by immune mediated graft-versus-leukemia effect of the transplanted cells that reduce the risk of relapse considerably and improve the relapse-free survival but also is associated with the increased risk of death and morbidity. Therefore, the alloSCT advantage has to be carefully balanced against the excess mortality (ranging between 10% and 40%) and morbidity due to transplant-related complications, such as infection and graft-versus-host disease that are typically connected with alloSCT and can diminish all of the benefit of a reduced risk of relapse. (Cornelissen et al., 2007). For this reason, allogeneic stem cell transplantation is usually avoided in a type of AML that has a pattern of cytogenetics with a relatively favorable prognosis, such as AML with the chromosomal translocations t(8;21) or inv(16)/t(16;16)(Marcucci et al., 2000; Perea et al.,2006). In the latter subtypes the risk of relapse is in the order of 35% to 40% or less. By contrast, a transplant is treatment of choice for all other patient whose leukemia cells bear a cytogenetic or molecular abnormality that predicts a high or intermediate risk of relapse after chemotherapy (Löwenberg et al., 2008b; Koreth et al, 2009). Exception could be done for two additional genotypically defined subsets of AML that are categorized as low-risk within the large category of CN-AML. Each of those entities has a risk of relapse of about 35%. The first genotype is defined by the presence of 'favorable' mutations in NPM1 and the absence of concurrent 'unfavorable' FLT3-internal tandem duplications (NPM1mut /FLT3-ITDneg).61 This genotype accounts for approximately 16% of all newly diagnosed patients younger than 60 years old. There is no demonstrable benefit from transplantation in patients with NPM1mut/FLT3-ITDneg AML. The second subset of AML with 'favorable' mutations in the transcription factor gene CEBPA (CEBPAmut) could not be analyzed in this way because of a lack of statistical power due to a limited number of cases. The latter low-risk subtype CEBPAmut accounts for 8% of all AML. Nevertheless, the available body of evidence suggests that these AMLs are unlikely to profit from an alloSCT (Schlenk et al., 2008).

Thus, it could be concluded that patients with AML with t(8;21), AML with inv(16)/t(16;16), AML with *NPM1*mut/ *FLT3*-ITDneg and AML with *CEBPA* mutations should not considered for alloSCT. Nevertheless, it is important to stress that sufficient evidence so far exist only for the AML with recurrent cytogenetic abnormalities and the benefits for the two additional genetic low-risk AML entities should be validated in the larger studies in the future (Schlenk et al., 2008).

In the near future these results will also need to be considered more specifically in the light of the extended scale of allogeneic stem cell transplantation strategies with respect to reduced-intensity conditioning regimens and in relationship to different transplant sources and donor types (matched unrelated and haploidentical donors, umbilical stem cell grafts).(Löwenberg et al, 2008a)

2. Motivation and aim of the study

Correct diagnosis of the diverse subtypes of acute myeloid leukemia (AML) and acute lymphoblastic leukemia (ALL) play a central role for individual clinical risk stratification and therapeutic decisions. Modern therapeutic concepts of AML are based on individual risk stratification at diagnosis and during follow-up. The ultimate test of any disease diagnostic algorithm approach is its usefulness in guiding the selection of effective treatment strategies. (Haferlach et al., 2007, Löwenberg et al, 2008b) As discussed above, cytogenetic as well as various genomic markers (gene mutations, gene overexpression) may provide input for algorithms for remission induction and post-remission treatment decisions. At the same time, it remains appropriate to realize that prognostic factors in fact remain a moving target and they are only relevant to therapies available at a given time. Algorithms that provide a basis for risk-adapted therapeutic choices may include immunological markers, cytogenetic factors, molecular markers as well as clinical parameters (e.g., age, attainment of an early or late complete remission) and hematological determinants (e.g., secondary AML, white blood cell count at diagnosis).

On the other hand, the more carefully AML is studied, the clearer it becomes that there is considerable heterogeneity between cases with respect to morphology, immunological phenotype, associated cytogenetic and molecular abnormalities and, more recently, patterns of gene expression. This is reflected in the substantially different responses to treatment. Some entities are becoming so distinct that they are regarded as different diseases with specific approaches to treatment.

In order to improve and simplify the diagnosis and management of AML patients that are diagnosed and treated at the at the University Clinic of Hematology-Skopje we conducted a prospective study to establish and standardize a diagnostic algorithm based on minimal screening tests which will facilitate risk adapted therapy for each single AML patient. The aims of our study were: first, to establish the correct lineage assignment of the blast cells, second, to evaluate the incidence of the favorable genetic markers PML/RARα, AML1/ETO and CBFβ/MYH11 among the AML cases, then to correlate the obtained results with the patient age, comorbidities, and performance status and consecutively to select the effective treatment strategy for each single acute leukemia patient.

3. Material and methods

3.1 Patients and samples

A total of 76 adult (>15 years) patients (from initially 77 tested) with acute leukemia who were consecutively admitted at the Clinic of Hematology-Skopje from January through December 2008 were enrolled in this study. The median age of the patients (41 men, 35 women) was 52 ± 18.66 years (range 16-80), and most of the patients 37 (48.7%) were between 55 and 75 years old. The diagnosis was made by standard morphological examination and cytochemical analyses of bone marrow smears according to the criteria established by the FAB Cooperative Study Group (Bennet et al, 1997) and confirmed by immunophenotyping of bone marrow aspirates and/or peripheral blood samples (Bain et al., 2002; Bene et al., 1995) following the criteria of the European Group for the Immunological Classification of leukemias (EGIL) and the British Committee for Standards in Hematology (BCSH) (Bain et al., 2002; Bene et al., 1995). Consecutively, patients were further stratified in the adequate genetic AML entities according to the results of the molecular analyses. The samples contained more than 20% of blast cells (most of which had more than 50%). All patients were tested for the presence of the fusion transcript of the mayor recurrent cytogenteic abnormalities in AML (PML/RARα, AML1/ETO, CBFβ/MYH11) by RT-PCR, according to standard procedures. (Gabert et al.2003; Beillardet al, 2003).

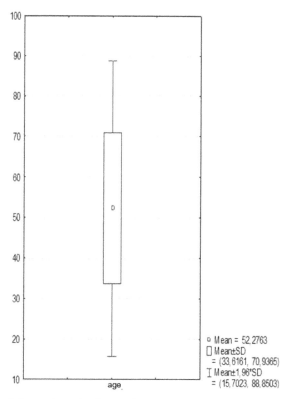

Fig. 1. Average age of the patients in the study group

3.1.1 Clinical data from the patients

Clinical data from the patients were collected according the internal protocol that was approved by the University Clinic of Hematology Institutional Review Board. All included patients had to sign a written consent.

3.2 Morphology

The morphology was analyzed by microscopic examination of >500 nonerythroid cells on May Gruenwald Giemza stained air-dried bone marrow smears (Bennet et al,1997; Döhner et al., 2010; Panovska-Stavridis et al., 2008).

3.3 Cytochemical analysis

Air-dried bone marrow smears were stained for MPO, non specific esterase (NSE) and periodic acid-Schiff (PAS) according to the manufacturers guidelines. The percentage of positive cells for either stain was assessed by microscopic examination of 200 nonerythroid cells (Bennet et al, 1997; Döhner et al., 2010; Panovska-Stavridis et al., 2008).

3.4 Immunophenotyping

The muliparameter flow cytometry (MPF) was performed at the beginning at the Institute for Immunobiology and Human Genetics, Faculty of Medicine-Skopje and then continued at the University Clinic of Hematology-Skopje. Immunophenotyping was done first, by using Cytomation (DAKO-Cytomation) flow-cytometer and than by BD FACSCanto™ II analyzer, on whole blood and/or bone marrow specimens using lysing solutions (BD-Bisciensies, San Jose.CA. USA)(Bain et al., 2002). We prepare the samples for simultaneous detection of three cytoplasmic/nuclear and membrane antigens. The first step involved immunostaining of cell suspension with multiple panels of tree monoclonal antibodies (McAb) labeled with fluorescein (FITC), phycoerythrin (PE) and phycoerythryn-Cy5 tandem complex (Pe-Cy5) as third color (Panovska-Stavridis et al., 2008). The slightly modified panel of monoclonal antibodies (McAb) against myeloid- and lymphoid-associated antigens as suggested by the EGIL was utilized (Bain et al., 2002; Panovska-Stavridis et al., 2008). The antibodies and their manufacturers are listed in Table 1.

	B-lineage	T-lineage	Myeloid markers	Non-lineage restricted
First line	CD19, cyt CD79b, cyt CD22	CD 2, CD7, cyt CD3	CD117,CD13, CD33,CD14, CD15, anti-MPO, anti-lisosyme	TdT, CD34, HLA-DR, CD 56
Second line	SmIg (kappa/lambda)**, cytIgM[2],CD138	CD1a,mCD3[1], CD4,CD5,CD8, anti TCR α/β, anti TCR γ/δ***	CD41, CD61, CD42,CD71 Anti-glycophorin A	CD38

All markers were manufactured by BD-Biosciences, except antilysozyme (DAKO); 1.cyt: cytoplasmic; 2.m: membrane *MPO: myloperoxidase;** SmIg:surface immunoglobulin;*** TCR:T cell receptor

Table 1. Panel of monoclonal antibodies (McAb) for diagnosis of acute leukemias

For the detection of cytoplasmic and nuclear antigens we used commercially available permeabilization/fixation solutions (FACS Permeabilization solution BDBiosciencies;San Jose.CA.USA) ((Bain et al., 2002).

We incubated 100ml of specimens (peripheral blood or bone marrow) and appropriate McAb for 15min at room temperature, than added the permeabilization solutions and/or lysing solution and repeated the incubation procedure. After the incubation we washed the samples three times with PBS-A, than re-suspended the cell with isotones solution and acquired the data. As control we used a lysed, but unstained sample (Panovska-Stavridis et al., 2008)

Acquired data were analyzed with software by using CD45 gating strategy (Borowitz et al, 1993). This technique involves incubation of all samples with fluorochrome - labeled CD45 McAb and with the McAb for which reactivity needs to be established with an alternative fluorochrome). In the initial step of the analyses, gating was set up on a CD45-positive versus light side-scatter dot plot. The procedure allowed the discrimination between the blast cell population and normal cells and the exclusion of platelets and debris. Thereafter, if necessary, it was possible to perform another gating, to separate the cells positive with the McAb under study (Borowitz et al, 1993). Leukemias were first screened by the primary panel and, if necessary, further characterized by the McAb of the secondary panel (Bain et al., 2002).

Antigen expression was considered positive if 20% or more blast cells reacted with a particular antibody, except reactivity of blasts cells with MPO. It was considered positive if 10% or more of mononuclear cells were MPO positive (Bain et al., 2002; Döhner et al., 2010).

3.5 Molecular analysis

Mononuclear cell preparation, RNA isolation, and cDNA synthesis were performed at the Department of Molecular Biology, Immunology and Pharmacogenetics, Faculty of Pharmacy-Skopje, according to standard procedures. Aliquots of 5 µL of cDNA (100 ng RNA equivalent) were used for Real-time Quantitative polymerase chain reaction (RQ-PCR) with primers and dual-labeled probes as described by Gabert et al. Positions and nucleotide sequences of the primers and probes are shown in Table 2.

The RQ-PCR reaction was performed in a 25-µl reaction volume using 12.5 µl (1x) Master Mix (Applied Biosystems), 300nM primers and 200nM probes on a Mx3005P(TM) QPCR System (Stratagene) under the following conditions: 95°C for 10min, followed by 50 cycles of 95°C for 15s, 50°C for 1min. In order to correct variations in RNA quality and quantity and to calculate the sensitivity of each measurement, a control gene (CG) transcript was amplified in parallel to the fusion gene (FG) transcript. Since ABL (Abelson) gene transcript expression did not differ significantly between normal and leukemic samples, ABL was used as a control gene in this study (24). Positions and nucleotide sequences of the primers and probe are shown in Table 2.

3.6 Statistical analysis

Statistical analyses were performed by using the statistical analyses software SPSS 18.0 and by applying the Descriptive statistics (cross tabulation, frequencies, descriptive ratio statistics), bivariate statistics (means, t-test, correlation (bivariate, partial, distances), nonparametric tests and linear regression statistical methods. The Level of probability for obtaining the null hypothesis, in accordance with the international conventions for bio-medical sciences was 0.05 or 0.01 (Armitage et al., 2002).

Transcript	EAC code[a]	Primer/probe localization, 5'-'3' position (size)	Sequence
AML1 /ETO	ENF701	AML1, 1005–1026 (22)	5'-CAC CTA CCA CAG AGC CAT CAA A-3'
	ENR761	ETO, 318–297 (22)	5'-ATC CAC AGG TGA GTC TGG CAT T-3'
	ENP747	AML1, 1049–295 (30)	FAM 5'-AAC CTC GAA ATC GTA CTG AGA AGC ACT CCA-3' TAMRA
PML /RARα	ENF905	PML, 1198–1216 (19)	5'-CCG ATG GCT TCG ACG AGT T-3'
	ENF906	PML, 1642–1660 (19)	5'-ACC TGG ATG GAC CGC CTA G-3'
	ENF903	PML, 1690–1708 (19)	5'-TCT TCC TGC CCA ACA GCA A-3'
	ENR962	RARA, 485–465 (21)	5'-GCT TGT AGA TGC GGG GTA GAG-3'
	ENR942	RARA, 439–458 (20)	FAM 5'-AGT GCC CAG CCC TCC CTC GC-3' TAMRA
CBFβ /MYH11	ENF803	CBFB, 389–410 (22)	5'-CAT TAG CAC AAC AGG CCT TTG A-3'
	ENR862	MYH11, 1952–1936 (17)	5'-AGG GCC CGC TTG GAC TT-3'
	ENR863	MYH11, 1237–1217 (21)	5'-CCT CGT TAA GCA TCC CTG TGA-3'
	ENR865	MYH11, 1038–1016 (23)	5'-CTC TTT CTC CAG CGT CTG CTT AT-3'
	ENPr843	CBFB, 434–413 (22)	FAM 5'-TCG CGT GTC CTT CTC CGA GCC T-3' TAMRA
ABL	ENF1003	ABL, 372–402 (31)	5'-TGGAGATAACACTCTAAGCATAACTAAAGGT-3'
	ENF1063	ABL, 495–515 (21)	5'-GATGTAGTTGCTTGGGACCCA-3'
	ENF1043	ABL, 467–494 (28)	FAM 5'-CCA TTT TTG GTT TGG GCT TCA CAC CAT T-3' TAMRA
[a]ENF = forward primer, ENR = reverse primer, ENP = TaqMan probe			

Table 2. Sequences and positions of the RQ-PCR primers and probes

4. Results

In the period of twelve months, between January and December 2008, 77 patients were submitted and tested for acute leukemia at the University Clinic of Hematology-Skopje. Cyto-morphological analyses showed that the average rate of the blast cells in the differential blood counts and in the bone marrow was 54.6%(3-99.0%) and 73,5%(20-98.0%) respectively. In 7 patients blast cells were not detected initially.

4.1 Results from the cytochemical analyses

Results from the cytochemical analyses and the images of peripheral smears with positive examples from different cytochemical staining are presented at Figure 2 and Photo 1 respectively.

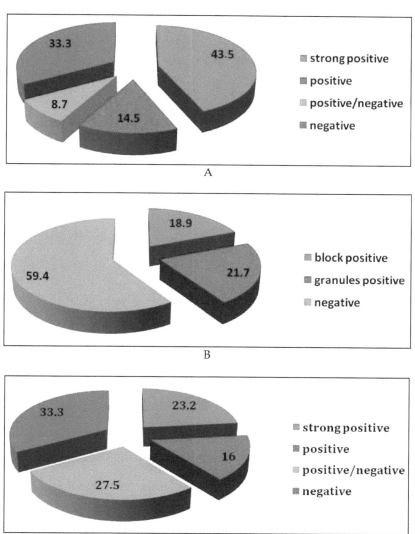

Fig. 2. Distribution of patients according to reactivity with different cytochemial staining.
A:Patient distribution according to MPO reactivity of the blasts cells. B: Patient distribution according to PAS reactivity of the blasts cells. C: Patient distribution according to NSE reactivity of the blasts cells.

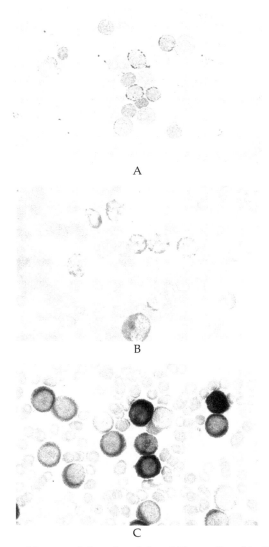

Photo 1. Images from positive reactivity of peripheral blast cells with different cytochemical staining , A: PAS reactivity, B: POX reactivity, C: NSE reactivity

Statistical analyses showed that there is a statistically significant correlation between the AML and MPO positivity (X^2 with Yates's correction=16.628 p<0.01)(Figure 2A). According to cross reaction ratio, MPO positivity presents statistically significant risk which improves the chance of AML diagnosis for 39 times (OR=392.1603 (4.177<0R<305.9796, CI 95%)). Also, a statistically significant correlation was noted between the PAS positivity and ALL (X^2 with Yates's correction=5.514 p<0.01)(Figure 2B). Strong PAS positivity was registered in 75% of ALL cases. Regarding the cytochemical stain NSE and AML no statistical correlation was

observed (X^2 with Yates's correction=2.456 p=0.117), expect for AML M4 and M5 entities
which showed statistically significant correlation (p<0, 05) (Figure 2C).
Morphology and cytochemistry established myeloid lineage in 57 (74.0%) cases and
lymphoid differentiation in 11 (14.3%) cases (Figure 2). Morphology and cytochemistry did
not establish lineage involvement in 9 (11.7%) cases. Basic morphological and cytochemical
analyses established the lineage assignment of the blasts cells in 68 (88.3%) patients.

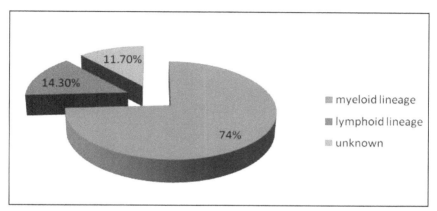

Fig. 3. Distribution of cases based on lineage assignment of blasts cells detected with basic
morphological and cytochemial analyses

4.2 Results from the immunological analyses

Immunological analyses with multi-parameter flow-cytometry were performed in all 77
patients. Further immunological analyses of cases in which lineage could not be assigned
based on morphology and cytochemistry established myeloid lineage in 4 patients, (AML-
M0) and one case indicated nonhematopoietic malignancy. In this case, immunophenotype
of the malignant cells (CD45-/CD56+/CD9+) indicated a neuroectodermal origin of the
malignant cells (Bain et al., 2002). Later neuroblastoma was diagnosed in this patient.
Immunological analyses change the assigned lineage based on morphology and
cytochemistry in 3(3.8%) of the patients from lymphoid to myeloid. The results of our study
showed that routine immunophenotyping improved diagnosis in 12 (15.5%) cases.
Consequently, based on FAB and immunologic criteria of EGIL and BTSH 64 acute
leukemias were classified as myeloid. Correlation between the antigen expressions with
FAB morphology of AML cases which confirmed the AML diagnosis in 83. 1% of the cases is
presented at Table 3. According to FAB criteria, the leukemias were classified as M0 (n=4),
M1 (n=8), M2 (n=20), M3 (n=5), M4 (n=17), M4-Eo (n=1), M5 (n=8), M6 (n=1).
Multivariate Cox-proportional regression analyses showed that in 89.7% of AML cases
lineage assignment is defined with the following five markers: CD13, CD33, CD117, HLA-
DR and anti-MPO. Most frequently detected maturation myeloid marker which was
expressed in 42.9% of AML case was CD15. Twenty three (35.9 %) of AML patients showed
expression of lymphoid antigens. Co-expression of two lymphoid markers was detected in
eleven (17.1%) cases, and most frequently co-expressed lymphoid marker was CD7 and was
detected in 28.5% of the cases.

	CD45	CD117	CD13	CD14	CD15	CD33	CD10	CD34	HLA-DR	MPO	Lysosime	TdT	CD2	CD7	CD19	CD56
Number of tested patients	64	64	64	64	64	64	64	64	64	64	64	64	64	64	64	64
Number of positive patients (%)	63 (98.4)	53 (82.8)	57 (89.2)	17 (26.7)	28 (43.7)	57 (89.2)	5 (7.8)	40 (62.5)	55 (85.9)	46 (71.8)	30 (46.8)	8 (12.5)	10 (15.6)	18 (28.1)	3 (4.6)	15 (23.4)
FAB morphology																
M0	4	2	1	0	0	2	0	4	4	4	0	2	0	1	0	0
M1	8	7	7	0	0	8	2	6	7	6	0	3	1	4	0	1
M2	21	20	19	1	6	18	1	16	17	18	6	1	0	0	2	7
M3	4	4	4	0	4	4	0	2	1	4	4	0	1	2	0	2
M4	17	14	15	8	8	16	4	9	16	12	12	0	5	6	0	3
M4E-0	1	1	1	1	1	1	0	0	1	1	1	2	0	1	1	0
M5	9	4	7	7	9	7	1	2	8	1	7	0	3	4	0	2
M6	0	1	1	0	0	1	0	1	1	0	0	0	0	0	0	0

Table 3. Correlation between the antigen expressions with FAB morphology of AML cases

4.3 Results from the molecular analyses

Molecular evaluation of AML cases demonstrated presence of the three major recurrent genetic abnormalities as follows: 5 patients were positive for the fusion transcript PML/RAR α (Figure 5), 3 patients were positive for AML/ETO1 and 7 for the fusion transcript CBFβ/MYH11 (Figure 4).

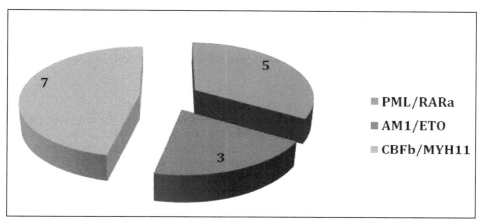

Fig. 4. Distribution of molecular abnormalities detected with the RQ-PCR assay in the group of AML patients;

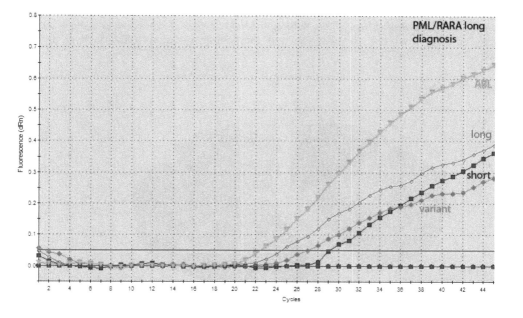

Fig. 5. Detection of fusion transcript PML/RARα using the RQ-PCR method

In 5 of the AML case PML/RARα fusion transcript was detected. Four of those patients had morphology and immunophenotype that correlate with AML-M3 diagnosis. The five patients were first diagnosed as AML-M2 and only after the positive result for PML/RARα the diagnosis was revised as AML-M3. In all those five patients target therapy with ATRA was initiated.

RT-PCR analysis also detected molecular abnormalities in the Core binding factor (CBF) in 10 AML patients; the presence of the AML/ETO1 fusion gene was confirmed in 3 patient and CBFβ/MYH11 in 7 patients.

Molecular analyses enabled 23.7% of the cases from our study to be classified in the adequate genetic entities of AML with different prognosis requiring different therapeutic approach.

4.4 Results from the analyses of the clinical data of the patients

We evaluate the distributions of the patients from our study group in the different grades of the Eastern Cooperative Oncology Group (EKOG) performance status scale (Oken et al. 1982)(Figure 6). All the patients with EKOG performance status higher than grade 2 and patients with serious co morbidities were not suitable candidates for alloSCT.

Furthermore, all the obtained results were correlated and consecutively effective treatment strategy for each single acute leukemia patient was selected.

5. Discussion

Modern diagnostic approach for acute leukemias combines cytomorphology, cytochemistry, multiparameter flow cytometry, chromosome banding analysis, accompanied by diverse fluorescence in situ hybridization techniques, and molecular analyses. The correct diagnosis is essential for classification of this heterogeneous complex of disorders and plays a central role for individual risk stratification and therapeutic decisions (Haferlach et al., 2007; Lichtman et al., 2010)

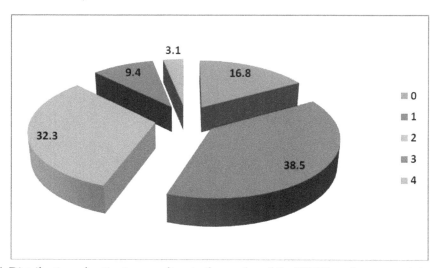

Fig. 6. Distribution of patients according to the grades of the EKOG performance status

5.1 Immunophenotyping in modern diagnosis of AML

Assignment of lineage is critical in the diagnostic evaluation of acute leukemia, as treatment for AML and ALL markedly differs. Myeloid and lymphoid lineage may be distinguished based on cellular morphology, cytochemical staining, and expression of lineage-specific antigens (Döhner et al., 2010). Analyses of diagnostic evaluation of acute leukemia in our study showed that immunophenotyping was necessary for lineage assignment in 4 (8.9%) cases that were morphologically and cytochemically undifferentiated, and also for correction of the lineage that was assigned based on morphology and cytochemistry in 3(3.8%) additional cases.

Flow cytometric immunophenotyping is a powerful technological tool that aids in the diagnosis, classification and monitoring of hematological malignances. It is essential in the diagnosis of AML, as it demonstrates a particular lineage involvement and has a prognostic significance in the majority of AML cases. We used the panel based on the recommendation of the EGIL group and BTSH. Our analyses comprised of a two step process with the first panel of markers being applied to all cases of acute leukemia and the second only in patients with AML that did not demonstrate a clear myeloid commitment. We also evaluated further lymphoid antigen positive AML cases by using the second panel of McAb (Stelzer & Goodpasture, 2000).

The second panel of McAb was aimed at identifying uncommon types of AML, such as those with megakaryocytic or elytroid differentiation and the exclusion or conformation of diagnosis of non-hematological malignancy. In our study, we applied the second AML panel in 27 cases; 4 which did not demonstrate clear myeloid commitment and 23 cases with lymphoid antigen positive AML cases. With our primary McAb we were able to differentiate AML form ALL in 96.8% of cases. Only in one patient (AML-M6-1.5%) lineage differentiation was assigned after staining with the secondary McAB panel and one case of non-hematological malignancy was confirmed.

Immunophenotyping was crucial in all cases of poorly differentiated myeloid leukemia (AML-M0), megakaryoblatstic leukemia (AML-M7) and in some case of monoblastic leukemia (AML-M5) and those with primitive erythroid cells as predominant leukemic cells (AML-M6). This is also important for recognizing an AML case that co-expresses lymphoid-associated antigens. In addition, immunophenotyping enables recognition of unusual forms of acute leukemia: designated acute biphenotypic or acute mixed lineage leukemia. The leukemia associated immunophenotype (LAIP) of the blast cells is a useful tool for detection of minimal residual disease in AML cases (Döhner et al., 2010; Stelzer & Goodpasture, 2000; Swerdlow et al., 2008).

In order to classify AML cases in the different AML entities we correlated the immunological data from immunophenotyping with the FAB morphological and cytochemical classification. One of the difficulties in knotting the flow cytometric data with traditional morphology is the lack of routine flow cytometric data analyses that would ensure correlation of the immunophenotyping data to abnormal morphologic counterpart. Our approach was based on the fact that complete eight-part differential of the myeloid lineage in the normal bone marrow could be done with correlations of the expression of CD45 expression versus light side scatter (SSC) characteristics of the cells. Extension of this technique to the analyses of leukemias allows abnormal cell to be recognized as independent clusters in CD45/SSC histograms with pattern of CD45 and SSC expression that correlate to the same pattern of the morphologically similar cells in normal bone marrow. Flow-cytometric analyses by using CD45 gating strategy reveled that leukemic myeloblasts demonstrate very similar CD45/SSC characteristics to normal myeloblasts, especially the early myeloblasts. In fact, leukemic cells generally demonstrate CD45/SSC characteristics that closely resemble their nearest normal morphological counterparts in the bone marrow. In the histograms the leukemic cells can be easily recognized as an abnormal cluster of cells in CD45/SSC „space" which is usually occupied by normal myeloid blasts. Using this method we define in our study group each category of AML as defined by FAB system (Stelzer & Goodpasture, 2000). Early myeloblasts are presented at Figure 6. Flow cytometric analyses show that those leukemic cells demonstrate low light forward and side scatter (FSC&SSC), which means that those cells are small and don't contain any granules. They also have low CD45 expression.

The predominant immunophenotype characteristics of early myeloblasts are an expression of all pan-myeloid antigens: CD13, CD33, CD117 and HLA-DR and lack expression of more mature myeloid antigens such as CD15 and CD14. Also, high proportion of the leukemic cells expresses CD34. With the maturation process of the blast cells, CD34 expression becomes more heterogeneous and weaker. The densest is at AML-M0 blasts, which typically express only one myeloid-associated antigen plus. Myeloid blasts that arise as a result of the genetic change in more mature myeloid progenitor lose the characteristics of the early myeloblasts. For example, AML-M3 blasts usually lack the expression of CD34 and HLA-DR.

At Figure 7 are presents more mature myeloblasts, M5 blast. It is obvious that they are bigger when compared with the AML-M1 blasts presented on Figure 6, and contain some more granules (have higher FSC&SSC). Immunophenotypically, they are characterized with expression of some more mature myeloid markers as CD14 and CD15, and in most of the case with lost CD34 expression.

The results from our study showed that routine immunophenotyping improved the diagnosis in 12 (15, 5%) cases with acute leukemia which was essential for more appropriate individual clinical stratification of the patient with acute leukemia. Our data demonstrate that flow cytometry in correlation with the morphological classification criteria for each subtype of AML can be used for initial classification of each FAB AML entities and and justify routine implementation of flow cytometry analyses in the diagnostic evaluation of AML cases.

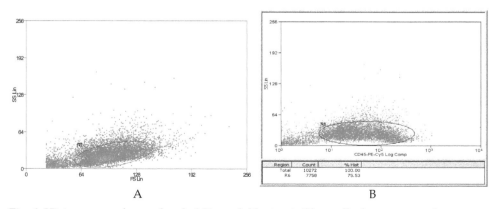

Fig. 6. Histogram analyses of early M1 myeloblasts ; A: Blast cells demonostrate low FSC&SSC, B:Blast cells have low CD45 expression

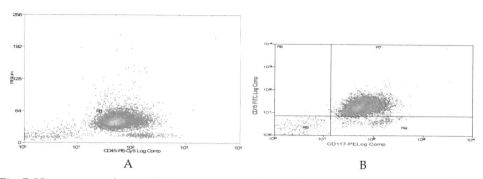

Fig. 7. Histogram analyses of M5-myloblasts; A: Blast cells are biger and more granular and
have higher CD45,B: Blasts cells express CD117 and the myeloid expression maturation
marker CD15

5.2 Molecular analyses in the modern diagnosis of AML

Results from the immunophenotying guided us to perform exact molecular analyses and
further define some specific genetic entities of AML. We tested our AML patients for the
presence of PML/RARα, AML1/ETO and CBFβ/MYH11 fusion transcripts, by using RT-
PCR method. Results from those analyses additionally improved the exact classification of
the AML subtypes and made target and specific therapy available for some of the specific
AML subtypes (Marcucci et al., 2000; Perea et al.2006; Wang et al., 2008)

Nonrandom chromosomal abnormalities are identified at the cytogenetic level in
approximately 55% of all adult primary or de novo AML patients and have long been
recognized as important independent prognostic indicators for achievement of complete
remission (CR), duration of first CR, and survival after intensive chemotherapy treatment.
Two of the most prevalent cytogenetic subtypes of adult primary or de novo AML are t (8;
21) (q22; q22) and inv (16) (p13q22). These abnormalities result in the disruption of genes
encoding subunits of the CBF, which is a αβ heterodimeric transcriptional factor involved in
the regulation of normal hematopoiesis and are collectively referred as CBF-AML. At the
molecular level, t(8;21)(q22;q22) and inv(16)(p13q22) result in the creation of novel fusion
genes, AML1/ETO and CBFβ/MYH11.Detection of t(8;21)(q22;q22) or inv(16)(p13q22) in
adult patients with primary AML is a favorable independent prognostic indicator for
achievement of cure after intensive chemotherapy or bone marrow transplantation, and may
serve as a as a paradigm of the risk-adapted treatment in AML (Döhner et al. 2010&
Marcucci et al., 2000).

In almost all studies of adult primary AML, the highest CR rate (approximately 90%) and
the longest disease free survival (DFS) at 5 years (approximately 50%) have been associated
with CBF-AML cases. It has been suggested that the superior outcome of AML patients with
CBF gene rearrangements compared with other AML patients may be attributed to an
increased sensitivity of the leukemic blasts to cytarabine that in combination with
anthracyclines represents the backbone of AML treatment. The collective analysis of all data
regarding the treatment of CBF-AML indicates that incorporation of multiple courses of
high dose of cytarabine as consolidation therapy should be considered as the therapeutic
standard for primary adult CBF-AML (Marcucci et al., 2001; Perea et al.2006).

The prognostic impact of the CBF gene rearrangements appears equally significant in the setting of BMT of AML patients in first CR. However, the iatrogenic morbidity and mortality of BMT suggest that patients with CBF-AML should not receive this therapeutic modality as initial treatment. The collective analysis of all data regarding the implementation of all SCT in AML treatment suggest that although allo SCT and auto SCT may have a potential role in the initial management of AML other than CBF-AML, the treatment-related morbidity and mortality of SCT represent a therapeutic limitation for treatment of CBF-AML patients. Considering the high probability of cure that these patients can achieve with intensive chemotherapy, it is reasonable to spare them the toxicity of SCT as consolidation in first complete remission (Löwenberg et al., 2008a; Koreth et al, 2009; Marcucci et al., 2000; Marcucci et al., 2001 & Perea et al.2006).

APL or AML-M3 is a distinct subtype of AML which is characterized by a t(15;17) translocation leading to a *PML-RARA* fusion gene. Historically, recognition of this form of AML as a separate entity was important for the clinicians, not because the chemotherapy used as treatment differed substantially from that used for the other subtypes of AML, but because the relatively common occurrence of life-threatening coagulopathy mandated special supportive maneuvers, including the use of low-dose heparin and aggressive blood product support. In the past, induction mortality was often significant, with some older series reporting an incidence approaching 50%. APL was typified with the worst features associated with leukemia: a fulminant disorder that struck primarily young people, had devastating effects on an individual's life, and resulted in death for a large number of patients during the initial phases of treatment. The last two decades have seen a fundamental shift from this paradigm, with APL now recognized as one of the most curable forms of acute leukemia. Introduction of the differentiation therapy with ATRA into the treatment of APL completely revolutionized the management and outcome of this disease, and presents the first model of targeted therapy for cancer. This agent represents one of the most spectacular advances in the treatment of human cancer, providing the first paradigm of molecularly targeted treatment. Treatment of APL with ATRA combined with anthracycline-based chemotherapy yields a CR rate of approximately 90% for newly diagnosed APLs. The relapse rate is approximately 20%, and with the development of new molecular target therapies such as arsenic trioxide, a cure can now be expected even for relapsed patients. After the advent of ATRA, the introduction of arsenic trioxide (ATO), probably the most biologically active single drug in APL has provided a valuable addition to the armamentarium and may have contributed to further improvements in the clinical outcome of this disease. Several treatment strategies using these agents, usually in combination with chemotherapy, have provided excellent therapeutic results with survival rates exceeding 70% in multicenter clinical trials. Cure of patients with APL depends not only on the effective use of combination therapy involving differentiating and classical cytotoxic agents, but also, critically, upon supportive care measures that take into particular account the biology of the disease and the complications associated with molecularly targeted therapies. Moreover, it is important to consider diagnostic suspicion of APL as a medical emergency (uncommon in AML) that requires several specific and simultaneous actions, including immediate commencement of ATRA therapy, prompt genetic diagnosis, and measures to counteract the coagulopathy (Grimwade et al., 2002; Wang et al., 2008).

5.2.1 Why we used RT-PCR method for detection of the genetic abnormalities?

RT-PCR methods for detecting the PML/RARα fusion transcript also provide the "gold standard" approach for confirming a diagnosis of APL. In addition to its high specificity and sensitivity, it is essential for defining PML breakpoint location thereby establishing the target for reliable monitoring of the minimal residual disease (MRD).

Standard cytogenetic analysis is currently the most common method for identifying the most common recurrent cytogenetic abnormalities t(8;2l)(q22;q22) and inv(16)(pl3q22) or t(16;16)(p13;q22) in AML patients. This technique also allows detection of secondary chromosomal abnormalities such as del (9q),-X and -Y which are frequently associated with t(8;21)(q22;q22), or +8 and +22 more often found with inv(16)(p13q22). Still, despite the recent improvements in the cytogenetic methodology and the use of complementary techniques such as fluorescence in situ hybridization and comparative genomic hybridization to increase the rate of successful karyotyping, the possibility that subtle structural chromosomal aberrations are missed remains (Marcucci et al., 2000). In t(8;21) (q22;q22) or inv(16) (p13q22), failure to detect submicroscopic (cryptic) rearrangements of the involved genes leads to false-negative results that may ultimately impact the correct stratification of this patient population in prognostic and risk-adapted therapy groups. Sensitive molecular methodologies such as RT-PCR have been successfully used to detect cryptic CBF abnormalities in diagnostic samples of AML patients with karyotypes that are otherwise negative for t(8;21)(q22;q22) or inv(16)(p13q22). Andrieu et al.,1997 reported detection of AML1/ETO fusion transcripts by RT-PCR in cases with unsuccessful cytogenetic studies, normal karyotypes, or karyotypes other than t(8:2 1)(q22;q22) such as del(8q), i(8)(q10) or del(9q). Langabeer et al., 1997 used a two-step RT-PCR to screen for the AMLI/ETO and CBFβ/MYHll fusion transcripts in AML patients entered into the U.K. MRC AML 10, 11, and 12 trials and compared the results with conventional cytogenetics. All patients with cytogenetic evidence of t(8;21)(q22;q22) or inv(16)(pl3q22) were positive by RT-PCR for the corresponding fusion transcripts. RT-PCR was also positive in 31 cases (19 cases of AML1/ETO and 12 cases of CBFβ/MYH11) without CBF cytogenetic abnormalities, increasing the overall detection rate of "t(8;21)(q22;q22)" and "inv(16)(p13q22)" from 8.1% to 12.9% and from 6.5% to 10.3%, respectively. The authors of these studies concluded that all primary AML should be routinely tested for the presence of the CBF fusion genes by molecular screening to improve genomic stratification of AML patients in risk-related treatment groups (Marcucci et al., 2000).

Although patients with CBF-AML have a relatively good prognosis, a substantial number of them relapse and eventually die of their disease. Because relapse after intensive treatment is likely to occur as the result of failure to completely eradicate the leukemic blasts, evaluation of MRD by a sensitive molecular technique such as PCR based techniques has been proposed to detect persistence of malignant clones and predict disease relapse in AML patients in CR. This strategy has been successful in CML (Radich et al.,1995) and acute promyelocytic leukemia (Grimwade et al., 2002; Wang et al., 2008), but its clinical applicability to other subgroups of acute leukemia remains controversial.

RQ-PCR provides the most sensitive parameters for AML with reciprocal gene fusions PML/RARα, CBFβ–MYH11, AML1–ETO (Haferlach et al., 2007). The score of gene expression of the respective fusion transcripts after consolidation therapy in relation to gene expression at diagnosis correlates significantly with prognosis [Haferlach et al., 2007]. The prognostic value of quantitative PCR in MRD diagnostics in these subgroups was demonstrated in several studies. Patients with an MRD level<1% after induction chemotherapy in relation to initial diagnosis had a relapse rate of 8% in contrast to 91% in the patients with MRD levels of ≥1% in the investigation on the CBF-leukemias by Krauter et al.,2003. Marcucci et al, 2000, were able to define a distinct transcript copy number in inv(16)/CBFB/ MYH11 below which relapse was unlikely and above which relapse occurred with high probability. A Gruppo Italiano Malattie Ematologiche Maligne dell' Adulto (GIMEMA) trial showed that molecular switch from CR to PML/RARα positivity was followed by hematologic relapse after a median time of 3 months in 95% of all APL cases (Diverio et al. 1998). Data from different studies indicate that of all AML subtypes, quantitative PCR monitoring could be best established for the reciprocal gene fusions.

Molecular analyses enabled 23.7% of the cases of our study to be classified in the adequate genetic entities of AML with different prognosis requiring different therapeutically approach.

5.3 Analyses of the clinical characteristics of the patients in the era of modern diagnosis of AML

5.3.1 Analyses of the EKOG performance status

Several studies support the use of the ECOG performance status as a measure of physical functioning and prognosis in patients with AML (Oken et al. 1982). A retrospective study of data from five Southwestern Oncology Group (SWOG) trials that included 968 patients with AML found that the mortality rate within 30 days of initiation of induction therapy is dependent upon both the patient's age and ECOG performance status at diagnosis. A second retrospective analysis of 998 patients age 65 or greater (range 65 to 89; median 71 years) who underwent intensive induction chemotherapy reported eight-week mortality rates of 23, 40, and 72 percent for patients with ECOG PS of zero to 1, 2, and 3 to 4, respectively. One-year overall survival rates for the same groups were 35, 25, and 7 percent, respectively. A third retrospective study of 2767 patients with non-APL AML from the Swedish acute leukemia registry also reported that older patients with an ECOG PS of zero to 1 had 30 day death rates after intensive chemotherapy of less than 15 percent, while patients with a PS of 3 or 4 had higher early death rates regardless of patient age ranging from 26 to 36 percent. Seventy percent of patients up to age 80 years had a PS of zero to 2. A prospective trial of induction chemotherapy with cytarabine plus daunorubicin in 811 older adults (median age 67 years, range 60 to 83 years) with ECOG PS of zero to 2 reported a 30-day mortality rate of 11 percent (Appelbaum et al, 2006). We used the EKOG performance status score in initial randomization of our AML patients for different induction and consolidation approaches, in order to avoid intensive induction and consolidation treatment for patient with EKOG performance status higher than 2. Only 8 (12.5%) patients from our study group have EKOG performance status higher than 2, but only 3 of those patients were younger than 60 years of age.

5.3.2 Analyses of the comorbidities

Comorbidity is an also a distinct additional clinical entity that exists or may occur during the clinical course of patient with a primary disease (i.e. AML). Comorbid conditions are poor prognostic factors especially in older patients with AML. Patients with age-related

chronic cardiac, pulmonary, hepatic or renal disorders or diabetes suffer greater acute
toxicity from chemotherapy. Older patients may also have decreased bone marrow
regenerative capacity, even after successful leukemia cytoreduction. Inability to tolerate long
periods of pancytopenia and malnutrition or the nephrotoxicity of drugs such as amino
glycosides or amphotericin remains a major barrier to successful treatment (Piccirillo et
al.2004; Sorror et al, 2005). Six 6(9,3%) patients from our study had seriouos comorbidities
which limited the aplication of intensive chemotherapy in their treatment. Five of them were
older than 60years.

5.4 Approach to AML diagnostic algorithms

Modern diagnostic approaches in the AML should be created as integral and basic parts of
optimized treatment concepts for the benefit of the each individual patient. The ultimate test
of any disease diagnostic algorithm approach is its usefulness in guiding the selection of
effective treatment strategies. Algorithms that provide a basis for risk-adapted therapeutic
choices may include immunological markers, cytogenetic factors, molecular markers as well
as clinical parameters (e.g., age, attainment of an early or late complete remission) and
hematological determinants (e.g., secondary AML, white blood cell count at diagnosis)
(Haferlach et al., 2007).

A comprehensive approach in diagnosis, classification, and treatment follow-up in patients
with acute leukemias can, therefore, be suggested by diagnostic algorithms, which also
show the relationship and the hierarchy between single methods. These standard guidelines
for AML mostly result from a combination of different methods and intend to add
prognostic information (Lowenberg 2008).

Our diagnostic algorithm for AML (as shown in Fig. 8) starts with cytomorphology and
cytochemistry. These methods should be performed in combination: cytomorphology and
cytochemistry allow rapid classification of the acute leukemias and further enables the
choice of the antibody panel for flow cytometric analyses. In case cytomorphology gives
indices for characteristic aberrations — in the FAB subtypes M3/M3v for t(15;17)/PML/
RARα, in FAB M4eo for inv(16)/CBFβ/MYH11, or in M1/2 with the characteristic long
Auer rods for the t(8;21)/AML1/ETO, PCR analyses for these rearrangements should be
promptly applied.

Especially in case of suspicion for APL due to clinical symptoms or due to the
morphological findings, RT-PCR for PML/RARα should be initiated as soon as possible
(Schoch et al., 2002). We think that, regardless of the morphological, cytochemical and
immunological futures of the blast cells, RT-PCR for the fusion oncogene PML/RARα are
recommendable in all AML cases. The RT- PCR method is the most sensitive and rapid
technique for detection of this oncogene and provides an optimal basis for MRD analyses.
Further we suggest all AML cases which are PML/RARα negative to be tested for the
presence of the reciprocal fusions genes that describe CBF-AML, AML1/ETO and
CBFβ/MYH11.Those analyses provides the basis for sub-classification of the AML cases in
prognostically relevant subclasses. This is the prerequisite for adequate individual clinical
risk stratification and therapeutic decisions.

Moreover, we correlated the obtained result for the applied multimodal diagnostic approach
with the patient age, EKOG performance status and comorbidities, which allowed us to
optimize the individual risk stratification for each AML patient.

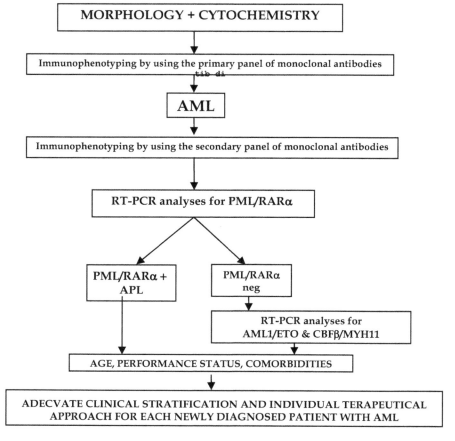

Fig. 8. Diagnostic algorithm and algorithm for risk adapted therapy in AML patients

6. Conclusions

A basis for every therapeutic decision in AML cases should be provided by a multimodal diagnostic approach. The optimal therapeutic conditions are based on exact classification and prognosis of the AML subtype at diagnosis and to delineation of sensitive markers for MRD studies during the complete hematologic remission. MRD methods have many potential applications in the clinical management of patients with acute leukemia. Today, a multimodal diagnostic approach which combines different diagnostic techniques is needed to meet these requirements. The diagnostic process is becoming more demanding with respect to experience, time and costs due to the expansion of methods and algorithms, which guide the diagnostic procedure from basic to more specific methods and which finally lead to results that are essential for modern diagnostics and therapeutic concepts. There are numerous overlaps between different diagnostic methods. These can be used for optimal pathways in the complex diagnostic proceedings and for validation of the results of single methods, which can be summarized in diagnostic algorithms. Basic morphological and cytochemical analyses performed in our study group established the lineage assignment of the blasts cells in 68 (88.3%) patients. Routine immunophenotyping improved the diagnosis in 12 (15.5%) more cases. Molecular analyses enabled 23.7% of the cases from our study to be classified in the adequate genetic entities of AML with different prognosis requiring different therapeutical approach.

The applied multimodal diagnostic approach consisted of minimal number of cytomorphological, cytochemistry, immunological and molecular analyses enables improved and more precise diagnosis and clinical stratification in 38.2% acute leukemia patients from our study. Moreover, when we correlate those results with the results obtained from the analyses of the EKOG performance status and the incidence of the serious comborbidities in our study group, an additional 12.5% of the patients were stratified to a different risk adapted therapy.

Our initial results are consistent with literature data and indicate that our applied multimodal diagnostic approach improved the diagnosis of the specific genetic entities of AML in which specific treatment approach is indicated and allows individual clinical stratification in treatment protocols of the patients.

7. References

Andrieu, V., Radford-Weiss, I., Troussard, X., Chane, C., Valensi, F., Guesnu, M., Haddad, E., Viguier, F., Dreyfus, F.; Varet, B.; Flandrin, G.; & Macintyre, E. (1997). Molecular detection of t(8;2 I)/AMLI-ETO in AML MI/M2: Correlation with cytogenetics, morphology and immunophenotype. *Br J Haematol,* Vol.4, No.92,(March 1996), pp. 855-865, ISSN 0007-1048

Appelbaum, F.R., Rowe, J.M., Radich, J., & Dick, J.E. (2001). Acute myeloid leukemia. *Hematology (Am Soc Hematol Educ Program),*(November 2001), pp. 62-86, ISSN 1520-4391

Appelbaum, F.R., Gundacker, H., Head, D.R., Slovak, M.L., Willman, C.L., Godwin, J.E., Anderson, J.E.,& Petersdorf, S.H. (2006). Age and acute myeloid leukemia. *Blood,*Vol. 107, No.9, (May 2006), pp.3481–3485,ISSN0006-4971

Armitage P., Berry G., & Matthews J.N.S.(2002) *Statistical Methods in Medical Research* (4th edition),Blackwell ISBN:978063052578,Oxford,UKBain, BJ, Barnet, D, Linch, D, Matutes, E, & Reilly, J.T. (2002).Revised guidelines on immunophenotyping in acute leukemias and chronic lymphoproliferative disorders. *Clin Lab Hem,*Vol. 24,(2002),pp.1-13, ISSN 0141-9854

Beillard, E., Pallisgaard, N., van der Velden, V.H., Bi, W., Dee, R., van der Schoot E., Delabesse E., Macintyre E., Gottardi E., Saglio G., Watzinger F., Lion T., van Dongen, J.J., Hokland, P., & Gabert, J.(2003). Evaluation of candidate control genes for diagnosis and residual disease detection in leukemic patients using 'real-time' quantitative reverse-transcriptase polymerase chain reaction (RQ-PCR) – a Europe against cancer program. *Leukemia,* Vol. 17, No. 12,(December 2003), pp 2474-2486, ISSN 0887-6924

Bene, M.C., Castoldi, G., Knapp, W., Ludwig, W.D., Matutes, E., Orfao, A., & van't Veer, M.B. (1995). Proposals for the immunological classification of acute leukemias. European Group for the Immunological Characterization of Leukemias (EGIL). *Leukemia,* Vol. 9, No. 10, (October 1995), pp.1783-1786, ISSN 0887-6924

Bennett, J.M., Catovsky, D., Daniel, M.T., Flandrin, G., Galton, D.A., Gralnick, H.R., & Sultan, C.(1976). Proposals for the classification of the acute leukaemias. French–American–British (FAB) Cooperative Group. *Br J Haematol,*Vol.33, No.4 (August 1976), pp.451–458, ISSN 0007-1048

Borowitz, M.I., Guenter, K.I., Shults, K.E., & Stelzer, G.T. (1993). Immunophenotyping of acute leukemia by flow cytometry analysis. Use of CD45 and right-angle light scatter to gate on leukaemic blasts in three colour analysis. *Am J Clin Pathol*, No.100,(November 1993), pp.534-540,ISSN 0002-9173

Byrd, J.C., Mrózek, K., Dodge, R.K., Carroll, A.J., Edwards, C.G., Arthur, D.C., Pettenati, M.J., Patil, S.R., Rao, K.W., Watson, M.S., Koduru, P.R., Moore, J.O., Stone, R.M., Mayer, R.J., Feldman, E.J., Davey, F.R., Schiffer, C.A., Larson, R.A., & Bloomfield, C.D.; Cancer and Leukemia Group B (CALGB 8461). (2002). Pretreatment cytogenetic abnormalities are predictive of induction success, cumulative incidence of relapse, and overall survival in adult patients with de novo acute myeloid leukemia: results from Cancer and Leukemia Group B (CALGB 8461).*Blood*, Vol. 100, No.13, (December 2002), pp. 4325-4336, ISSN 0006-4971

Cornelissen, J.J., van Putten, W.L., Verdonck, L.F., Theobald, M., Jacky E., Daenen, S.M., van Marwijk-Kooy, M., Wijermans, P., Schouten, H., Huijgens, P.C., van der Lelie, H., Fey, M., Ferrant, A., Maertens, J., Gratwohl, A.,& Lowenberg, B. (2007). Results of a HOVON-SAKK donor versus donor analysis of myeloablative HLA-identical sibling stem cell transplantation in first remission acute myeloid leukemia in young and middle aged adults: benefits for whom? *Blood*, Vol.109, No. 9, (May 2007), pp. 3658-3666,ISSN 0006-4971

Diverio D., Rossi V., Avvisati G., De Santis S., Pistilli A., Pane F., Saglio G., Martinelli G., Petti M.C., Santoro A., Pelicci, P.G., Mandelli, F., Biondi, A., & Lo Coco, F.(1998). Early detection of relapse by prospective reverse transcriptase-polymerase chain reaction analysis of the PML/RAR alpha fusion gene in patients with acute promyelocytic leukemia enrolled in the GIMEMA-AIEOP multicenter "AIDA" trial. GIMEMA-AIEOP Multicenter "AIDA" Trial. Blood, Vol. 92, No.3, (August 1998), pp.784-789, ISSN 0006-4971

Döhner, H., Estey, E.H., Amadori, S., Appelbaum, F.R., Büchner, T., Burnett, A.K., Dombret, H., Fenaux, P., Grimwade, D., Larson, R.A., Lo-Coco, F., Naoe, T., Niederwieser, D., Ossenkoppele, G.J., Sanz, M.A., Sierra, J., Tallman, M.S., Löwenberg, B.,& Bloomfield, C.D.; European Leukemia Net. (2010). Diagnosis and management of acute myeloid leukemia in adults: recommendations from an international expert panel, on behalf of the European Leukemia Net. *Blood*, Vol.115, No.3, (January 2010), pp.453-474, ISSN 0006-4971

Fernandez, H.F. (2010). New Trends in the Standard of Care for Initial Therapy of Acute Myeloid Leukemia. *Hematology (Am Soc Hematol Educ Program)*, (November 2010), pp. 62-86, ISSN 1520-4391

First MIC Cooperative Study Group. (1986). Morphologic, immunologic, and cytogenetic (MIC) working classification of acute lymphoblastic leukemias: report of the workshop held in Leuven, Belgium, April 22-23, 1985. *Cancer Genet Cytogenet*, Vol. 23, No.3, (November 1986), pp.189-197, ISSN 0165-4608

Freeman, S.D., Jovanovic, J.V., & Grimwade, D. (2008). Development of minimal residual disease-directed therapy in acute myeloid leukemia. *Semin Oncol*, Vol. 34, No.4, (August 2008), pp.388-400, ISSN 0093-7754

Gabert, J., Beillard, E., van der Velden, V.H., Bi, W., Grimwade, D., Pallisgaard, N., Barbany, G., Cazzaniga, G., Cayuela, J.M., Cavé, H., Pane, F., Aerts, J.L., De Micheli, D., Thirion, X., Pradel, V., González, M., Viehmann, S., Malec, M., Saglio, G., & van Dongen, J.J. (2003). Standardization and quality control studies of 'real-time' quantitative reverse transcriptase polymerase chain reaction of fusion gene

transcripts for residual disease detection in leukemia – A Europe Against Cancer
   Program. *Leukemia,* Vol.17, No.12, (December 2003), pp.2318–2357, ISSN 0887-6924
Grimwade, D. (2001). The clinical significance of cytogenetic abnormalities in acute myeloid
   leukaemia. *Best Pract Res Clin Haematol,* Vol. 14, No. 3, (September 2001), pp. 497-
   529, ISSN 1521-6926
Grimwade, D. & Lo Coco, F. (2002). Acute promyelocytic leukemia: a model for the role of
   molecular diagnosis and residual disease monitoring in directing treatment
   approach in acute myeloid leukemia. *Leukemia,* Vol.16, No.10,(October 2002),
   pp:.1959–1973, ISSN 0887-6924
Haferlach, T., Bacher, U., Kern, W., Schnittger, S., & Haferlach, C. (2007). Diagnostic
   pathways in acute leukemias: a proposal for a multimodal approach. *Ann Hematol,*
   Vol. 86, No. 5, (May 2007), pp.311–327, ISSN 0939-5555
Haferlach, T. (2008). Molecular Genetic Pathways as Therapeutic Targets in Acute Myeloid
   Leukemia. *Hematology (Am Soc Hematol Educ Program),*(November 2008), pp.401-
   411, ISSN 1520-4391
Koreth, J., Schlenk, R., Kopecky, K.J., Honda, S., Sierra, J., Djulbegovic, B.J., Wadleigh, M.,
   De Angelo, D.J., Stone, R.M., Sakamaki, H., Appelbaum, F.R., Döhner, H., Antin,
   J.H., Soiffer, R.J.,& Cutler, C. (2009). Allogeneic stem cell transplantation for acute
   myeloid leukemia in first complete remission: systematic review and meta-analysis
   of prospective clinical trials. *JAMA,* Vol. 301, No. 22, (June 2009), pp.2349-2361,
   ISSN 0098-7484.
Krauter, J., Gorlich, K., Ottmann, O., Lubbert, M., Dohner, H., Heit, W., Kanz, L., Ganser, A.,
   & Hei,l G. (2003). Prognostic value of minimal residual disease quantification by
   real-time reverse transcriptase polymerase chain reaction in patients with core
   binding factor leukemias. *J Clin Oncol,* Vol. 21, No.23, (December 2003), pp.4413-
   4422, ISSN 0002-9173
Langabeer, S.E., Walker, H., Rogers, J.R., Burnett, A.K., Wheatley, K., Swirsky, D.,
   Goldstone, A.H., & Linch, D.C. (1997). Incidence of AMLl/ETO fusion transcripts
   in patients entered into the MRC AML trials. *Br J Haematol,* Vol. 99, No. 4,
   (December 19970), pp.925-928, ISSN 0007-1048
Langabeer, S.E., Walker, H., Gale, R.E., Wheatley, K., Burnett, A.K., Goldstone, A.H., &
   Linch, DC.(1997). Frequency of CBFβ/MYHII fusion transcripts in patients entered
   into the UK MRC AML trials. The MRC Adult Leukaemia Working Party.*Br J
   Haematol,* Vol. 96, No. 4, (March 1997), pp. 736-739, ISSN 0007-1048
Lichtman, M.A.; Kipps, T.J.; Seligsohn, U.; Kaushansky, K.; & Prchal, J.T. (2010). *Williams
   Hematology,* Eighth Edition, The McGraw-Hill Companies, Inc., ISBN 978-0-07-
   162144-1, China
Löwenberg, B. (2008a). Diagnosis and prognosis in acute myeloid leukemia: the art of
   distinction. *N Engl J Med,* Vol. 358, No. 18, (May 2008), pp. 1960-1962, ISSN 0028-4793
Löwenberg, B. (2008b). Acute Myeloid Leukemia: The Challenge of Capturing Disease
   Variety. *Hematology (Am Soc Hematol Educ Program),* (November 2008), pp.1-11,
   ISSN 1520-4391
Marcucci, G., Caligiuri, M.A., Döhner, H., Archer, K.J., Schlenk, R.F., Döhner, K., Maghraby,
   E.A., & Bloomfield, C.D. (2001).Quantification of CBF beta/MYH11 fusion
   transcript by real time RT-PCR in patients with inv(16) acute myeloid leukemia.
   Leukemia, Vol. 15, No.7, (July 2001), pp. 1072–1080, ISSN 0887-6924
Marcucci, G., et al. (2000). Molecular and Clinical Advances in Core Binding Factor Primary
   Acute Myeloid Leukemia: A Paradigm for Translational Research in Malignant
   Hematology. *Cancer Investigation,* Vol.18, No. 8, (2000), pp.768-780, ISSN 0735-7907

Oken, M.M., Creech, R.H., Tormey, D.C., Horton, J., Davis, T.E., McFadden, E.T., & Carbone, P.P. (1982). Toxicity And Response Criteria Of The Eastern Cooperative Oncology Group. *Am J Clin Oncol*, Vol.5, No.6, (December 1982), pp.649-655, ISSN 0002-9173

Panovska-Stavridis, I., Cevreska, L., Trajkova, S., Hadzi-Pecova, L., Trajkov, D., Petlickovski, A., Srbinovska, O., Matevska, N., Dimovski, A., & Spiroski, M. (2008). Preliminary results of introducing the method multiparameter flow cytometry in patients with acute leukemia in the Republic of Macedonia. *Macedonian Journal of Medical Sciences*, No.1(2), pp:36-43, ISSN 1857-5749

Perea, G., Lasa, A., Aventín, A., Domingo, A., Villamor, N., Queipo, de Llano, M.P., Llorente, A., Juncà, J., Palacios, C., Fernández, C., Gallart, M., Font, L., Tormo, M., Florensa, L., Bargay, J., Martí, J.M., Vivancos, P., Torres, P., Berlanga, J.J., Badell, I., Brunet, S., Sierra, J., & Nomdedéu, J.F.; Grupo Cooperativo para el Estudio y Tratamiento de las Leucemias Agudas y Miel.(2006). Prognostic value of minimal residual disease (MRD) in acute myeloid leukemia (AML) with favorable cytogeneticst(8;21) and inv(16)]. *Leukemia*, Vol. 20, No.1, (January 2006), pp.87-94, ISSN 0887-6924

Piccirillo, J.F., Tierney, R.M., Costas, I., Grove, L., & Spitznagel, E.L. Jr.(2004). Prognostic importance of comorbidity in a hospital-based cancer registry. *JAMA*, Vol. 291, No. 20, (May 2004), pp.2441-2447, ISSN 0098-7484

Radich, J.P., Gehly, G., Gooley, T., Bryant, E., Clift, R.A., Collins, S., Edmands, S., Kirk, J., Lee, A., Kessler, P., et al. (1995). Polymerase chain reaction detection of the BCR-ABL fusion transcript after allogeneic marrow transplantation for chronic myeloid leukemia: Results and implications in 346 patients. *Blood*, Vol. 85, No. 9, (May 1995), pp.2632-2638, ISSN 0006-4971

Schlenk, R.F., Döhner, K., Krauter, J., Fröhling, S., Corbacioglu, A., Bullinger, L., Habdank, M., Späth, D., Morgan, M., Benner, A., Schlegelberger, B., Heil, G., Ganser, A., & Döhner, H.; German-Austrian Acute Myeloid Leukemia Study Group. (2008). Mutations and treatment outcome in cytogenetically normal acute myeloid leukemia. *N Engl J Med*. Vol. 358, No. 18, (May 2008), pp.1909–1918, ISSN 0028-4793

Schoch, C., Schnittger, S., Kern, W., Lengfelder, E., Löffler, H., Hiddemann, W., & Haferlach, T. (2002). Rapid diagnostic approach to PML–RAR alpha-positive acute promyelocytic leukemia. *Hematol J*,Vol.3, No.5, (2002), pp.259–263, ISSN 1466-4860

Sorror, M.L., Maris, M.B., Storb, R., Baron, F., Sandmaier, B.M., Maloney, D.G., Storer, B.(2005). Hematopoietic cell transplantation (HCT)-specific comorbidity index: a new tool for risk assessment before allogeneic HCT. *Blood*. Vol. 106, No.8, (October 2005), pp.2912-2919, ISSN 0006-4971

Stelzer, G.T., & Goodpasture, L. (2000). Use of multiparameter flow cytometry and immunophenotyping for the diagnosis and classification of acute myeloid leukemia, In *Immunophenotyping*, Stewart C,S & Nicholson J.K.A.,pp.215-238,Wiley-Liss, ISBN 0-471-23957-7, United States of America

Swerdlow, S.H.; Campo, E.; Harris, N.L.; Jaffe, E.S.; Pileri, S.A.; Stein, H.; Thiele, J.; Vardiman, J.W. (2008). *WHO Classification of Tumours of Haematopoietic and Lymphoid Tissues*, Fourth Edition, IARC, WHO Press, ISBN 9789283224310, Geneva, Switzerland

Vardiman, J.W., Thiele, J., Arber, D.A., Brunning, R.D., Borowitz, M.J., Porwit, A., Harris, N.L., Le Beau, M.M., Hellström-Lindberg, E., Tefferi, A., & Bloomfield, C.D.(2009). The 2008 revision of the WHO Classification of Myeloid Neoplasms and Acute Leukemia: rationale and important changes. *Blood*, Vol. 114, No.5, (July 2009), pp. 937–951, ISSN 0006-4971

Wang, Z.Y., & Chen, Z. (2008). Acute promyelocytic leukemia: from highly fatal to highly curable. *Blood*, Vol. 111, No. 5 (March 2008), pp.2505-15, ISSN 0006-4971

10

Radio-Photoluminescence Glass Dosimeter (RPLGD)

David Y.C. Huang[1] and Shih-Ming Hsu[2]
[1]Memorial Sloan-Kettering Cancer Center
[2]China Medical University
[1]USA
[2]Taiwan (ROC)

1. Introduction

Radiation is a type of the energy transport. It produces ionization, scintillation, and luminescence when radiation interacts with matter. By detecting these phenomena from the response of the dosimeter after exposure, one can acquire an understanding on the types and the intensity of the radiation.

Solid state dosimeters can be divided into two categories, active dosimeters and passive dosimeters. When radiation interacts with medium inside the dosimeter, the active dosimeter transfers radiation intensity into the pulse of electric signals. Based on those signals, users can determine the types and the intensity of the radiation. As for passive dosimeters, radiation interaction is detected through certain physical processes after radiation interacts with medium in the dosimeter. From the physical processes, users can also determine the types and the intensity of the radiation. Active dosimeters are used for dose measurements in areas with unknown radiation level to gather the radiation information immediately. Therefore, the proper radiation protection actions can be initialized. The common active dosimeters in the market are gas-filled counters, scintillation counters, and semi-conductor detectors...etc. On the other hands, passive dosimeters are often used as periodic radiation monitor for people work in the radiation environment to monitor the cumulated dose and the types of radiation. They can be used as personal dose measurement, long-term environmental radiation dose monitor...etc. The film badge, Thermoluminescence Dosimeter (TLD), Optically Stimulated Luminescence Dosimeter (OSLD), and Radio-photoluminescence Glass Dosimeter (RPLGD) are commonly used passive dosimeters. In clinics, many different kinds of dosimeters are applied in the procedures to verify dose delivery accuracy, to obtain dose to critical areas or organs, and to verify machine output for QA purposes.

For TLD, OSLD, and RPLGD, when radiation interacts with the medium in the dosimeters, part of the absorbed energy are first stored in a metastable energy state of the medium. Then some of this energy can be recovered later as visible light after proper physical process, such as heating.

2. Radio-Photoluminescence Glass Dosimeter (RPLGD)

OSLD is made of the same luminescent material as one used in TLD. The only differences are different excitation source and different readout technique used. However, RPLGD uses glass compound as the luminescent material and applies different excitation method along with different readout technique. In 1949, Wely, Schulman, Ginther, and Evans manufactured the first RPLGD system (Yokota). Schulman applied this system in radiation dose measurement in 1951 (Yasuda, Troncalli). The luminescent material used by Schulman was a compound glass of 25% of KPO_3, 25% of Ba $(PO_3)_2$ and 50% of Al $(PO_3)_2$, with proper amount of $AgPO_3$ to form silver activated phosphate glass. It is very difficult to measure dose under 1 mGy with Schulman's RPLGD system, because it has a high pre-dose (residual dose). Pre-dose is the phosphorescence light emitted from RPLGD without any irradiation and excitation process. It is the minimum radiation can be measured with RPLGD. Besides, because of the pre-mature luminescence measurement technique and the poor quality of excitation source for color centers, the measurement accuracy with Schulman's RPLGD is very poor. Therefore, RPLGD is not a popular dosimeter in day to day applications in those days.

However, there are many researchers continue to devote in the developments of RPLGD and its readout system; including people at Asahi Techno Glass Corporation (ATGC) in Japan, at Toshiba Corporation in Japan, and at Karlsruhe Nuclear Research Center (KNRC) in Germany. The developments of new generation RPLGD and readout system were completed in 1990 (Piesch). Table 1 shows the types and compositions of the glass luminescent material developed by ATGC and Toshiba. The excitation source was changed from ultra-violet into pulse ultraviolet laser. The improvements in the glass material and in readout system make the RPLGD capable for lower dose (10 μGy) measurement with excellent accuracy (A. T. G., Corporation Chiyoda Technol).

TLD is still the major dosimeter used for personal dose monitor and for dose verification in diagnostic radiology and in radiotherapy in nowadays. The major problem with TLD is its non-repeatable readout for the measurements. Based on the preliminary report by Hsu et al on the study of the characteristics of RPLGD in radiation measurement, it proves that the radiation detection characteristics of RPLGD are superior to that of TLD (Hsu). Therefore, in the near future, RPGLD will become one of the important dosimeters for dose measurement and radiation detection in the field.

The work on the radiation measurement with self-manufactured RPLGD by Schulman in 1951 opened the history of RPLGD applications in dose measurement (Yasuda, Troncalli). After exposed to radiation, stable color centers are formed in the glass and more color centers are formed with increasing radiation intensity. After irradiated by ultraviolet light, color centers are excited and emit 600 nm to 700 nm visible orange light (Burgkhardt). It is called radio-photoluminescence phenomenon. The amount of orange light emitted from RPLGD is linearly proportional to the radiation received; therefore, it is suitable for long term personal dose monitor or environmental radiation monitor. RPLGD is used in Japan for over 80% of radiation workers as an external dosimeter (Corporation Chiyoda Technol).

3. Principle of RPLGD and its readout methods

The basic principle of RPLGD is that the color centers are formed when the luminescent material inside the glass compound exposed to radiation and fluorescence are emitted from the color centers after irradiated with ultra-violet light. The excited electrons generated from the color centers return to the original color centers after emitting the fluorescence. This process is called radio-photoluminescence phenomena. Because the electrons in the color centers return to the electron traps after emitting the fluorescence, it can be re-readout for a single irradiation.

glass series	composition ratios (mol%)							
	Li	Na	P	O	Al	Ag	Mg	Ba
FD-1	3.7	-	33.4	53.7	4.6	3.7	-	0.9
FD-3	3.6	-	34.5	53.5	5.1	3.3	-	-
FD-4	3.5	-	34.0	52.7	5.0	4.8	-	-
FD-5	-	9.0	33.1	51.3	6.1	0.5	-	-
FD-6	-	6.6	33.2	51.4	5.5	1.4	1.9	-
FD-7	-	11.0	31.5	51.2	6.1	0.2	-	-

Table 1. The types and compositions of silver activated phosphate glass

Figure 1 shows the old RPLGD readout technique (Piesch). The pre-dose M_0 (M_0 (t_0) = I_2 x Δt) was obtained with photomultiplier tube (PMT) first. After RPLGD irradiated by the radiation, the total light intensity is M_1 (M_1 = I_1 x Δt). The "actual" light intensity from the irradiation, M, is M_1 - M_0 = (I_1 x Δt) – (I_2 x Δt). The radiation dose can then be estimated from M. The traditional way to calculate the light intensity is to subtract the pre-dose reading (M_0) from the total reading (M). With the traditional readout technique, if the glass surface is covered with dust or other material the pre-dose reading (M_0) and the total dose reading (M) are both affected and results in a large error for dose estimation. Therefore the old RPLGD readout technique will not measure the dose accurately.

In 1990, a new RPLGD readout system was developed by the cooperation of ATGC (Japan) and KNRC (Germany). The major modification in this new system is to use pulse ultra-violet laser as excitation source, instead of ultra-violet light. The intensity, the excitation time and position of the pulse ultra-violet laser can be accurately controlled. Traditionally, it takes seconds for the unit to count the excitation time; however, it has changed to micro second (μs) for the new system. The readout time is decreased rapidly with the new system. Furthermore, with a collimated laser beam, the laser can be delivered to the exact position in the glass. The radiation energy can also be estimated accurately with the energy compensator filter.

With the pulse ultra-violet laser excitation system, decay curve of fluorescence can be divided into three portions according to the fluorescence decay time of RPLGD. They are (1) pre-dose or the light signal emitted from the impurity covering the glass surface, (2) the light signal from color centers formed by radiation, and (3) the light signal emitted from pre-dose after long time decay.

Any signal detected within the fluorescence decay time between 0 to 1 μs, the readout system mark it as the light signal from pre-dose or from the impurity on the glass surface.

The readout system takes light signal emitted in the fluorescence decay time between 1 to 40 µs as the signal from radiation exposure. For light signal emitted in the fluorescence decay time up to 1 ms, the readout system takes it as the signal produced by pre-dose with long decay time characteristics. The characteristics of the fluorescence decay curve are illustrated in figure 2.

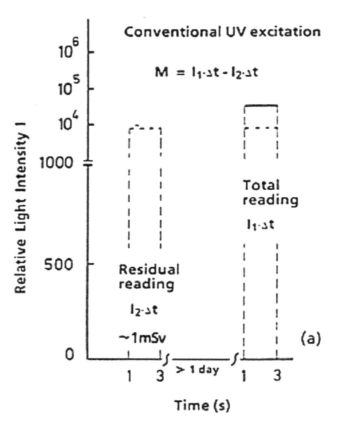

Fig. 1. Old readout technique for RPLGD (Piesch)

In figure 3, the area of F_1 is the integral of fluorescence decay curve between t_1 (1 µs) and t_2 (40 µs) and it is the luminescence signal produced by radiation. However, there are pre-dose signals included in the lower half part of F_1, therefore, one should subtract this portion from F_1 to obtain the "actual" luminescence signal emitted by exposure. The way to subtract the pre-dose signal is to find F_2 from the longer fluorescence decay curve of pre- dose. The area of F_2 is the integral between t_3 and t_4 where time between t_3 and t_4 and t_1 and t_2 is the same, 39 µs. From the proportional relationship of trapezium area, it shows the area of pre-dose in F_1 is $F_2 \times f_{ps}$ (f_{ps} is the conversion factor for trapezium area). Therefore, the actual luminescence signal from the color centers is $F_1 - F_2 \times f_{ps}$. The exposure received by RPLGD can be obtained from the luminescence signal emitted.

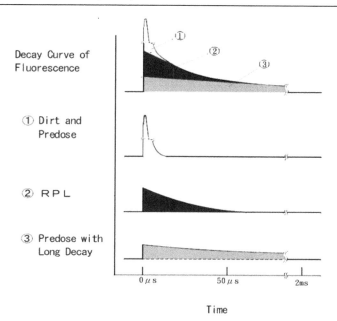

Fig. 2. The luminescence decay curve of RPLGD (A. T. G.)

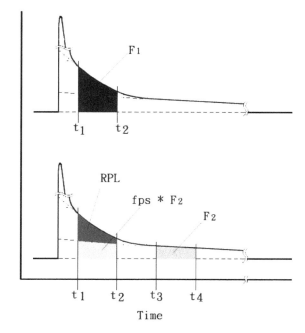

Fig. 3. The readout technique with pulse ultra-violet laser (A. T. G.).

4. Chemical characteristics of the silver ions

The color centers were structured at the silver activated phosphate glass. The numbers of ionic silver relate to energy levels in color centers and the numbers of electron trap(s). The numbers of electron trap(s) increase with increasing numbers of ionic silvers. However, excessive numbers of ionic silver decrease the penetration efficiency of the pulse ultra-violet laser and increases energy dependence. Therefore, a proper ratio of ionic silver is required for the best luminescence and excitation efficiency (Yokota).

At present, the most common type of glass in RPLGD for radiation dose measurement is FD-7. The $AgPO_4$ in silver activated phosphate glass of FD-7 can be viewed as Ag^+ and PO_4^-. When the tetrahedron of PO_4^- is exposed to the radiation, it loses one electron and forms a "positron hole". The electron released from the PO_4^- will combine with Ag^+ to form an Ag^0. Similarly, hPO_4 ("hole" formed after PO_4^- loses one electron) will combine with Ag^+, and then gains a "positron hole" to become an Ag^{2+}. Both Ag^0 and Ag^{2+} can form color centers as shown in Figure 4.

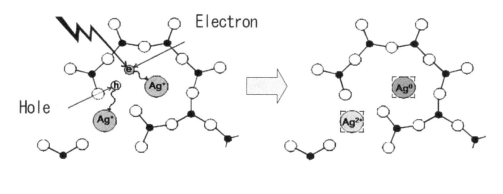

$$Ag^+ + e^- \longrightarrow Ag^0 \ (\text{electron trap})$$
$$Ag^+ + hPO_4 \longrightarrow PO_4 + Ag^{2+} \ (\text{hole trap})$$

Fig. 4. The color centers formation mechanism of FD-7 (A. T. G.)

After exposure, the Ag^+ at valence band of silver activated phosphate glass combines with electron released from both PO_4^- and hPO_4 (formed by PO_4^-) to become color centers (Ag^0 and Ag^{2+}). When these color centers excited by 337.1 nm pulse ultra-violet laser, the electrons in Ag^0 and Ag^{2+} excited to higher energy levels and emit 600 – 700 nm visible orange light, then return to the original color centers. Energy gained by electrons from the pulse ultra-violet laser is not high enough to let electron escape from color centers. Therefore these electrons will not return to the valence band of the glass material directly. For electrons to gain enough energy to return to the valence band, we need to anneal RPLGD at 400°C for one hour. The color centers won't disappear after readout; hence, RPLGD can be read repeatedly. Figure 5 shows the energy levels of RPLGD.

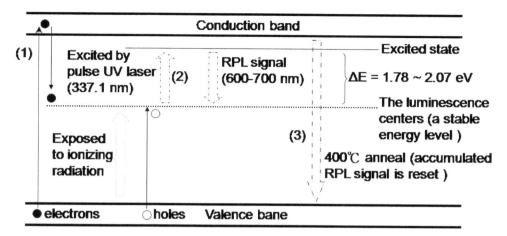

Fig. 5. The energy levels of RPLGD. (1) After RPLGD being exposed, Ag^+ at the valence band combines with electron released from PO_4^- and hPO_4 formed by PO_4^- to become a color center. (2) After electron at color center excited by 337.1 nm pulse ultra-violet laser, it will be excited and emits 600 – 700 nm visible orange light, then return to the original color centers (3)After annealing at 400°C for one hour, the electron at color centers returns to the valence band of luminescence material (Hsu).

5. The radio-photoluminescence model

The luminescence materials used in either TLD or OSLD have an ordered crystal structure with lattice defects. From the glow curve, which is generated after annealing, one has the information on the electron distribution functions at different energy trap(s). The luminescence models for TLD and OSLD are developed based on this information. However, RPLGD is a mixture of inorganic amorphous solid and does not have lattice structure and lattice luminescence centers. Therefore we cannot get the information on electron trip(s) distribution function to establish the luminescence model for RPLGD. We can only establish the radio-photoluminescence model based on the energy of the excitation source and the energy of the released visible light.

After excited with 337.1 nm pulse ultra-violet laser, RPLGD emits 600 – 700 nm visible lights. From the emitted lights we know the energy gap between the excited energy levels which electrons jump to and the energy levels at color centers is between 1.78 and 2.07 eV. Becker assumed there are many continuous energy levels at the color centers of the RPLGD (Becker), as shown in Figure 6. It shows the electrons in the valence band are excited to the conduction band after irradiation. When electrons return to the valence band, portions of electrons are captured by the electron trap(s) located at P shell and Q shell, and then form color centers. After excitation, the electrons in color centers jump to higher energy level, emit fluoresce, then return to the original color centers. RPLGD is manufactured via the process of melting various compounds under high temperature, different from the manufacture process of TLD or OSLD which is via process of long-crystal formation. Hence, the color centers of PRLGD are not built at the lattice. There are no formal reports on the luminescence model for RPLGD. We believe that the color centers of RPLGD may be structured among the orbital electrons in the compound. The various continuous energy levels are formed with different bonding structures among elements. Those energy levels can store free electron energy which is produced by the excitation process. Therefore, its excitation energy gap has a continuous value (from 1.78 to 2.07 eV) which releases 600 nm – 700 nm visible lights.

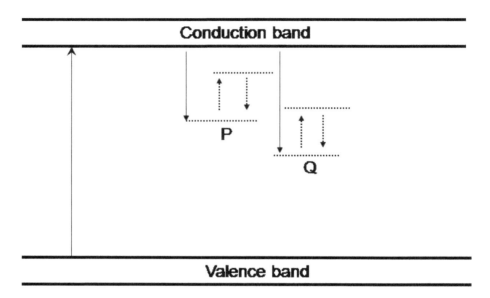

Fig. 6. There are many continuous energy levels in RPLGD color centers.

6. Physical characteristics of radio-photoluminescence glass dosimeter

The pulse ultra-violet laser excitation system improves the readout accuracy of RPLGD and also shortens the readout time. The improvement in the luminescent material lowers the detectable dose limit. These improvements make the applications of RPLGD in radiation measurements growing rapidly. There are three major types of RPLGD in the market; the SC-1 for environmental radiation dose monitor; the GD-450 for personal external radiation dose monitor; and the Dose Ace for research purposes. All those three types use FD-7 glass, manufactured by Asahi, Japan, as shown in Figure 7.

The SC-1 is a plate-type RPLGD with outside capsule volume of 30 x 40 x 9 mm³.The dimension of FD-7 glass inside the capsule is 16 x 16 x 1.5 mm³. There are two layers of tin filters, one on the top and another at the bottom, over of the capsule with a dimension of 0.75 mm and 3 mm respectively. These tin filters are used as energy compensator to estimate the radiation energy and to lower the energy dependence effect. The FD-7 in GD-450 has a dimension of 33 x 7 x 1 mm³. There are five different types with different thickness of filters in the capsule of GD-450; namely, 0.2 mm acrylic plate; 0.5 mm acrylic plate; 0.7 mm aluminum filter; 0.2 mm copper filter; and 1.2 mm tin filter. The functions of these filters in

GD-450 are the same as that of SC-1; to estimate radiation energy and to lower the energy dependence effect. The GD-450 dosimeters are the major personal dosimeters used in Japan.

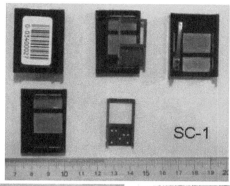

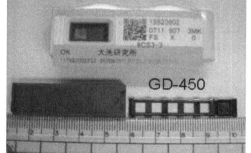
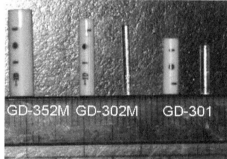

Fig. 7. Three types of RPLGD; above: SC-1 system for environmental radiation monitor; below left: GD-450 system for personal dose monitor; and below right: small volume Dose Ace system for research

The Dose Ace type RPLGD is mainly for research purposes. It is a cylindrical shape with three different models; GD-302M, GD-352M, and GD-301. The GD-302M and GD-352M have a length of 12 mm and a diameter of 1.5 mm, while GD-301 has a length of 8.5 mm and a diameter of 1.5 mm. GD-301 and GD-302M, without filters in capsule, are used to measure the dose of high energy photons as in radiotherapy. However, there is a Tin filter in the capsule for GD-352M to lower the energy dependence effect. The GD-352M can be used for measuring the dose from low energy photons as in diagnostic radiology. In the process of dose readout, based on the dose values, the dose ranges are divided into two categories, low dose range (10 μGy – 10 Gy) and high dose range (1 Gy - 500 Gy).The readout system can automatically distinguish the dose range according to different readout magazine used by the users. On the top of that, there are different readout areas in RPLGD for different dose ranges too. The readout area for high dose range is located at between 0.4 mm and 1 mm, a total length of 6 mm and a total volume of 0.47 mm³, from the non-series end in the readout area (as shown in Figure 8); while the low dose range is located from 1 mm to 6 mm with a volume of 0.47 mm³. The high dose readout area can be used for the measurement of dose with high gradient too. The Table 2 shows the characteristics of various RPLGDs.

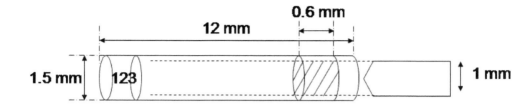

Fig. 8. The high dose readout area for GD-320M; the series end is located on the left side, the readout area is located at 0.4 mm to 1.0 mm from the non-series end, the diameter of incident pulse ultra-violet laser is 1 mm (Hsu).

Type	SC-1	GD-450	Dose Ace
Effective atomic number	12.04	12.04	12.04
The dose linearity range	10 µGy - 10 Gy	10 µGy - 10 Gy	10 µGy - 10 Gy 1 Gy - 500 Gy
Energy dependency (20 keV / ^{137}Cs)	1.2（with energy compensator filter）	1.2（with energy compensator filter）	3.4（w/o energy compensator filter）0.8（with energy compensator filter）
Fading effect	< 5 % / yr	< 5 % / yr	< 5 % / yr
Repeatable readout	yes	yes	yes
Angular dependency	± 8% (0 ~ 80 degree)	± 3% (0 ~ 80 degree)	0 (0 ~ 80 degree)

Table 2. The characteristics of RPLGD

In Figure 9, it shows the readout reproducibility for GD-352M and TLD-100H respectively with a C.V. (coefficient of variation) of 0.46 – 3.11 for GD-325M and C.V. of 0.71 – 3.87 for TLD-100H. The figure shows that the C.V. is smaller for RPLGD as compared to that of TLD because of different manufacture methods. Each RPLGD is made after glass material melted at high temperature and results in a smaller variation among each RPLGD. On the other hand, the TLD is made with growing crystal, therefore the variation is greater.

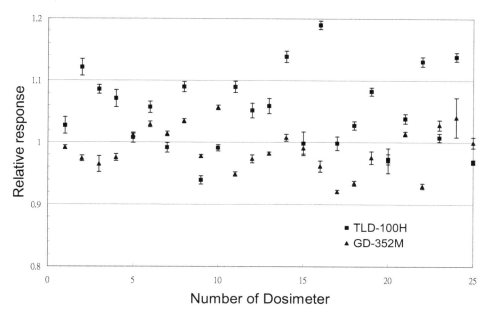

Fig. 9. The readout reproducibility of GD-352M and TLD-100H

Figure 10 shows the dose linearity for GD-352M and TLD-100H respectively in a range of 0.105 mGy and 50.4 mGy. The measured dose points are at 0.105 mGy, 0.168 mGy, 0.672 mGy, 1.05 mGy, 2.1 mGy, 6.3 mGy, 25.2 mGy, and 50.4 mGy with five RPLGDs for each measured point. The correlation coefficient is close to unity for both GD-325M and TLD-100H. It shows that the dose irradiated is proportional to the dose estimated from readout.

Figure 11 shows the energy dependence for GD-302M, GD-352M, and TLD0-100H respectively. The values shown in figure 11 are normalized to the readout from Cs-137 irradiation. When un-filtered GD-302M irradiated with low energy photons, the interactions between photons and RPLGD are increased because of the photoelectric effect. Therefore the luminescence signal is increased too. For filtered GD-352M, the Tin filter can stop the low energy photons; hence, the energy dependence effect is less.

Table 3 shows the characteristics comparisons of different passive dosimeters. It demonstrates that the physical characteristics of OSLD are better than that of TLD. And the physical characteristics of RPLGD are better than that of OSLD because of different readout system and different luminescence material. Therefore, RPLGD could become one of the important dose measurement tools in the future.

	TLD	OSLD	RPLGD
Principe of measurement	luminescence signal	optically stimulated luminescence signal	radiophotoluminescence signal
Luminescence material	crystal	crystal	glass
Excitation source	heat	visible light	ultra-violet laser
Sensitivity	material-dependent	material-dependent	good
Repeatable readout	no	yes, but intensity reduced	yes, with the same intensity
Range of measurement	material-dependent (10μGy - 10 Gy)	material-dependent (10μGy - 10 Gy)	10μGy - 10 Gy 1 Gy - 500 Gy
Geometrical shape	chip and powder	powder	various shapes
Fading effect	material-dependent (5 - 20 % / quarter)	material-dependent (0 - 10 %/year)	less than 5%/year
Energy dependence	material-dependent	material-dependent	± 20% (having energy compensation filter)
Capability to distinguish the types of radiation	yes	yes	yes
Re-useable	yes	no	yes

Table 3. The characteristics comparisons of TLD, OSLD, and RPLGD

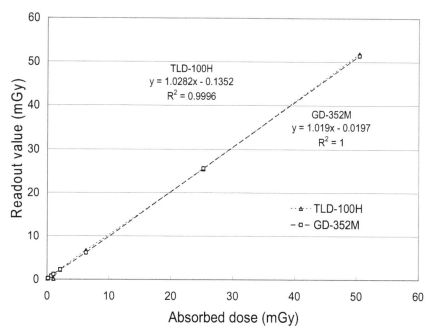

Fig. 10. The dose linearity curves for GD-352M and TLD-100H, both C.V.s are less than 3.

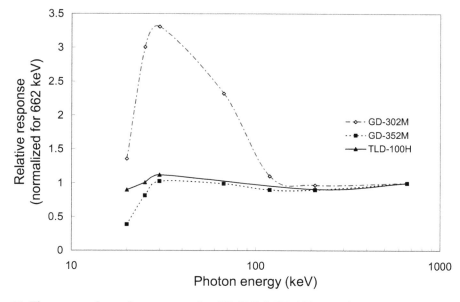

Fig. 11. The energy dependence curves for GD-302M, GD-352M, and TLD-100H

7. Characteristics of RPLGD for clinical applications

The clinical applications of RPLGD characteristics are summarized in the followings:
1.   Repeatable readout
The luminescence signal does not disappear after readout; therefore, repeated readout for a single exposure is possible for RPLGD.
2.   Small difference in individual sensitivity
The readout variation between different PRLGDs with the same exposure is small. RPLGD is manufactured with melted glass; therefore, its individual sensitivity is small as compared to that of either TLD or OSLD.
3.   No correction factor needed
The luminescence single can be converted to the exposure dose directly without the need of correction factors. The exposure dose can be determined with the help of readout from reference PRLGD built-in to the readout system.
4.   Small energy dependence
The energy dependence existed in FD-7 glass, if there is no energy compensator filter with it. However, energy dependence can be reduced with energy compensator filter.
5.   Small fading effect
The stability of color centers in RPLGD is high. Hence the effects of environment conditions such as humidity and temperature have very little impact to color centers, hence low fading effects for RPLGD.
6.   Better reproducibility
By using pulse ultra-violet laser as excited source, the accuracy of repeated readout can be maintained. Therefore, RPLGD has a very good reproducibility.
7.   Wide measurable dose range
The dose linearity range for RPLGD is 0 – 500 Gy. This range covers the dose range used in the medical field. RPLGD can therefore be applied for dose verification in radiotherapy as well as in diagnostic radiology. RPLGD is also desirable for high dose gradient area, such as IMRT (Intensity Modulated Radiotherapy) procedures or HDR (High Dose Rate Remote Afterloader) procedures because of its small effective readout area.
8.   Feasibility of personal dose monitor tools
The characteristics, physical and chemical, of RPLGD are equal to or better than that of TLD and OSLD because of its luminescence material and readout technique. Hence, RPLGD can be used as dose monitor for radiation field worker.

8. Applications of RPLGD

Araki applied the RPLGD system in Stereotactic Radiosurgery (SRS) procedure for dose measurements, including Gamma Knife, Cyberknife etc (Araki, Arakia). The results of output factors are comparable with the results from Hi-p Si Stereotactic field detector and Mote Carlo calculation. It shows RPLGD can be used for small field radiation measurements effectively. Nose designed a tube to hold RPLGDs for dose measurements for head and neck patients to verify the delivery dose against the calculated dose from treatment planning system (Nose). Although the maximum dose variation can be as high as 15%; however, those differences are mostly from the positioning errors. Based on the RPLGD physical characteristics study, the error from the RPLGD system stability is less than 3% (out of 15%). Yasuda and Iyogi applied RPLGD in space and environment radiation monitor (Yasuda, Iyogi). Hsu et al. also applied RPLGD in prostate HDR (High Dose Rate Remote Afterloader) procedure to study the dose distributions (Hsu). Many institutes in US and Europe devote into the developments and the researches in the new luminescence material and readout techniques for RPLGD (Yasuda, Araki, Arakia, Nose, Iyogi, Norimichi ,Hsu).

With its small volume, RPLGD can be used in in-vivo dose measurements; e.g. dose evaluation in animal irradiation study. RPLGD can also be placed in the anthropomorphic phantom to evaluate dose received during the clinical procedures for diagnostic radiology and radiotherapy. With its characteristics of repeatable readout and small effective readout area, RPLGD can also be used in brachytherapy procedures to evaluate the dose delivery accuracy for each procedure as well as for entire course. On the top of that, with the help of dedicated tube to hold RPLGD, one can apply RPLGD in the area of adjacent critical organs to monitor the organ dose to avoid the dose exceeding the tolerance during the radiotherapy procedure. It can improve the patient life quality after radiotherapy.

9. References

[1] Yokota R., Nakajima S., Improved fluoro-glass dosimeter as personnel monitoring dosimeter and micro-dosimeter. Health phys.11, 241; 1965.

[2] Yasuda H., and Ishidoya, T., Time resolved photoluminescence from a phosphate glass (GD-300) irradiated with heavy ions and gamma rays. Health Phys. 84, 373 ; 2003.

[3] Yasuda H., and Fujitaka K., Efficiency of a radio-photoluminescence glass dosemeter for low-earth-orbit space radiation. Radiat Prot Dosimetry. 100, 545 ; 2002.

[4] Troncalli A. J., and Chapman J., TLD linearity vs. beam energy and modality. Med Dosim. 27, 295 ; 2002.

[5] Piesch E., Burgkhardt B., Vilgis M., Photoluminescence dosimetry: progress and present state of art. Radiat Prot Dosimetry. 33, 215; 1990.

[6] Corporation, A. T. G., RPL glass dosimeter / Small element system Dose Ace ; 2000.

[7] Corporation Chiyoda Technol, Personal monitoring system by glass badge ; 2003.

[8] Hsu S.M., Yeh S.H., Lin M.S. and Chen W.L., Comparison on Characteristics of Radio-photoluminescent Glass Dosimeters and Thermoluminescent Dosimeters. Radiat. Prot. Dosim. 119, 327 ; 2006.

[9] Burgkhardt B., Festag J. G., Piesh E., and Ugi S., New aspects of environmental monitoring using flat phosphate glass and thermoluminescence dosimeters. Radiat Prot Dosimetry. 66, 187 ; 1996.

[10] Yokota R., Muto Y., Silver-activated phosphate dosimeter glasses with low energy dependence and higher sensitivity. Health phys. 20, 662: 1971.

[11] Becker K., High r-dose response of recent silver-activated phosphate glasses. Health phys. 11, 523: 1964.

[12] Araki F., T. Ikegami, Measurements of Gamma-Knife helmet output factors using a radio-photoluminescent glass rod dosimeter and a diode detector. Med Phys. 30, 1976; 2003.

[13] Arakia F., Moribe N., Dosimetric properties of radio-photoluminescent glass rod detector in high-energy photon beams from a linear accelerator and cyber-knife. Med Phys. 31, 1980; 2004.

[14] Nose T., Koizumi M., Yoshida K., Nishiyama K., Sasaki J., Ohnishi T., Peiffert D., In vivo dosimetry of high-dose-rate brachytherapy: study on 61 head-and-neck cancer patients using radio-photoluminescence glass dosimeter. Int J Radiat Oncol Biol Phys. 61, 945: 2005.

[15] Iyogi T., Ueda S., Environmental gamma-ray dose rate in Aomori Prefecture, Japan. Health Phys. 82, 521; 2002.

[16] Hsu S.M., Yeh C.Y., Yeh T.C., Hong J.H., Tipton Annie Y.H., Chen W.L., Sun S.S., D.Y.C. Huang, Clinical application of radio-photoluminescent glass dosimeter on dose verification for prostate HDR procedure. Med. Phys. 35, 5558: 2008.

[17] Norimichi Juto. The large scale personal monitoring service using the latest personal monitor glass badge. Paper of proceedings of AOCRP-1-Korea, 2003.

Permissions

The contributors of this book come from diverse backgrounds, making this book a truly international effort. This book will bring forth new frontiers with its revolutionizing research information and detailed analysis of the nascent developments around the world.

We would like to thank Dr. Hala Gali-Muhtasib, for lending her expertise to make the book truly unique. She has played a crucial role in the development of this book. Without her invaluable contribution this book wouldn't have been possible. She has made vital efforts to compile up to date information on the varied aspects of this subject to make this book a valuable addition to the collection of many professionals and students.

This book was conceptualized with the vision of imparting up-to-date information and advanced data in this field. To ensure the same, a matchless editorial board was set up. Every individual on the board went through rigorous rounds of assessment to prove their worth. After which they invested a large part of their time researching and compiling the most relevant data for our readers. Conferences and sessions were held from time to time between the editorial board and the contributing authors to present the data in the most comprehensible form. The editorial team has worked tirelessly to provide valuable and valid information to help people across the globe.

Every chapter published in this book has been scrutinized by our experts. Their significance has been extensively debated. The topics covered herein carry significant findings which will fuel the growth of the discipline. They may even be implemented as practical applications or may be referred to as a beginning point for another development. Chapters in this book were first published by InTech; hereby published with permission under the Creative Commons Attribution License or equivalent.

The editorial board has been involved in producing this book since its inception. They have spent rigorous hours researching and exploring the diverse topics which have resulted in the successful publishing of this book. They have passed on their knowledge of decades through this book. To expedite this challenging task, the publisher supported the team at every step. A small team of assistant editors was also appointed to further simplify the editing procedure and attain best results for the readers.

Our editorial team has been hand-picked from every corner of the world. Their multi-ethnicity adds dynamic inputs to the discussions which result in innovative outcomes. These outcomes are then further discussed with the researchers and contributors who give their valuable feedback and opinion regarding the same. The feedback is then collaborated with the researches and they are edited in a comprehensive manner to aid the understanding of the subject.

Apart from the editorial board, the designing team has also invested a significant amount of their time in understanding the subject and creating the most relevant covers. They scrutinized every image to scout for the most suitable representation of the subject and create an appropriate cover for the book.

The publishing team has been involved in this book since its early stages. They were actively engaged in every process, be it collecting the data, connecting with the contributors or procuring relevant information. The team has been an ardent support to the editorial, designing and production team. Their endless efforts to recruit the best for this project, has resulted in the accomplishment of this book. They are a veteran in the field of academics and their pool of knowledge is as vast as their experience in printing. Their expertise and guidance has proved useful at every step. Their uncompromising quality standards have made this book an exceptional effort. Their encouragement from time to time has been an inspiration for everyone.

The publisher and the editorial board hope that this book will prove to be a valuable piece of knowledge for researchers, students, practitioners and scholars across the globe.

List of Contributors

Varisa Pongrakhananon
Chulalongkorn University, Department of Pharmacology and Physiology, Faculty of Pharmaceutical Sciences, Bangkok, Thailand

Varisa Pongrakhananon and Yon Rojanasakul
West Virginia University, Department of Basic Pharmaceutical Sciences, Morgantown, West Virginia, USA

Isabelle Fakhoury and Hala Gali-Muhtasib
American University of Beirut, Lebanon

O'Leary D.P., Neary P.M. and Redmond H.P.
Department of Academic Surgery, Cork University Hospital, Ireland

Zhixia Zhou, Cai Zhang, Jian Zhang and Zhigang Tian
Institute of Immunopharmacology & Immunotherapy, School of Pharmaceutical Sciences, Shandong University, China

Jose Francisco Zambrano-Zaragoza
INSERM, UMR 891, CRCM, Institut Paoli-Calmettes, Universite Medierranée, Marseille, France

Jose Francisco Zambrano-Zaragoza
Universidad Autónoma de Nayarit, Ciencias Químico Biológicas y Farmacéuticas, Tepic Nayarit, Mexico

Nassima Messal, Sonia Pastor, Yves Guillaume, Jacques Nunes, Marc Lopez and Daniel Olive
INSERM, UMR 891, CRCM, Institut Paoli-Calmettes, Universite Medierranée, Marseille, France

Emmanuel Scotet, Marc Bonneville and Crystelle Harly
Centre de Recherche en Cancerologie de Nantes Angers, IRT UN, INSERM UMR 892, Nantes France

Danièle Saverino
Department of Experimental Medicine-Section Human Anatomy, University of Genova, Italy

Marcello Bagnasco
Medical and Radio metabolic Therapy Unit, Department of Internal Medicine, University of Genova, Italy

Pierre Pontarotti
Université Aix Marseille 1, UMR 6632 Marseille, France

Jaroslav Vorlíček, Barbora Vrbova and Jan Vrba
Czech Technical University, Czech Republic

Brent Herron, Alex Herron, Kathryn Howell, Daniel Chin and Luann Roads
PSL Medical Center, Denver, USA

Tahir H. Shah, Elias Siores and Chronis Daskalakis
Institute of Materials Research and Innovation (IMRI), University of Bolton, United Kingdom

Irina Panovska-Stavridis
University Clinic of Hematology, Skopje, Republic of Macedonia

David Y.C. Huang
Memorial Sloan-Kettering Cancer Center, 1USA

Shih-Ming Hsu
China Medical University, Taiwan (ROC)

Printed in the USA
CPSIA information can be obtained
at www.ICGtesting.com
JSHW011811301024
72690JS00002B/50

9 781632 411327